BONE REGENERATION IN IMPLANTOLOGY: TOOTH AS A GRAFT

ELIO MINETTI

BONE REGENERATION IN IMPLANTOLOGY: TOOTH AS A GRAFT

Andrea Casasco
Marco Casasco
Stefano Corbella
Edoardo Giacometti
Henry K.L. Ho
Andrea Palermo
Paolo Savadori
Silvio Taschieri

Edited by Flavio Pisani

Spec in Oral Surgery, MSc in Periodontics, MSc in Implant Dentistry
Senior Clinical Lecturer in Periodontology
Programme Lead MSc in Clinical Periodontology
University of Central Lancashire (UK)

edra

Original title
Elio Minetti – Il dente come materiale da innesto

ISBN: 978-88-214-5353-3

Book Publishing Manager: Costanza Smeraldi
Paper, Printing and Binding Manage: Michele Ribatti
Translation: Elio Minetti
Copyediting: ALTER EDOM s.r.l., Noventa Padovana (PD), Italy

ISBN: 978-88-214-5534-6
eISBN: 978-88-214-5441-7

Edra S.p.A.
Via G. Spadolini 7, 20141 Milano
Tel. 02 881841
www.edizioniedra.it

Printed by "Starprint" S.r.l., May 2021

(*) Edra S.p.A. a LSWR GROUP company.

Authors

Elio Minetti, DDS

Dentist
Adjunct Professor, Department of Biomedical, Surgical and Dental Sciences, University of Milan, Italy
Postgraduate in Implantology and Oral Surgery, New York University
Private dentist, Milan, Italy

Andrea Casasco, MD

Medical Surgeon, Specialist in Odontostomatology
Full Professor of Histology, University of Studies of Pavia
Head of the Section of Histology and Embryology, Department of Public Health, Experimental and Forensic Medicine, University of Pavia
Chief Medical Officer of Centro Diagnostico Italiano

Marco Casasco, MD

Medical Surgeon, Specialist in Odontostomatology
Researcher, University of Pavia
Professor of Histology and General Embryology, Degree Course in Dentistry and Dental Prosthetics, University of Pavia
Lecturer in Cytology, Degree Course in Medicine and Surgery, University of Pavia

Stefano Corbella, DDS

Dentist
Academy Researcher, Department of Biomedical, Surgical and Dental Sciences, University of Milan - IRCCS Istituto Ortopedico Galeazzi, Milan
Visiting Professor, Sechenov University, Moscow
PhD in Innovative Techniques in Oral Implantology, University of Milan

Edoardo Giacometti, MD

Medical surgeon
Adjunct Professor, University of Genoa Postgraduate in Implantology and Oral Surgery, New York University
Freelance, Turin

Henry K.L. Ho, DDS

Dentist
Adjunct Professor, University of Frankfurt, Titu Maiorescu University of Bucharest, University of Naples Federico II
Master in Dental Surgery, National University of Singapore
Member of the Royal College of Surgeons, Edinburgh
Private dentist, Singapore

Andrea Palermo, DDS

Dentist
Associate Professor, College of Medicine and Dentistry, Birmingham
Adjunct Professor, University of Bari "Aldo Moro"
Postgraduate in Implantology and Oral Surgery, New York University
Private dentist, Lecce

Paolo Savadori, BSC

Doctor of Biotechnology
Head of the Research Histology Service, IRCCS Istituto Ortopedico Galeazzi, Milan
PhD in Tooth Histology and bone tissue, University of Milan

Silvio Taschieri, MD

Medical Surgeon, Specialist in Odontostomatology
Associate Professor, Department of Biomedical, Surgical and Dental Sciences, University of Milan - IRCCS Istituto
Ortopedico Galeazzi, Milan
Associate Professor, Sechenov University, Moscow

Acknowledgements

I would like to thank all those who made possible the realization of this book, in particular Prof. Aldo Bruno Giannì and Prof. Carlo Maiorana, the friends and colleagues who participated in the drafting of the book and our whole group, in alphabetical order:

Tomás Beca Campoy (Spain)
Fulvio Bromuri (Italy)
Andrea Casasco (Italy)
Marco Casasco (Italy)
Martin Celko (Czech Republic)
Marcello Contessi (Italy)
Stefano Corbella (Italy)
Ugo Gambardella (Italy)
Edoardo Giacometti (Italy)
Simon Haan (Singapore)
Henry K.L. Ho (Singapore)
Mauro Libertucci (Italy)
Andrea Palermo (Italy)
Jesus Santillana (Spain)
Paolo Savadori (Italy)
Johannes Schmitz (Italy)
Silvio Taschieri (Italy)

Foreword

Regenerative therapy in implant dentistry, especially that involving bone grafting materials, has been the subject of extensive clinical and laboratory research for many decades. As clinical implant procedures have become more technically advanced, placing implants in sites that are moderately to severely compromised, the need for new and improved regenerative materials has increased exponentially.

While autogenous bone has provided positive outcomes for our grafting procedures, it does not come without a number of negative factors. While providing the basics of osteoinduction, osteoconduction, and osteogenesis, the negative factors of the need for additional surgical sites for harvesting, and the increase in post-operative patient morbidity are well known. Added to this is the fact that autogenous bone is a poor space maintainer, due to its quite high early resorption rate.

To resolve this deficiency, many bone replacement grafts have been developed, all being osteoconductive with varying resorption rates. The bottom line is that most of these grafting materials have proved successful in producing bone that allowed for successful integration of dental implants. The volume of bone produced, however, varied with the resorption rates of the graft material chosen. Additionally, to reduce the length of the regenerative time period, growth factors (platelet or laboratory-sourced) were often added. The cost of these combined regenerative materials by this time had become quite expensive.

These combined negatives resulting from the utilization of these non-autogenous bone replacement grafts led to interesting research in another grafting material pathway. The utilization of an autogenous grafting material derived from the patient's extracted teeth. Specifically chosen was the dentin fraction of these teeth known to be quite similar in composition to bone.

Thus, followed years of scientific and clinical research to both develop the safety, efficacy, and potential of dentin grafts and the development of a delivery system to turn the extracted teeth into a functional bone graft.

This textbook walks us through the basics of bone regeneration from vascular supply to bone anatomical structure. It then shows how autogenous dentin very well fulfills the requirements of an autogenous bone graft through a comprehensive review of how the tooth is processed chairside to turn it into a safe and effective grafting material.

The final chapter reviews the cyto-histology of bone tissue followed by data from ongoing studies on the use of dentin grafts. The chapter ends with the presentation of 20 clinical cases of alveolar ridge preservation, sinus grafts, and periodontal applications.

This well-written and comprehensive textbook should be read by all those interested in providing a well-researched, inexpensive, autogenous bone grafting solution to their patients.

Stephen S. Wallace, DDS
Associate Professor, Columbia University, Division of Periodontics
Diplomate: International Congress of Oral Implantologists
Fellow: Academy of Osseointegration

Foreword to the Italian edition

The text by Elio Minetti and Co-authors represents an important effort in addressing the specific topic of the use of dental tissue as bone reconstruction material in implantology.

In the last twenty years, research has spent a great deal of time identifying materials that, alongside the autologous bone tissue, could satisfactorily recreate the ideal support for osseointegrated implants, in the light of the concept of prosthetically guided implantology.

The systematic way in which the Authors dealt with the use of dental tissue as a bone graft substitute is based on the high level of histological and microscopic evidence. It makes use of the knowledge of the scientific literature and the aids currently in use to obtain the graftable preparation with a description of their strengths and it focuses on the detailed description of the preparation procedures.

Finally, a series of clinical cases transforms the concepts expressed into reality that are easily usable by operators who are well aware of the regenerative and reconstructive problems in osseointegration.

Our appreciation goes to Elio Minetti and Co-authors, who with passion and rigor bring to the scientific community a valid contribution that opens up new operational possibilities in the field of peri-implant tissue reconstruction.

Carlo Maiorana
Director of the School of Specialization in Oral Surgery
University of Milan

Aldo Bruno Giannì
Director of the Department of Biomedical, Surgical and Dental Sciences
University of Milan
Director of the UOC of Maxillo-facial Surgery and Odontostomatology
Fondazione IRCCS Ca' Granda Ospedale Maggiore Policlinico, Milan

Foreword to the Italian edition

Regenerative medicine today represents a fundamental and essential discipline in almost all medical specialties. Regenerating lost organs and tissues, in order to restore the functions compromised by degenerative pathologies, has always represented an ideal goal, very often utopian, for medicine. Thanks to the progress of research in biomaterials and biotechnology, deriving from synergistic collaborations between doctors, biologists, bioengineers, and the advent of "tissue engineering", in recent decades, more and more effective regenerative treatments have been developed and are predictable. Among the most studied tissues there is bone, that has the ability to completely regenerate the damaged parts without leaving scars and to guarantee a *restitutio ad integrum* of the original shape and function. Obviously, this ability is subject to some conditions, actually well known by orthopedists, that have engaged the pioneers of research on bone regeneration mechanisms for decades. Among these, inside the defect to be filled, the presence of a scaffold- an osteoconductive implant capable of giving three-dimensional support to the growing tissue-, of the osteogenic cells capable of generating new bone tissue and of various types of signal molecules (such as platelet growth factors and differentiation factors [BMPs]) which attract the progenitor cells, transform them into osteogenic cells and guide the various phases of the regenerative process step by step. All this work must be supported by an adequate oxygen and nutrient supply via the vascular flow, which must also grow from scratch within the tissue being formed, through the porosity of the support scaffold.

Since the dawn of research on bone regeneration, researchers have understood that the ideal material with which to fill the bone defects, being in possession of all the necessary properties, was the autogenous bone tissue, which was taken from other skeletal areas and implanted in the defect. However, this involved a second surgery for bone removal, increasing the morbidity of the surgery, pain and discomfort for the patient. To avoid resorting to autogenous bone, numerous types of alternative materials, or "bone substitutes", have been developed, deriving from various sources (corpses, animals, laboratory synthesis). Although many of these materials have been found to be effective in promoting bone regeneration, all of them lack some properties with respect to autogenous grafting; the majority have osteoconductive properties only, few have extremely long resorption times and others pose safety risks, not to mention the costs, which are often unjustified.

In the search for the "Holy Grail" of bone regeneration, some researchers have tested not only single materials, but various combinations, in some cases even mixing low-absorbable materials (to ensure mechanical support) with rapidly resorbable materials (to make space for newly bone formed), adding a scent of growth factors (recombinant or contained in platelet concentrates), a pinch of recombinant BMPs and, why not, also some mesenchymal stem cells (appropriately grown in the laboratory).

Even assuming that these cocktails are effective, it is not feasible today to apply them routinely in daily practice, for a variety of reasons, not only economic.

Other lines of research have been oriented towards a return to natural methods, rediscovering and exploiting the regenerative potential contained within ourselves. Hence the success of autologous platelet concentrates, which enhance the healing process in a natural way using our own blood. However, their effectiveness for bone regeneration is controversial as they are unable to provide the necessary mechanical support. And therefore, we asked ourselves: is there an autogenous material capable of regenerating bone in a natural way, without having to take a bone harvest from another site? The answer is in this book. The classic texts on histology, in use for decades in biomedical faculties, already told us that the tooth has a composition extremely similar to the bone tissue and also the dentin matrix contains BMPs, as demonstrated by the famous pioneering researches of Urist (the "father" of the BMPs) in the 1960s. As if there was somehow a predestination. Hence the ingenious intuition that the extracted teeth, instead of ending up in the bin could be reused to regenerate the missing bone. Why buying expensive biomaterials, processed and packaged biomaterials when Mother Nature can provide us with the solution? Of course, even here a little technology is necessarily required to process the tooth and make it suitable for the purpose, but the raw material provided by the patient themself, guarantees safety, harmlessness and above all reduced costs.

The tooth as a grafting material is an extremely hot topic and an increasing number of preclinical and clinical research demonstrates its effectiveness in various situations, from the preservation of the post-extraction socket, to the sinus lift, to GBR, etc.

This extremely comprehensive and enjoyable book provides an overview of all the aspects of bone regeneration, focusing on the benefits of using the tooth as a bone graft material to promote regeneration. The various devices available on the market are presented and compared, the main in vitro and histological studies are summarized, the current scientific evidence on the subject is discussed and numerous clinical cases are presented. Among the authors there are doctors, dentists and biotechnologists, academics and professionals, researchers who are passionate about this topic and transmit their experience to the reader in an effective, rigorous and at the same time pleasant way. This text certainly represents a valid support for all those who want to approach the use of the tooth as graft material in their daily clinical practice or even just to deepen the topic. For me the reading was very pleasant and full of ideas, and I hope it will be the same for all the users.

Massimo Del Fabbro
Associate Professor of the Department of Biomedical,
Surgical and Dental Sciences
University of Milan

Preface

Why do we use grafting materials and what are their key properties?

The regeneration revolution was born in the late 1980s thanks to the observations of Dahlin and Lindhe. It was soon realized that the materials used to fill the defect were just as important as the covering membranes and the surgical technique. Numerous bone substitutes have been proposed and used, but the gold standard has always been the autologous bone tissue.

A graft material must be safe, biocompatible and must not lead to immune reactions or disease transmission. It must maintain space for the vessels and allow for the formation of new ones.

These characteristics are determined by the chemical composition, the micro-surface, the crystallinity and the size of the crystals. The latter are essential for the adhesion of cells to the surface and for the production of new bone. The cohesion characteristics of the material are also fundamental for easy handling during the surgical phases.

87% of the market is composed of materials from animals or synthetic with osteoconductive properties.

In 2014, we began studying a new field of research: the possibility of using the tooth as a graft material, as it is supposed to have osteoinductive properties.

This volume collects our experiences in this new field, with all the limitations deriving from temporal, economic and numerical factors. We are convinced that the future of regeneration can go in this direction. The results obtained so far make clear that the possibilities of what until recently was considered a waste material are very good and that probably in the future we will be able to have even greater successes.

Not everything is positive, in fact to date there are limitations in the use of the tooth as, for example, the conservation of the extracted teeth has just begun or the cleaning of the tooth before use is still manual - even if research towards the automation in tooth cleaning are in place. It will probably take a few more years to have fully mechanized systems. To date, only one device is able to automate the subsequent stages of the process, which are *the conditio sine qua non* to guarantee the reproducibility and scientificity of the preparation.

But what are the reasons for choosing to use the tooth as a grafting material?

The *tooth graft procedure* arises from the observation of the root resorption of the replanted teeth. This phenomenon is well documented in the literature. The real cause, however, can only be understood by reading the definition of "dentin" in the books of Histology. The tooth is "mineralized bone", which, in direct contact with the bone itself, becomes part of the normal bone remodeling process. The tooth is made up of, like bone, an inorganic part and an organic part. The inorganic part is composed of hydroxyapatite and the organic part of collagen and non-collagenic proteins. The part of the tooth that is of great interest is the organic component capable of osteoinduction and its maintenance after treatment is the real target of the use of this type of graft material.

To all intents and purposes, the tooth, being made up of hydroxyapatite and autologous collagen, can also be an excellent osteoconductive material. All manufacturers of grafting materials try to collagen their products. The tooth is naturally collagenated and is autologous. But our aim is to also use the remaining non-collagen proteins, which are about 4% of the tooth and which guarantee osteoinduction.

How can this "bone" be used in regeneration? The literature is surprisingly large, with studies beginning as early as the 1970s. However, the use of a tooth presents numerous unknowns: in particular, the size of the material, its cleanliness and its demineralization treatment. Should the tooth be used in the form in which it is or should some treatment be carried out to improve its effectiveness?

We hope, with this text, to be able to give some answers. Numerous other studies and insights will be needed to build and improve understanding of this research field. This is our first brick.

Elio Minetti

Contents

Vascular anatomy of the maxillaries in relationship to bone regenerative procedures

S. Taschieri, S. Corbella

Introduction

Bone grafts have been the pillar of bone defect reconstruction for more than a century.[1]

The Research[2–8] has highlighted the advantages of graft vascularization. When compared with non-vascularized bone graft for reconstruction of critical size bone defects, the vascularized bone exhibits earlier blending and more solid biomechanical integrity,[2,4] as well as an improved resistance to a progressive resorption and higher chances to recover from local infection or from the irradiation. This can be learnt from the current understanding of osteogenesis, fracture healing and tissue perfusion.

Wagels and colleagues, in 2013,[1] specified that when a critical but not yet defined size of the defect is reached, the results of non-vascularized bone grafting are unpredictable.

After Taylor's description of the fibula flap technique in 1975,[6] numerous types of bone flaps have been described.

Yet, unlike when it happened for soft tissue reconstruction, it appears that anatomical models of bone vascularization have not, for a long time, typically been applied to the selection or manipulation of the bone component of a flap.

Subsequently, other researchers have put much effort[9–15] in performing anatomical studies that have facilitated understanding of the bone vascularization model. Designing reliably vascularized bone can often be neglected at the expense of intended reconstruction, leading to increased clinical failures.

From the aforementioned studies it could be inferred that success in reconstructing critical sized bone defects should require adequately vascularized and morphologically similar bone.

Thanks to the modern biomaterials and the autologous bone grafting, it is currently possible to undertake regenerative procedures even in patients with an important deficit of the same area, provided that suitable surgical techniques are used and favorable anatomical conditions are present. However, it must be considered that their removal is very invasive, sometimes not simple in the technique and very complicated to adapt to the recipient bone.

Other disadvantages are represented by both the quality of postoperative life and the resorption that usually occurs with the use of autologous bone blocks. In dentistry, except in rare cases of extreme bone dehiscences of the jaws, it is currently preferred to use grafts consisting of granules of bio-compatible materials (allografts or xenografts).

Many scientific researches have shown that these grafts are able to be vascularized by the angiogenesis that follows the operative trauma.[16,17]

This event is of the utmost importance for graft maturation and new bone formation. In addition, the particulate graft adapts to all surface irregularities.

Their use, however, is not without complication, since these grafts must be "immobilized" and often need to be completely covered with the use of membranes.[18] The membranes that are used, both resorbable and non-resorbable, with different resorption times, are designed to allow the passage of both regenerative cells and new vessels deriving from the new angiogenesis. Any uncovering of them during the regeneration phases may lead to a clinical failure and possible graft infections.

It must also be taken into account that the neo-vascularisation occurs and acts for few millimeters starting from the bone substrate and that the portion of biomaterial that most distracts will mature more slowly and often incompletely.[19]

For this reason, large granular grafts require adequate positioning, i.e. as much as possible between bone walls and close to the blood vessels.

Carotid artery

The common carotid artery has a different origin in the right and left side of the body. On the right side, it originates from the brachiocephalic artery, while on the left side it comes directly from the aortic arch. The common carotid artery begins laterally to the trachea and then to the larynx up to the height of approximately the superior margin of the thyroid cartilage, where it divides into the internal carotid artery and the external carotid artery. The internal carotid artery goes up to the "Rocca petrosa" of the temporal bone; here it enters the cranial cavity, passes through the cavernous sinus and ends under the anterior perforated substance. Its terminal portions are the anterior cerebral artery and the middle cerebral artery. During its course, it gives ramifications which also contribute to the vascularization of part of the nasal cavity and of some upper regions of the face.

Almost all the arteries of the oral cavity and neighboring regions are made up of branches deriving from the external carotid artery.

The external carotid artery begins between the third and fourth cervical vertebrae, below the anterior border of the sternocleidomastoid muscle; subsequently it moves upwards, reaches the lower margin of the digastric muscle and the stylohyoid muscle, crosses the most posterior part of the submandibular triangle and then enters the retromandibular fossa and, finally, near the angle of the mandible, it changes direction becoming ascending and running parallel to the posterior margin of the mandible, through the retromandibular fossa. At the level of the neck of the mandible, it bifurcates into its two terminal branches: the superficial temporal artery and the maxillary artery.

The branches of the external carotid are: anterior, posterior, medial and terminal. Those that mostly affect the vascularization of the grafts are the further branches of these vascular trunks and its terminal branch.[20]

In this chapter those of greatest interest will be dealt with.

Maxillary artery

This artery originates from the external carotid artery under the mandibular neck, in the thickness of the parotid gland, then it follows a course in an anterior direction, slightly upward and medially, through the infratemporal fossa. This fossa, also known as the zygomatic fossa, is a space located in the lateral wall of the face, posterior to the jaw and located inferiorly and medially to the zygomatic arch, homologous to the subtemporal fossa (or window) of other vertebrates. It appears as the direct downward continuation of the temporal fossa. The artery, during its journey, is located on the internal surfaceof the mandible. The relationship with the external pterygoid muscle is variable; in fact, in half of the cases, it is found external to this muscle after it has passed between the mandible and the sphenomandibular ligament; in the rest of the cases it is found medial to the external pterygoid muscle. Once the artery has reached the antero-superior end of the infratemporal fossa, it passes through the pterygopalatine fissure, or pterygopalatine hiatus, entering its fossa and, consequently, dividing into its terminal branches.

In a schematic way, the maxillary artery can be divided into four parts.

- The first part is called the *mandibular tract* and corresponds to the short tract located medial to the neck of the mandible; between its collateral branches (the deep auricular artery, anterior tympanic, middle meningea), the *inferior alveolar artery*, which descends on the medial aspect of the mandible branch. It provides *a mylohyoid branch* for the muscle of the same name and penetrates, together with the inferior alveolar nerve, into the mandibular canal. It runs through this canal up to the height of the first premolar where it divides into an *incisional branch* that continues in the anterior portion of the alveolar canal and anastomoses with the homonymous branch of the opposite side providing *alveolar branches* and a *mental branch* that exits through the mental foramen distributing to the chin.
- The second tract is the *pterygoid or muscular artery* which is the longest among the four and it is related to the homonymous external muscle. Its collateral branches are: deep temporal arteries, irregular pterygoid branches, masseterin artery and bucinatory artery.
- The third part, also called *maxillary*, is related to the posterior surface of the maxillary bone (1.1). Numerous collateral branches, often considered in surgical procedures, originate from this branch. In fact, apart from the pharyngeal branch and the artery of the petrogopalatine canal, these are the following branches:
  - the *superior posterior alveolar artery*, which descends on the maxillary tuberosity and divides into numerous branches which penetrate the alveolar canals and are distributed to the roots of the upper molars and premolars, to the gums and to the maxillary sinus;
  - the *infraorbital artery*, which enters the orbital cavity through the inferior orbital fissure, runs through the sulcus and the infraorbital canal together with the infraorbital nerve, it emerges in the face through the infraorbital foramen and, behind the upper lip elevator muscle, it resolves into a tuft of slender branches;
  - in the infraorbital canal, the artery supplies the *orbithal branches* for the lower rectus and the lower oblique muscles of the eyeball and for the lacrimal sac and the *anterior superior alveolar branches* that descend into the anterior alveolar canals to distribute to the canines and the upper incisors, to the gums and to the mucous membrane of the maxillary sinus. Some terminal branches of this artery go up in the face, up to the inner corner of the eye and to the lacrimal sac; others descend towards the upper lip (1.2);
  - the *greater palatine artery* (or *descending palatine artery*), which descends through the pterygopala-

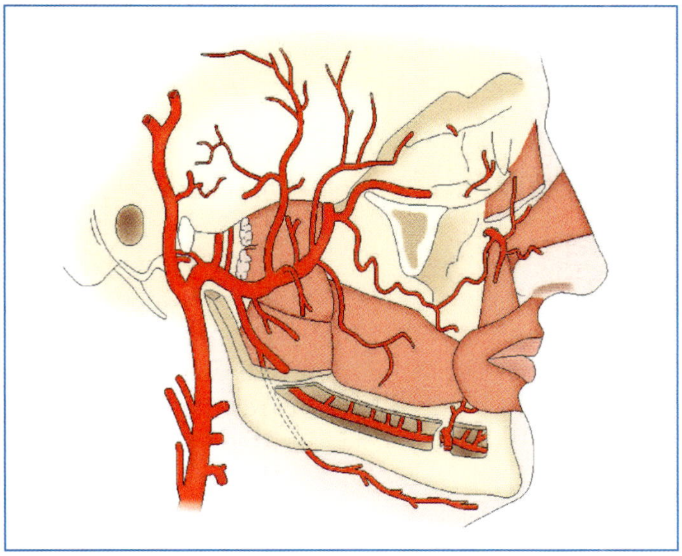

1.1 Course of the maxillary artery.

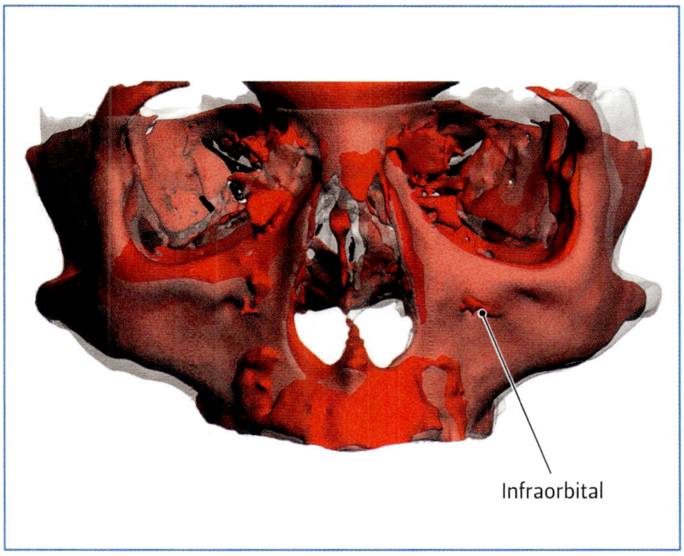

1.2 Infraorbital artery spraying area. (Image by S. Taschieri.)

tine canal with the posterior palatine nerve, originating from the sphenopalatine ganglion, and it supplies two or three minor palatine arteries which cross the palatine canals (1.3) and terminate in the soft palate and in the tonsil; it then emerges on the vault of the palate through the greater palatine foramen and it moves forward, along the alveolar process of the maxilla, to give branches to the bone and the palatine mucosa, to the minor glands in the palate and to the gums; it ends by anastomosing with a branch of the sphenopalatine artery that, through the incisive canal, descends into the palate.

- Finally, the fourth and last portion, also called terminal or sphenopalatine, divides into its terminal branches in the homonymous space from which it penetrates through its fissure, the sphenopalatine canal, into the nasal cavity where it divides into the *posterior medial nasal arteries* or *septum* and *posterior lateral nasal arteries*; the former are distributed to the nasal septum, the latter are carried to the horns, the walls of the foramina and the paranasal sinuses.[20]

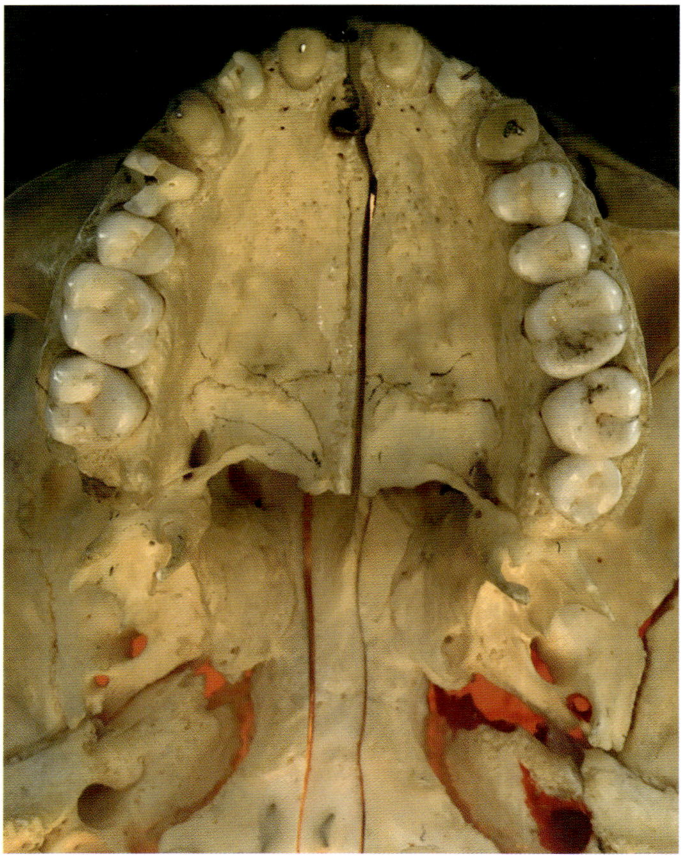

1.3 Crossing of the palatine canals by the palatine arteries. (Image by S. Taschieri.)

Upper and lower jaw

The interest in dentistry is aimed at two structures: the upper jaw and the lower jaw (mandible).

The maxilla consists of a central body, comparable to a triangular pyramid with the base facing the nasal cavity and the apex that continues in the zygomatic process, and by four processes:

1. the *frontal process*, which rises from the anterior-medial angle of the body and moves upwards, joining with the frontal bone;
2. the *zygomatic process*, which corresponds to the lateral angle of the body and is joined to the zygomatic bone;
3. the *palatine process*, which originates from the lower edge of the medial face of the central body and runs horizontally, joining the homologous process of the other maxilla, thus constituting the main part of the anterior portion of the hard palate;
4. the *alveolar process*, which projects downwards and presents the alveoli for the teeth of the upper arch.

On the contrary, the mandible is made up of a horseshoe-shaped body that continues on each side in a branch directed upwards and backwards.

Both the anatomical structures mentioned above contain and are delimited by numerous noble anatomical structures, for example the arterial and the venous vessels, the nerve trunks and the cavities, which must be known in detail by the oral surgeons.

The regenerative techniques of the upper and lower jaw involve a sound knowledge of the vascularization of the relevant anatomical areas.

Vascularization of the maxillary sinus

The maxillary sinus is certainly one of the areas of greatest interest due to the tendency of the residual bone crest, especially following the loss of dental elements, to undergo a resorption process.

The maxillary sinus can be compared to a triangular pyramid with a base or internal wall corresponding to the lower half of the nasal cavity, an upper or orbital face, an antero-lateral face, a posterior or pterygopalatine face and a corresponding external part to the zygomatic process of the maxilla (1.4).

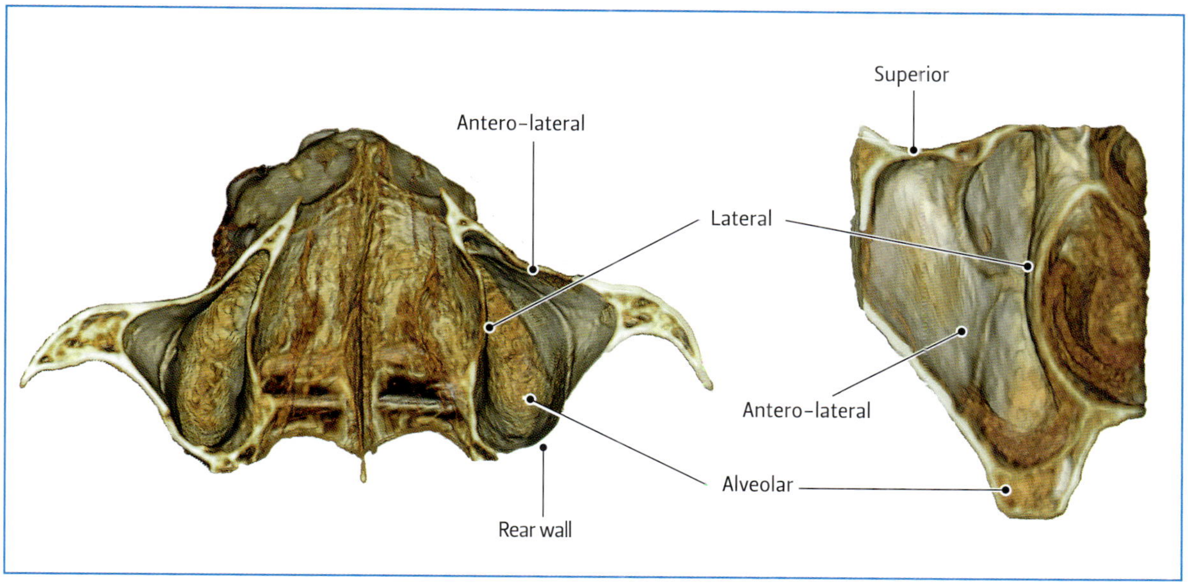

1.4 Maxillary sinus. (Image by S. Taschieri.)

The **antero-lateral wall** is depressed due to the presence of the canine fossa, it has a rectangular shape that looks forward and outward and corresponds, in turn, to the lateral wall of the maxillary bone. This wall is crossed by a partially intraosseous vascular anastomosis between the dental branch of the posterior-superior alveolar artery (PSAA), better known as the alveol-antral artery,[20-22] and the infraorbital artery (IOA).

Knowing this vascular anastomosis, detected in 100% of the cases (Solar and colleagues in 1999[23]) and in the dissective study by Rosano and colleagues, in 2009,[21] it is a clinically important consideration for all clinicians practicing oral surgery.

This anastomosis, when possible, should be preserved during the lateral sinus lift surgery, considering it as a vessel, albeit small in size (between 0.5 and 3 mm), capable of providing vascular support to the graft. This anatomical evidence is supported by its path which is often in the position in which the antrostomy is to be performed or in a neighboring position. Furthermore, this anastomosis is always intraosseous in the first millimeters of its course upstream and downstream, and then it continues at the vestibular level inside a channel formed in the bone wall and internally leaning directly on the Schneider's membrane (1.5).

The **upper or orbital wall** is triangular in shape and with the apex corresponding to the orbital process of the palatine bone; it constitutes a large part of the orbital floor.

This wall is bordered: anteriorly by the lower orbital edge and the lacrimal bone; inside, from the lower edge of the orbital lamina of the ethmoid; on the outside, from the zygomatic-maxillary suture in the anterior third and from the inferior orbital fissure in the posterior two thirds.

This wall, although optimally vascularized, is not important for the regeneration of any grafts aimed at increasing the bone volume within the maxillary sinus, but it has a higher value for the periodontal/periapical tissue regeneration of the upper jaw.

In fact, it is thanks to the lower orbital fissure that the infraorbital artery penetrates the orbit and then runs anteriorly, firstly contained in the infraorbital sulcus and then in the infraorbital canal. At this level, before

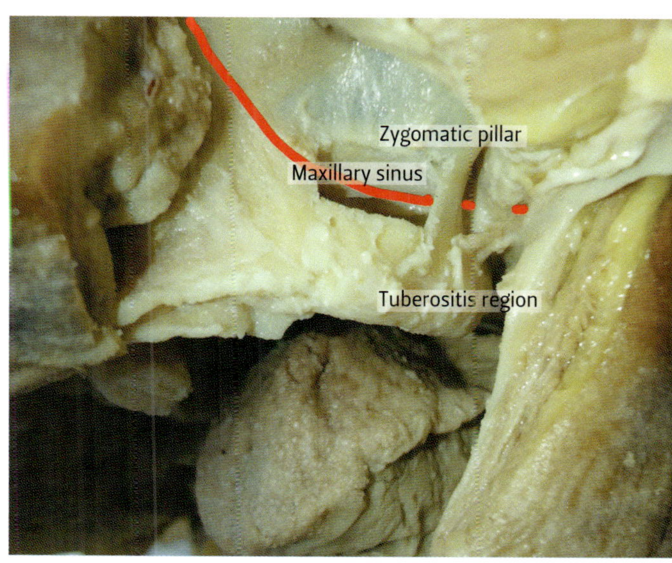

1.5 Course of the vascular anastomosis in the lateral wall of the maxillary bone. (Courtesy of A. Cardarelli.)

emerging at the infraorbital foramen, the infraorbital vessel gives off three branches or sometimes three groups of branches; these branches are the alveolar vessels (posterior, middle and anterior).

The **internal or nasal wall** has a rectangular shape and constitutes the bone septum that separates the maxillary sinus from the nasal cavity; its inferior portion corresponds to the inferior meatus of the nasal cavity.[24]

This wall, at a vascular level, is characterized by a multitude of small vascular tracts deriving from the posterior lateral artery of the nose, which perforate the wall and vascularize the mucous membrane of the maxillary sinus. The same wall is also vascularized by the posterior lateral arteries of the nose which, after having vascularized the superior and median concha, pass through the aforementioned wall with an antero-posterior direction supplying the sinus mucosa.[21] The presence of these numerous vascular branches makes this wall important for the angiogenesis of any graft placed. When it is possible and it is indicated based on the position of the graft, it is better that it is in contact or in a close proximity to this wall.

The **posterior wall** corresponds to the tuberosity of the maxilla and it is in relation to the infratemporal fossa, posteriorly and externally, and the pterygopalatine fossa posteriorly. The posterior-superior alveolar artery has a course extremely close to the maxillary tuberosity and many of its small vascular branches radiate into the complexity of its structure and participate in its vascularization. In addition, a close proximity can be seen between the posterior wall of the sinus, the descending palatine artery and the sphenopalatine artery.[21]

From what has been described, it is clear that the rich vascularization present in this anatomical area brings a consequent importance in the eventual angiogenesis for the maturation of a bone graft. It is therefore preferable that the graft positioning is performed by reaching the posterior wall either to give a correct and more suitable three-dimensional volume to accommodate the implants grafted in the right position or for its maturation.

Vascularization of the anterior jaw

Surgical procedures at the level of the anterior mandible require a high level of knowledge of its vascularization. In fact, any neurovascular damage can lead to serious postoperative sequelae. In the literature there are many cases of bleeding complications in the hours following surgery, especially implant surgery. The resulting hematoma expanding in volume, causes the lingual floor and the tongue itself to rise over time, sometimes so broadly that it obstructs the respiratory tract with consequent danger to the patient's vital parameters. To understand the possible hemorrhagic event, it is necessary to consider the presence of the rich para-symphyseal plexus to which the branches deriving from the anastomosis of the sublingual arteries coming from the right and left side belong. These arteries, which derive from the lingual arteries, penetrate inside the anterior area of the mandible both above and below the genus apofix in a variable number (in the literature there are up to 4/5 foramina with a common average of 1 to 3). Before their penetration, they often anastomose. Once penetrated, they are distributed within intrabony terminal branches giving support to the bone and dental vascularization by anastomosing with the central alveolar vessels between the two lower canines.

The presence of the genii apophyses prevents the formation of the anastomosis between the sublingual arteries and the inferior alveolar arteries.[20]

However in some studies an important presence at the level of vascularization that originates from the terminal derivation of the submental artery is reported, although with a wide variability in percentage. The artery penetrates through the mylohyoid muscle and it anastomoses itself in the same anatomical region.

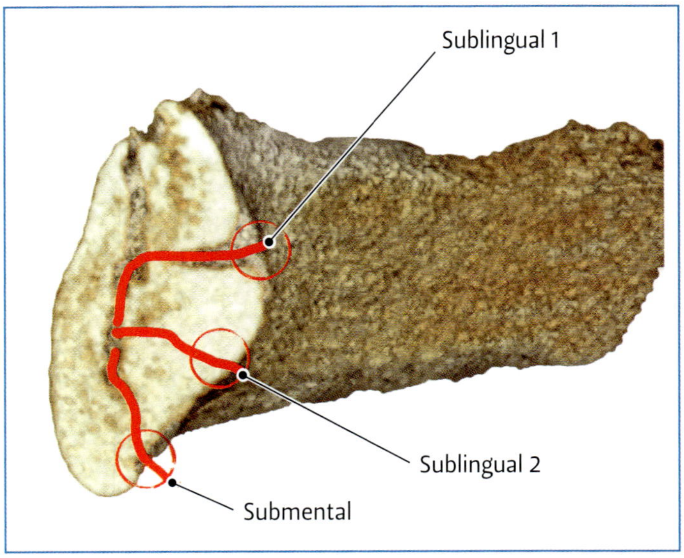

1.6 Course of the sublingual arteries and the submental artery in the anterior area of the mandible. (Image by S. Taschieri.)

In the literature its importance in the vascularization of the anterior area of the mandible varies considerably, from being the main one to being supplementary to that deriving from the sublinguals. Nakajima and colleagues, in 2014,[25] highlighted the wide variability with which the submental and the sublingual artery, respectively derived from the facial and lingual arteries, can originate from the main vascular trunks above mentioned, an origin which may be sometimes common. This subdivision essentially derives from the relationship that these vascular branches have with respect to their passage through the mylohyoid muscle (1.6).

The above mentioned complexity and the vascular number gives an idea of how complicated it is, on a surgical emergency level, to be able to stop the bleeding with ligatures up to the vascular derivation, but also it gives an idea of the angiogenic possibilities of this anatomical portion.[26]

REFERENCES

1. Wagels M, Rowe D, Senewiratne S, et al. History of lower limb reconstruction after trauma. ANZ J Surg 2013; 83(5):348-53.
2. Ostrup LT, Fredrickson JM. Distant transfer of a free, living bone graft by microvascular anastomoses. An experimental study. Plast Reconstr Surg 1974;54(3):274-85.
3. Ostrup LT, Fredrickson JM. Reconstruction of mandibular defects after radiation, using a free, living bone graft transferred by microvascular anastomose. An experimental study. Plast Reconstr Surg 1975;55(5):563-72.
4. Weiland AJ, Phillips TW, Randolph MA. Bone grafts: a radiologic, histologic, and biomechanical model comparing autografts, allografts, and free vascularized bone grafts. Plast Reconstr Surg 1984;74(3):368-79.
5. Berggren A, Weiland AJ, Dorfman H. Free vascularized bone grafts: factors affecting their survival and ability to heal to recipient bone defects. Plast Reconstr Surg 1982;69(1):19-29.
6. Taylor GI, Miller GD, Ham FJ. The free vascularized bone graft. A clinical extension of microvascular techniques. Plast Reconstr Surg 1975;55(5):533-44.
7. Taylor GI, Townsend P, Corlett R. Superiority of the deep circumflex iliac vessels as the supply for free groin flaps. Clinical work. Plast Reconstr Surg 1979;64(6):745-59.
8. Wood MB, Cooney WP. Vascularized bone segment transfers for management of chronic osteomyelitis. Orthop Clin North Am 1984;15(3):461-72.
9. Brookes M, Revell WJ. The blood supply of bone. London, Springer-Verlag 1998.
10. Rhinelander FW. Tibial blood supply in relation to fracture healing. Clin Orthop Relat Res 1974;(105):34-81.
11. Huggins C, Wiege E. The effect on the bone marrow of disruption of the nutrient artery and vein. Ann Surg 1939;110(5):940-7.
12. Kofoed H, Sjøntoft E, Siemssen SO, et al. Bone marrow circulation after osteotomy. Blood flow, pO_2, pCO_2, and pressure studied in dogs. Acta Orthop Scand 1985;56(5):400-3.
13. Gur E, Chiodo A, Pang CY, et al. The vascularized pig fibula bone flap model: effects of multiple segmental osteotomies on growth and viability. Plast Reconstr Surg 1999;103(5):1436-42.
14. Morgan JD. Blood supply of growing rabbit's tibia. J Bone Joint Surg Br 1959;41-B(1):185-203.
15. Simpson AH. The blood supply of the periosteum. J Anat 1985;140 (Pt 4): 697-704.
16. Khan SN, Cammisa FP, Sandhu HS, et al. The biology of bone grafting. J Am Acad Orthop Surg 2005;13(1):77-86.
17. Azi ML, Aprato A, Santi I, et al. Autologous bone graft in the treatment of post-traumatic bone defects: a systematic review and meta-analysis. BMC Musculoskelet Disord 2016;17(1): 465.
18. Wessing B, Lettner S, Zechner W. Guided bone regeneration with collagen membranes and particulate graft materials: a systematic review and meta-analysis. Int J Oral Maxillofac Implants 2018;33(1):87-100.
19. Mercado-Pagán ÁE, Stahl AM, Shanjani Y, et al. Vascularization in bone tissue engineering constructs. Ann Biomed Eng 2015;43(3):718-29.
20. Gaudy JF. Anatomie Clinique. Rueil-Malmaison, Éditions CdP, 2003.
21. Rosano G, Taschieri S, Gaudy JF, et al. Maxillary sinus vascularization: a cadaveric study. J Craniofac Surg 2009; 20(3):940-3.
22. Rosano G, Taschieri S, Gaudy JF, et al. Maxillary sinus vascular anatomy and its relation to sinus lift surgery. Clin Oral Implants Res 2011;22(7):711-5.
23. Solar P, Geyerhofer U, Traxler H, et al. Blood supply to the maxillary sinus relevant to sinus floor elevation procedures. Clin Oral Implants Res 1999; 10:34-44.
24. Chanavaz M. Maxillary sinus: anatomy, physiology, surgery and bone grafting related to implantology. Eleven years of surgical experience (1979-1990). J Oral Implantol 1990;16(3):199-209.
25. Nakajima K, Tagaya A, Otonari-Yamamoto M, et al. Composition of the blood supply in the sublingual and submandibular spaces and its relationship to the lateral lingual foramen of the mandible. Oral Surg Oral Med Oral Pathol Oral Radiol 2014;117(1): e32-8.
26. Rosano G, Taschieri S, Gaudy JF, et al. Anatomic assessment of the anterior mandible and relative hemorrhage risk in implant dentistry: a cadaveric study. Clin Oral Implants Res 2009; 20(8):791-5.

Fundamentals of oral implantology

S. Corbella, S. Taschieri

Introduction

Bone-integrated implantology is the branch of dentistry aimed at creating clinical conditions for the placement of dental prostheses by the insertion of dental implants that are precisely "osseointegrated", that is, an intimate anatomical and functional connection with healthy bone tissue when prosthetically loaded. In general, the use of osseointegrated implants is necessary in all clinical conditions in which the dental elements have been lost or when, following periodontal pathology, caries, trauma or other pathological conditions, it is not possible to maintain the natural dentition.

Osseointegrated implantology began with pioneering work.[1,2] For a long time the humans have tried to find solutions to edentulism, by the placement of "exogenous" devices inside the oral cavity, even implanted in the maxillary bones in a completely analogous way, although with obviously inadequate materials and techniques compared to what happens in the modern osseointegrated implantology. The evolution and the development of materials and techniques, as well as of scientific research, have led to the current situation in which osseointegrated implantology represents an excellent therapeutic option, supported by a large and valid scientific literature. While considering the fact that the clinical results of implant treatments are encouraging, it should be remembered that the fundamental aim of dental treatments is generally represented by the maintenance of healthy natural dental elements and therefore the evaluation between tooth and implant cannot be without a complete diagnostic and prognostic evaluation, not only about the dentition but about the entire subject, analyzing and knowing the expectations and the patient's possibilities of adhering to the therapeutic project to be implemented.

Modern and contemporary implantology, in general, does not ignore osseointegration. The achievement and maintenance of this intimate functional contact between bone and implant depends on a wide variety of factors that belong either to the subject to be treated (anatomical characteristics, characteristics of the bone in terms of volume and composition, systemic actions, socio-economic conditions, flawed habits, etc.), or to the operator and to the characteristics of the treatment that has been agreed.

The purpose of this chapter will be to treat these aspects in an analytical way and to offer a general overview of the current techniques and procedures related to implantology, without neglecting the possibilities of prevention and management of the technical and biological complications of the treatment.

Characteristics of the subject

The characteristics of the subject who needs to receive an implant treatment must fundamentally influence the choice and implementation of the treatment plan, identifying and considering, in each phase, the particular characteristics of the patient.

Systemic factors

Generally speaking, systemic conditions are one of the factors that most significantly influence the choice and implementation of the implant treatment plan.

The pre-surgical evaluation of a patient who will undergo implant treatment must include, in addition to an overall extraoral and intraoral evaluation, a general systemic evaluation of the state of health (2.1) and, in the first instance, it may be useful the assessment of the ASA status (Society of American Anesthesiologists) which allows to discriminate in an immediate and sustainable way from a medico-legal point of view, the subjects who can be eligible for treatment and the subjects for whom such treatment is contraindicated. From this point of view it is not indicated to suggest implant surgery to a decompensated patient, while subjects ASA-1 and ASA-2 (i.e. healthy or with systemic pathologies or compromises compensated) can always access the treatment. Following this general evaluation, the presence of systemic pathologies or conditions that may have some influence should be specifically assessed not about surgery or implant treatment in general. The presence of dys-metabolic pathologies such as diabetes, represents a surgical risk factor and an aspect that can affect the onset of biological complications at the level of the implants themselves, so it is essential that a pre-surgical and systemic monitoring over time should be in place. At the moment, there is no solid evidence that the presence of osteoporosis can limit the efficiency of the treatment of osseointegrated implantology.

In the general population, the increase in the average age has allowed a greater number of elderly subjects to have access to implant treatments. Although it has been confirmed by numerous scientific studies that age in itself does not represent a risk factor for immediate complications or over time,[3] it is correct to consider that often these subjects can present comorbidity and they frequently take medications that can affect treatment outcomes. It is not the purpose of this chapter to explore this topic, but certainly this category of patients must be considered with greater attention by referring them to a medical specialist. People who take drugs that affect the blood clotting process (anticoagulants, including so-called new oral anticoagulants, and anti-aging agents) and drugs used for bone diseases, including osteoporosis, such as bisphosphonates, can undergo treatment only after a careful evaluation of the risks and benefits, since they can experience severe complications following the trauma induced by the surgery itself. Among subjects who are taking drugs or who are undergoing systemic treatments, implant treatment is contraindicated in subjects undergoing anticancer chemotherapy or radiotherapy in the head and neck areas, including previous ones.

Local factors

The process of bone atrophy that always follows the extraction or loss of tooth elements was first described by Atwood in 1963.[4] This process is particularly intense during the first year and then gradually decreases in the following years and affects both jaws without distinction with different dynamics, in which usually the posterior region of the jaws is subject to a faster and more important resorption.

Obviously, the presence or the absence of an adequate bone volume for the placement of implants is a critical factor in the pre-surgical and prognostic evaluation of the treatment. The most famous classification proposed for bone atrophies (and therefore for the available bone volume) was presented by Misch and Judy in 1987[5] (2.1). This classification allows for a subdivision by complexity of implant cases and a pre-surgical evaluation aimed at the possibility of planning a guided regeneration intervention to increase the available bone volume. In fact, the presence of a type C or D bone volume cannot be separated from bone regeneration operations.

Bone volume must obviously be considered when choosing the diameter and length of the implants. These factors significantly influence the prognosis and the quality of the treatment since it is always necessary to consider, as suggested by the scientific literature, that in a mesio-distal direction the implant margin should be positioned at least 1.5 mm from the adjacent tooth and at least 3-4 mm from any nearby implant. Considering the thickness (intended as a bucco-lingual measurement of the bone), it is usually believed that there must be a

2.1 Evaluation checklist for suitable implant surgery patients

Extraoral examination	Intraoral examination	General systemic examination
Face aesthetics analysis	Dental aesthetics analysis	ASA state
Examination of soft tissues	General dental check (periodontal, orthodontic, conservative, endodontic, prosthetic)	Drugs taken
Position of the smile line	Level of oral hygiene	Concomitant systemic diseases
	Characteristics of the maxillary bone	Bad habits such as cigarette smoking and drugs
	Gnathological evaluation	Current or previous radiotherapy or chemotherapy
	Presence of parafunctions	State of pregnancy or breastfeeding

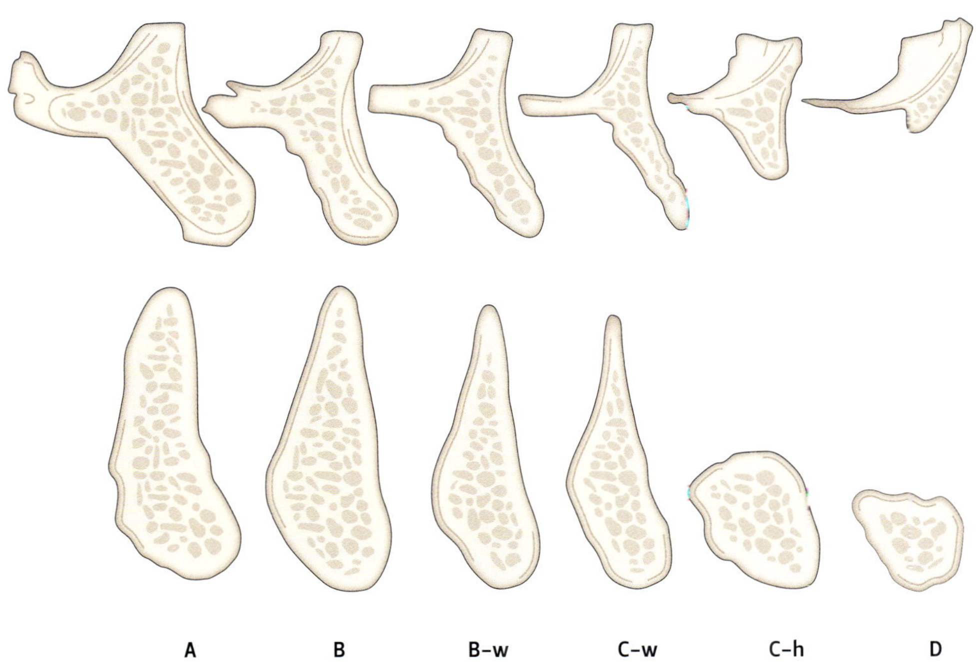

2.1 Classification of bone atrophy according to Misch & Judy. **A**: abundant bone in all dimensions; **B**: decrease of the vestibular bone theca; **B-w**: reduction in thickness of the residual crest (which makes implantation techniques difficult), moderate atrophy; **C-w**: reduction in thickness (which is inadequate for implantation techniques), advanced atrophy; **C-h**: inadequate reduction even in height; **D**: total loss of the alveolar process and maintenance of the basal bone only.

quantity of available buccal or lingual bone of at least 1-1.5 mm[6] (2.2). Using these parameters, it is safe to have a bone thickness of at least 6-7 mm, for example, to accommodate a 4 mm diameter implant. In view of this, it is frequently necessary to make interventions to increase the available bone volume, the principles of which will be described in the following chapters.

Alongside the considerations made regarding the need to have sufficient bone volume available for the insertion of an implant, it must be emphasized that a determining factor for the stability and success of implant treatments in the long term is represented by the bone density. While leaving to other chapters the description of the anatomical and histological characteristics of the bone tissue, it is advisable to observe how the maxillary bones have an extremely variable bone density, which is a fundamental factor in carrying out the implant treatment. Following the classification proposed by Misch,[7] it is possible to distinguish a bone D1, broadly corticalized and with a compact medulla, typical of the median region of the mandible, from a D2 bone, with a well represented cortical bone and less compact medullary part, typical of the anterior and posterior mandible, from a D3 bone, with poorly represented cortical bone and poorly represented medullary component (anterior and posterior superior maxilla) and a D4 bone, typical of

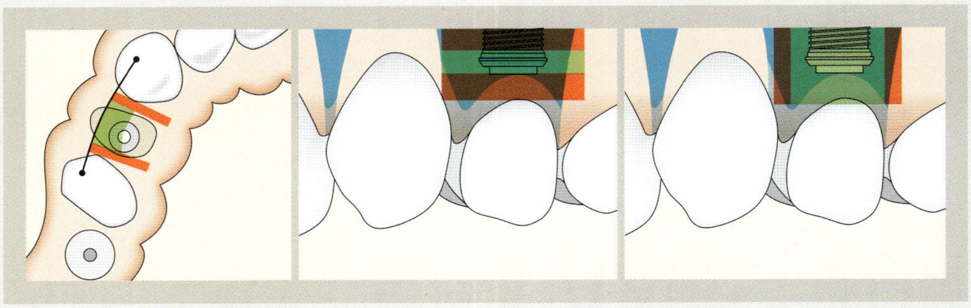

2.2 The distance between the implant and the adjacent tooth should be approximately 1.5–2 mm. In the apico-coronal sense, the implant should be positioned approximately 3–4 mm from the gingival margin of the future restoration, at least 2 mm apical with respect to the line joining the enamel-cementum junctions of the adjacent teeth. The buccal portion of the implant should be 1–2 mm palatal with respect to the emergence profile of the adjacent tooth.

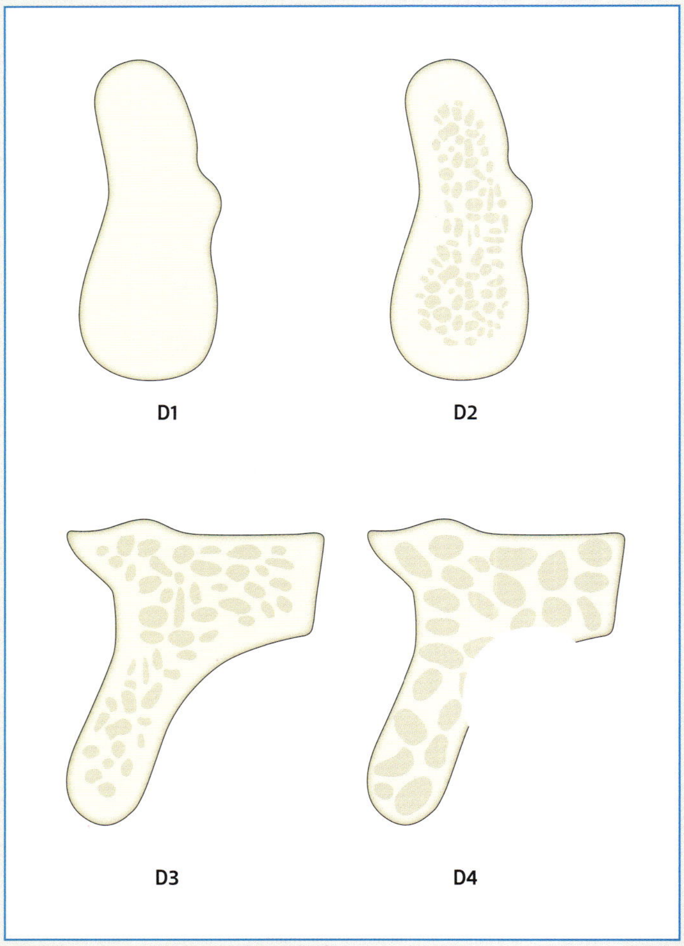

2.3 Misch classification of maxillary bone density.

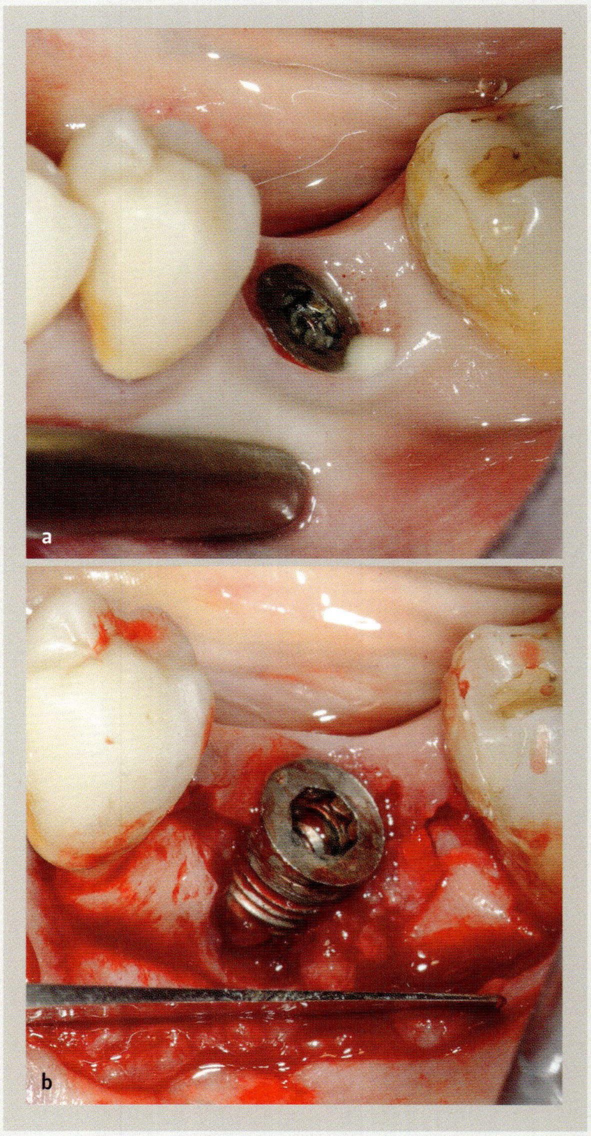

2.4 **(a,b)** Case of peri-implantitis.

the posterior maxillary region, little or no corticalized and with the medullary that frequently has large lacunae (📷 2.3). The bone density, due to anatomical and genetic characteristics, is determined by the possibility, after the extraction of the tooth, to allow and to facilitate an adequate healing of the socket, by the stimulation of local growth factors and with the use, where necessary, of biocompatible bone substitute biomaterials. The density of the bone itself is a fundamental prerequisite for obtaining the primary stability of the dental implant, reducing the chance of complications and favouring adequate post-surgical healing. In fact, it affects the percentage of contact between the implant and the bone (also influenced by the healing of the post-extraction socket) and the resistance to mechanical stress by the entire structure consisting of the implant and the prosthesis that it supports.

Factors related to other conditions or bad habits

Among the conditions that can influence the success of an implant treatment as a whole, we can mention bruxism, which is a condition in which the subject unconsciously grinds their teeth, especially at night. This situation involves a transmission of large forces at the level of the implant restoration (and consequently of the implant itself) which can cause a significant increase in the chance of the occurrence of prosthetic and mechanical complications in general.[8]

Cigarette smoking and the presence of untreated periodontitis are among the factors that can most frequently compromise the success of implant treatments.

Cigarette smoking acts as one of the factors most closely related to implant failure. On one hand, cigarette smoking involves direct physical (excessive heat) and chemical trauma to the mucosal tissues, inducing a local inflammatory process capable of providing the prerequisite for the development of biological complications; on the other hand, smoking can considerably reduce peripheral vascularization and therefore the ability of the peri-implant tissue itself to react to exogenous bacterial insults. The smoker must be informed about the increased risk herein described and therefore invited to quit this habit.

The presence of untreated periodontitis (of any stage and grade) is an absolute contraindication to implant treatment, since it represents one of the most certain and recognizable risk factors for implant failure and peri-implantitis. In addition to an accurate overall assessment of the health condition of the oral cavity, the implant treatment must always be preceded by a complete periodontal treatment.

In addition to these factors, which are easily objectified, it is necessary that our observation is also directed to those characteristics of the subject that pertain to the psychological background and that find expression in the motivation of the subject and their attitude towards the treatment itself.

Surgical procedure

As described in the previous paragraphs, implant treatment cannot ignore an overall assessment of the subject to be treated, either from a systemic or a local point of view. It has already been observed that the volumetric and anatomical characteristics of the available bone are a fundamental parameter to be evaluated and, in addition to the clinical examination, this evaluation is performed by the use of radiographs. Commonly, in the implant field it is advisable, in many conditions, to have three-dimensional images available, which allow a clear visualization of the anatomical structures and the available bone volume. Except in special cases, these images are obtained through the use of the so-called CBCT (Cone-Beam Computed Tomography), a particular type of three-dimensional radiography specifically designed for the dental field (📷 2.4). Through these images, and an adequate processing, it is also possible to obtain the creation of diagnostic or surgical stents or guides.

The pre-surgical control of the subject's systemic conditions may include the modification of the systemic therapeutic regimens in place and the administration of an antibiotic prophylaxis (2 grams of amoxicillin per os one hour before surgery or, in subjects with an allergy or hypersensitivity to beta-lactams, 500 mg of clarithromycin one hour before surgery) in patients who are eligible for as, for example, subjects who have undergone a heart transplant or with a history of previous bacterial endocarditis.[9]

Once the infiltrative local anaesthetic (LA) has been performed (generally it is better to avoid any nerve block) and a muco-periosteal flap in the region of implant insertion has been elevated, it is necessary to verify the size of the available bone volumes by direct visualization and measurement.

In general terms, the technique of positioning a dental implant involves the preparation of an implant site in the context of the identified bone volume. The preparation of the implant bed usually takes place through the use of calibrated cylindrical or conical spiral burs with gauge indications. This procedure must be performed with instruments and with movements that are not very traumatic to the bone and soft tissues to reduce the onset of complications. Since overheating of the site due to inadequate preparation or unsuitable instruments can represent an important cause of peri-implant bone resorption and failure, it is always recommended to implement when high speeds are adopted (higher than 600-800 revolutions per minute), a cooling of the osteotomy site with sterile physiological solution and an intermittent movement of "up and down" until the desired length is reached. Both the drill preparation procedure and the implant placement can be facilitated by the presence of bone consisting of D1-D3 density.

The positioning within the prepared site must be carried out by limiting any stress and with an insertion force that is not excessive, but at the same time adequate to allow sufficient stability to the implant itself. Typically, this procedure is performed at a low speed (15-20 revolutions per minute), without irrigation with saline, with a dynamometric device used manually or mounted on a handpiece.

Once the implant has been placed and the surgical treatment has been completed with suture placement, the patient must be instructed to avoid hot, irritating or hard food, preferably a semi-solid or liquid not hot diet for at least the first two days after surgery. Furthermore, the patient must be asked to avoid any trauma at the wound level and to limit the use of cold packs, for example, ice, for very short periods (5 minutes maximum) and only during the first 24 hours. The wound cleansing must be carried out with the aid of topical disinfectant (chlorhexidine 1% gel or 0.2% mouthwash) for at least 7 days from the date of the intervention, avoiding induced trauma from normal home oral hygiene devices. The administration of systemic drugs should be limited to analgesic or anti-inflammatory products, while the administration of antibiotics in the post-surgical period should be restricted to cases for which there is an indication and carefully evaluated case by case.

Timing of implant placement

All the considerations made previously relate to implants placed in native bone or in any case in healed bone following a dental extraction or a trauma. This reflects the desire to wait for a sufficient period for the complete maturation and healing of the bone before proceeding with the implant placement. This period does not have a defined duration, since there are no objective parameters to evaluate the end of the healing process but, on the basis of histological studies, it is assumed not to be less than 2 months for the mandible and 3 months for the maxilla, due to the different anatomical characteristics in the two districts.

However, with a view to some patient's needs it is possible to immediately place an implant at the same time of the extraction. The concept of an immediate post-extraction implant (or simply immediate implantation) has therefore found wide application especially in the frontal sextants of the upper jaw, for aesthetical concerns.

The literature has defined three keystone times for placing an integrated bone implant following the extraction of a dental element:[10]

1. immediately after extraction (immediate implantation);
2. early, that is, during the healing phase of the alveolus ("early");
3. after a complete healing of the extraction site (postponed or delayed).

In recent times, the possibility of placing implants immediately after the extraction of the dental element has greatly increased to accommodate requests for reducing treatment times.

From the existing scientific literature point of view it is possible to state that, in conditions of integrity of the post-extraction socket, the success rate of immediate implants is about 95%, although they still have a higher failure rate than implants placed in native bone.[11]

In short, the surgical procedure for immediate implants involves, after a thorough revision of the post-extraction socket to remove all the infected material, the preparation of the implant site in the context of the socket itself provided a careful evaluation of the anatomical conformation of the alveolus. If, as the immediate implant has been placed, there is a "gap" between the surface of the implant and the internal wall of the socket greater than 2 mm, the contextual positioning of a bone substitute as a filler is strictly indicated to reduce the physiological re-absorption process of the buccal bone.

In general terms, immediate implants turn out particularly indicated in all cases of implant placement in the anterior sectors of the upper jaw (from premolar to premolar mainly), if there is an aesthetic or organizational need to significantly reduce treatment times and the appropriate anatomical conditions are in place. Where it is necessary to perform bone regeneration interventions, or there is a marked resorption of the walls of the socket itself after an inflammatory process, or there has been a fracture of the bony walls of the alveolus, a delayed approach may be indicated and staged in multiple surgeries. A relative contraindication is represented by the presence of an infection at the level of the extracted element; this condition has been correlated with a higher rate of implant failures.[12]

General characteristics of the prosthesis and timing of prosthetic loading

Bone-integrated implants offer a chance to replace lost and missing dental elements by their ability to support a variety of dental prostheses. It is not the purpose of this chapter to offer a detailed description of the prosthetic options in the field of implantology but, in order to carry out an implant treatment, guided as much as possible by the rehabilitation, which will be positioned ("prosthetically" guided implantology) and which the treated subject will benefit from a functional and aesthetic point of view, an overview of the prosthetic available options is provided here.

In general, a distinction is made between removable and non-removable supported implant prostheses.

The first are, in general, total rehabilitations of entire arches which have an implant anchorage that provides stability during the chewing and speech functions, but which can be removed by the patient in order to carry out home oral hygiene procedures. The so-called "overdenture" prostheses belong to this category: they are total prostheses with implant anchorage but which also have a mucous support, which is fundamental.

Non-removable implant prostheses offer an adequate solution for partial and total edentulousness of both arches and are classified, according to the fixation method of the prosthesis itself to the implant, in cementum-retained prostheses (similar to traditional prostheses on teeth) and screw-retained prostheses. The latter appear to be more recommended today, since they are easily removed by the clinician in the event of the onset of complications; however, cemented prostheses still maintain broad indications.

The first historical approach to implantology provided that the prosthesis was placed after a certain period of "healing" following the implant placement. Currently, three different prosthetic loading times can be distinguished:[13]

1. "conventional" load, which occurs at a distance of at least two months from the placement of implants;
2. "early" loading that occurs in a period between the first week and two months of the "conventional" load;
3. "immediate" loading that occurs within the first week of implant treatment, ideally in the first hours.

The assumption through which an immediate prosthetic load can be implemented, mainly concerns the opportunity to obtain a primary stability, that is the stability of the implant at the placement, that would be sufficient to guarantee the absolute fixation to the structure.

Clearly this factor is dependent on the insertion torque and, therefore, on all the factors that influence it, which are represented by the implant morphology, the precision of the site preparation, the bone density at the site of the operation (the primary stability of an implant in bone D1 or D2 will certainly be greater than implants placed in bone D3 and D4) and, in general, by the surgical technique, with regards to the immediate implants. Immediate loading can be indicated in all regions of the maxillary arches, but is particularly suitable, where it is possible to implement it, in aesthetic regions and in cases of complete edentulism, in which the positioning of temporary restorations could be difficult to be realised.

In terms of implant success and survival rate, in general, the immediate loading has slightly lower percentages than conventional loading and this aspect, in the medium and long term, must be considered together with the indications and contraindications to the treatment.[14]

Implant complications

Implants and, in general, implant-prosthetic rehabilitations are obviously subject to early or late complications, i.e. technical or biological.

Technical complications relate to the prosthetic and implant device itself, and they can include fractures of any type of the prosthetic veneer, fractures of the fixation screw, of the implant, of the prosthetic abutment or of the entire prosthetic structure and a series of less serious problems, such as unscrewing or de-cementation of the prosthesis or the partial loss of material that can be solved easily.

Biological complications are divided into early and late ones depending on the timing of onset. Early complications occur less than 12 months after implant placement and include all immediate postoperative complications related to infection of the implant placement site, which can cause treatment failure. Early complications can also arise following the cementation of the restoration, due to the dispersion of cementum in the peri-implant tissues and can be easily solved through the identification and removal of the cementum itself, or as a result of an inadequate and excessive load that can, in extreme cases, lead to peri-implant bone resorption.

Late biological complications are represented by inflammatory diseases based on infections that affect the peri-implant soft tissues. Unlike periodontal tissues, peri-implant soft tissues lack a real attachment of connective fibers to the implant surface and the tissue is overall weaker against the insults caused by bacterial aggregation of the biofilm, if compared to the gingival tissues around natural dental elements. From a clinical point of view, we can distinguish peri-implant mucositis, a reversible inflammation of the peri-implant soft tissue without involvement of the peri-implant bone tissue, and peri-implantitis, in which we encounter the clinical signs of inflammation (edema, redness, bleeding on probing and possibly purulent exudate) alongside the radiological evidence of peri-implant bone resorption.

From the diagnostic point of view, the diagnosis of perimplantitis shows evidence of:

- bleeding or suppuration on probing;
- increase of the probing depth compared to previous measurements;
- presence of bone resorption in addition to changes in crestal bone tissue resulting from initial remodeling.[15]

If no previous findings are available, to make a diagnosis of peri-implantitis it is necessary to observe:

- a probing depth greater than or equal to 6 mm;
- an evidence of a bone level of at least 3 mm apical than the intraosseous portion of the implant (📷 2.4).

Thanks to these clinical characteristics it is possible to carry out an early diagnosis of peri-implant pathology which, therefore, cannot be separated from the planning of an adequate and calibrated maintenance protocol according to the characteristics of the patient who presents a clinical evaluation alongside an accurate radiographical evaluation.

The prevalence of peri-implant inflammatory pathology in the population is extremely high, involving on average 22% of implants placed with peri-implantitis and 43% of implants with peri-implant mucositis, and this occurs substantially for all types of rehabilitation.[16] Cigarette smoking and the presence of periodontitis are easily recognizable among the risk factors most easily correlated to perimplantitis, topics which are covered in greater detail in the previous paragraphs.

Since peri-implant mucositis is an easily treatable and reversible pathology, the approach strategy towards this event must include the prevention and early diagnosis before it can progress to peri-implantitis. Faced with a case of diagnosed peri-implantitis, the therapeutic protocol may include non-surgical treatment (with the use of local or systemic antibiotics, subgingival instrumentation, and use of disinfectants) aimed at reducing symptoms and short-term treatment. Later it can be associated to both regenerative and resective surgical treatment aimed at the removal of the inflammatory tissue in the pocket (or peri-implant lesion), the detoxification (through various techniques) of the implant surface and the treatment of the bone defect.

Although surgical therapeutic strategies against peri-implantitis have shown a certain efficacy, the pathology is to be considered a severe complication and therefore an adequate protocol for the prevention and management of the reversible phases of the pathology is always recommended.

REFERENCES

1. Adell R, Hansson BO, Brånemark PI, et al. Intra-osseous anchorage of dental prostheses. II. Review of clinical approaches. Scand J Plast Reconstr Surg 1970;4(1):19-34.
2. Brånemark PI, Adell R, Breine U, et al. Intra-osseous anchorage of dental prostheses. I. Experimental studies. Scand J Plast Reconstr Surg 1969;3(2):81-100.
3. Heitz-Mayfield LJ, Aaboe M, Araujo M, et al. Group 4 ITI Consensus Report: risks and biologic complications associated with implant dentistry. Clin Oral Implants Res 2018;29(Suppl 16):351-8.
4. Atwood DA. Postextraction changes in the adult mandible as illustrated by microradiographs of midsagittal sections and serial cephalometric roentgenograms. J Prosthet Dent 1963; 13 (5):810-24.
5. Misch CE, Judy KW. Classification of partially edentulous arches for implant dentistry. J Oral Implantol 1987;4(2): 7-13.
6. Chen ST, Buser D. Clinical and esthetic outcomes of implants placed in postextraction sites. Int J Oral Maxillofac Implants 2009;24(Suppl):186-217.
7. Misch CE. Bone character: second vital implant criterion. Dent Today 1988; 7(5): 39-40.
8. Salvi GE, Brägger U. Mechanical and technical risks in implant therapy. Int J Oral Maxillofac Implants 2009; 24(Suppl):69-85.
9. American Dental Association (ADA). For the dental patient...: antibiotics and your heart: new guidelines from the American Heart Association. J Am Dent Assoc 2007;138(6):920.
10. Hämmerle CH, Chen ST, Wilson TG Jr. Consensus statements and recommended clinical procedures regarding the placement of implants in extraction sockets. Int J Oral Maxillofac Implants 2004;19(Suppl):26-8.
11. Cosyn J, De Lat L, Seyssens L, et al. The effectiveness of immediate implant placement for single tooth replacement compared to delayed implant placement: a systematic review and meta-analysis. J Clin Periodontol 2019;46(Suppl 21):224-41.
12. Lee J, Park D, Koo KT, et al. Comparison of immediate implant placement in infected and non-infected extraction sockets: a systematic review and meta-analysis. Acta Odontol Scand 2018;76(5):338-45.
13. Esposito M, Grusovin MG, Maghaireh H, et al. Interventions for replacing missing teeth: different times for loading dental implants. Cochrane Database Syst Rev 2013;(3):CD003878.
14. Chen J, Cai M, Yang J, et al. Immediate versus early or conventional loading dental implants with fixed prostheses: a systematic review and meta-analysis of randomized controlled clinical trials. J Prosthet Dent 2019;122(6): 516-36.
15. Berglundh T, Armitage G, Araujo MG, et al. Peri-implant diseases and conditions: consensus report of workgroup 4 of the 2017 World Workshop on the Classification of Periodontal and Peri-Implant Diseases and Conditions. J Clin Periodontol 2018;45 (Suppl 20):286-91.
16. Derks J, Tomasi C. Peri-implant health and disease. A systematic review of current epidemiology. J Clin Periodontol 2015;42(Suppl 16):158-71.

Guided bone regeneration: rationale and fundamental concepts

E. Minetti

Development and structure of bone. Types of bone and structural organization

Bones can be classified according to their shape, **mode of development** and **microscopic structure**.

Form-based classification

The bones can be long, short, flat and irregular.

- **Long bones.** The long bones are those in which the length prevails over the width and they are present mainly in the upper limbs (humerus, radius ulna) and in the lower ones (femur, tibia, fibula). They have a central part, called body or diaphysis, and two ends, called epiphyses. On a cross section, the body looks thick and compact with a central canal called the medullary canal. The ends are formed of spongy bone surrounded by a layer of compact bone.
- **Short bones.** They have almost the same length, width and thickness. Examples are vertebrae, carpal bones, etc. In section they appear to be made up of spongy tissue delimited externally by a layer of compact tissue.
- **Flat bones.** They are characterized by a lesser thickness than the length and width. They consist of two sheets of compact tissue with a layer of spongy tissue in between. One example is the skull bones.[1]
- **Irregular bones.** They have complicated forms that cannot be classified in the previous categories. These include bones such as the ethmoid, the sphenoid, the pelvic bones, etc.

Development-based classification

According to their development, bones can be of two types: endochondral and intramembranous.

- **Endochondral bones.** These bones are formed by the replacement of hyaline cartilage by the bone. The bones of the base of the skull, spinal column, pelvis and limbs are preceded by a cartilaginous outline which serves as a model for the subsequent development. The cartilage model is then destroyed and replaced by bone tissue.
- **Intramembranous bones.** These bones are formed by a replacement of the connective tissue by the bone. They are mainly the flat bones and the jaws. The ossification process begins in the so-called ossification centers, in

which the mesenchyme condenses and its cells proliferate, transforming them into an osteoid tissue which soon calcifies. The subsequent growth occurs by an apposition pattern. The osteoblasts arranged around the primitive trabeculae process a new layer of osteoid tissue which is added to what has already formed previously. Some osteoblasts remain included in the matrix and become osteocytes.

In primitive bone tissue the lamellae are arranged randomly, which is why it is called non-lamellar bone tissue. Initially it is always spongy, but it thickens in those areas committed to develop into compact bone.

Classification based on microscopic structure

Histologically we can distinguish between mature bone and immature bone.

- The **mature bone** is divided into:
  - **cortical bone**, which consists of a dense, solid bone formed by lamellar bone;
  - **medullary bone**, which consists of a honeycomb structure with large cavities, spaces and trabeculae in the form of bars or strings.
- The **immature bone** (*woven bone*) is made up of bone with irregularly oriented collagen fibers and constitutes the first healing phase of a bone defect. It will later turn into mature lamellar bone.

Composition of the bone

Bone is a connective tissue composed of cells, fibres and amorphous substance. The intercellular substance is made up of an organic and an inorganic part, consisting of minerals (3.1).

The **inorganic part** (61%) is formed by a mineral, the hydroxyapatite crystals, which however contain a low Ca/P ratio compared to pure hydroxyapatite. The bone crystals are in the form of thin plates or leaf structures and they are compacted with respect to the long axis almost parallel to the collagen fibrils. The space between the fibres contains water and organic macromolecules.

The **organic part** (39%) is made up of 90% collagen, of which 95% is type I collagen and the remaining 5% is type III, V and XII collagen. Collagen guarantees resilience and elasticity to bones, making them resistant to fractures. The remaining 10% is made up of non-collagen proteins produced by the bone cells.[2]

Bone cells

Bone cells are represented by osteoblasts, osteoclasts and osteocytes (3.2).

OSTEOBLASTS

They are small mononuclear cells of mesenchymal derivation which secrete the organic macromolecules which

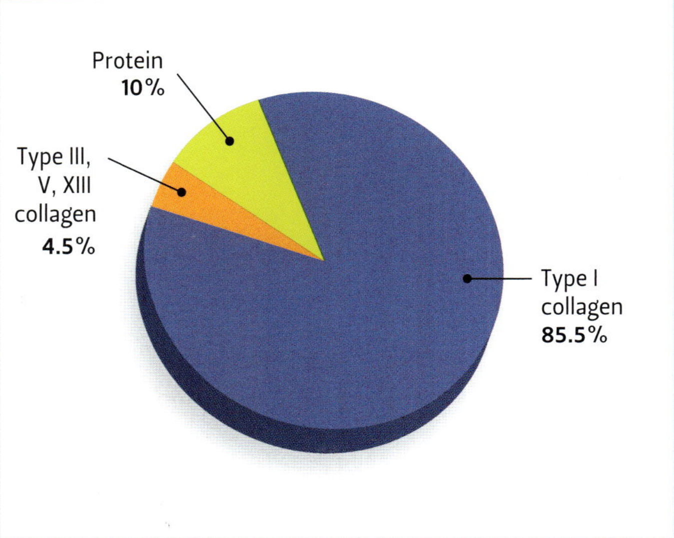

3.1 Schematic composition of the bone.

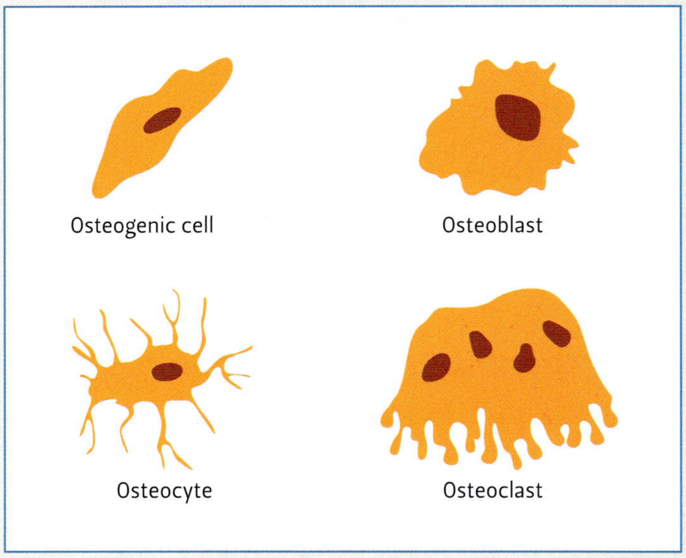

3.2 Bone cells.

constitute the bone matrix (3.3). The calcium and phosphorus salts will then settle on this collagen matrix, creating hydroxyapatite. These cells derive from mesenchymal osteoprogenitor cells present in the bone marrow, in other connective tissues and in the periosteum. They have a cuboid shape. They produce an organic matrix consisting mainly of type I collagen and non-collagenic proteins (3.1).

Osteoblasts release proteins along the mineralization front, where they also participate in the deposition of the mineral part. The cells adhere to each other and this allows them to connect through microfilaments that act as an information exchange system (3.4).

Osteoblasts arise from totipotent undifferentiated mesenchymal cells that can be divided into two types:

- **determined osteogenic precursor cells** (DOPCs), present in the bone marrow, endosteum and periosteum that differentiate into osteoblasts under the influence of BMPs (Bone Morphogenetic Protein);
- **inducible osteogenic precursor cells** (IOPCs), mesenchymal cells present in other organs and tissues that can be transformed into osteoblasts when stimulated.

The regulation of osteoblasts occurs by the action of various hormones including PTH (ParaThyroid Hormone), vitamin D, estrogenes, and glucocorticoids (3.2).

When they finish their function, they get trapped in the bone tissue and turn into osteocytes.

3.1 Main proteins present in the bone

· GLA protein (osteocalcin)
· Osteopontin
· Osteonectin
· Proteoglycans
· BMP (Bone Morphogenetic Protein)
· PDGF (Plateled Derived Growth Factor)
· FGF (Fibroblast Growth Factor)
· IGF (Insulin-like Growth Factor)
· Lysyl oxidase
· TRAMP (Tyrosine Rich Acidic Matrix Protein)

OSTEOCYTES

When the osteoblasts are trapped in the same bone structure they had produced, they turn into osteocytes (3.5).

Their average life is about 25 years and it is considerably longer than the osteoblasts', which is about 3 months.

Within the lacuna, the osteocyte decreases in size and creates a small space around itself, called osteocytic lacuna. Canaliculi depart from this lacuna through which cells communicate with adjacent cells by means of microfilaments in the direction of the

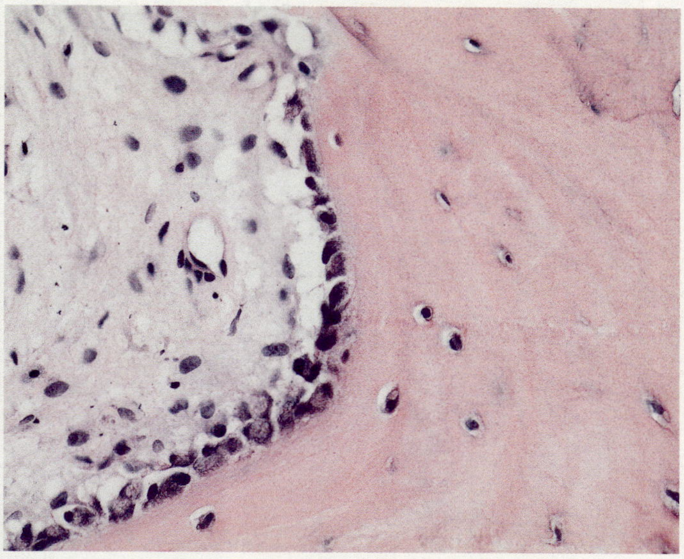

3.3 Osteoblasts online.

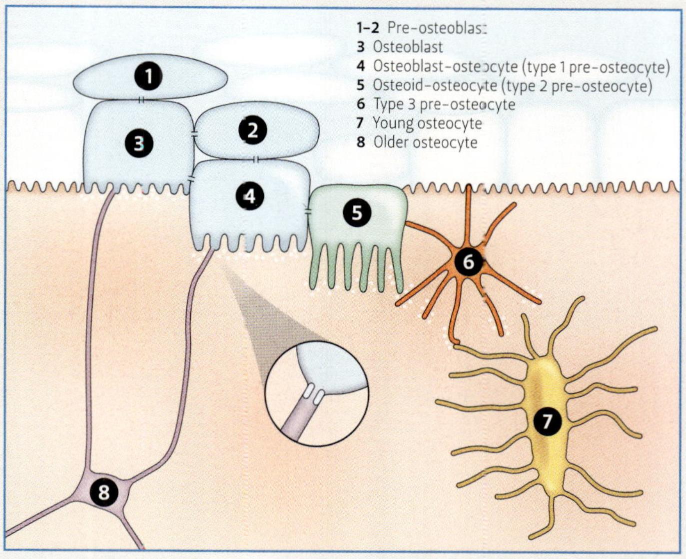

3.4 Evolution of osteoblasts.

3.2 Factors that favor the formation of osteoblasts

Differentiating factors	Adjustment factors	Local and systemic factors
• Wnt/ β-catenin • Cbfa1 • Osterix	• Runx-2	**Bone morphogenetic proteins (BMP)** • BMP2, BMP4, BMP6 **Cell growth factors** • Fibroblast Growth Factors (FGF) • Insulin-like Growth Factor (IGF 1-IGF 2) • Transforming Growth Factor β (TGFβ) • Platelet Derived Growth Factor (PDGF) **Hormones** • Parathyroid hormone (PTH) • Insulin • Growth hormone • Vitamin D3 • **Glucocorticoids** • **Cytokine-IL6**

osteoblast line on the surface (*see* 3.4). These channels also allow the diffusion of nutrients and waste, creating a connection system that allows to maintain the bone integrity.[3]

OSTEOCLASTS

They are cells that remove the bone tissue by eliminating the mineralized matrix; they are large and polynucleated (3.6). They have receptors for the parathyroid hormone and the calcitonin, both hormones acting on bone resorption control.

On their edge there are vesicles that acidify the contact environment and cause the lysis of the bone matrix. The organic component is dissolved by enzymes and the inorganic component by the pH variation. They have amoeboid-type movement skills (3.7).

The remodeling aims to rebuild the bone tissue following the load lines and the release of calcium ions contributes to the balancing of calcium.[4,5]

Bone matrix. Cortical bone, medullary bone, lamellar bone, immature bone

Osteoblasts synthesize a tissue called osteoid which is made up of a matrix of collagen and non-collagenic proteins. This tissue is converted into mineralized bone. The bone matrix is a compound blend of water, minerals, collagen and non-collagenic macromolecules.[6,7] Collagen, in addition to its structural role, also performs a morphogenetic function by acting as a reserve of non-collagenic proteins and support the deposition of mineral crystals. Then, during the tissue repair steps, growth factors are released both from the cells involved in the repair and from the bone matrix. The same growth factors are released during the resorption process by the osteoclasts.[8]

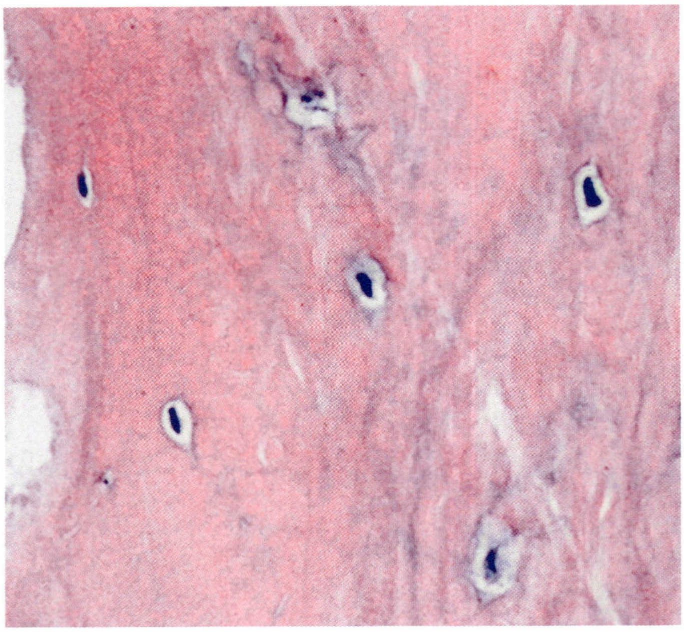

3.5 Osteocytes.

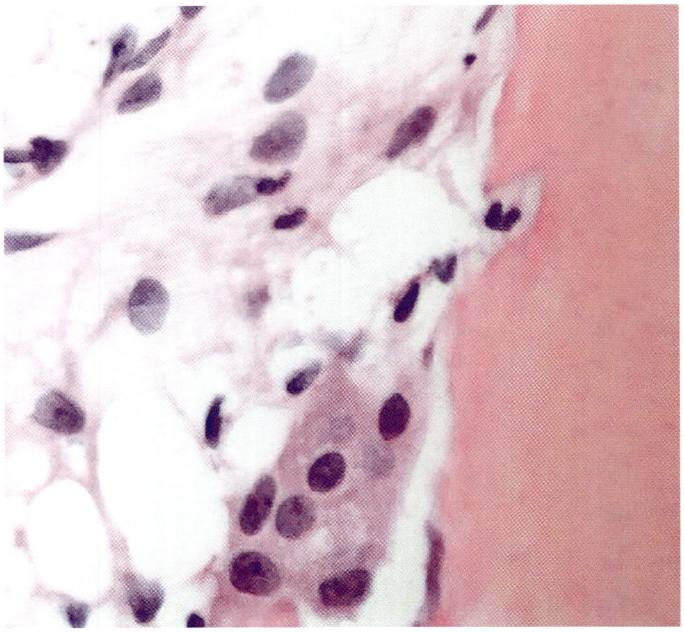

3.6 Osteoclast.

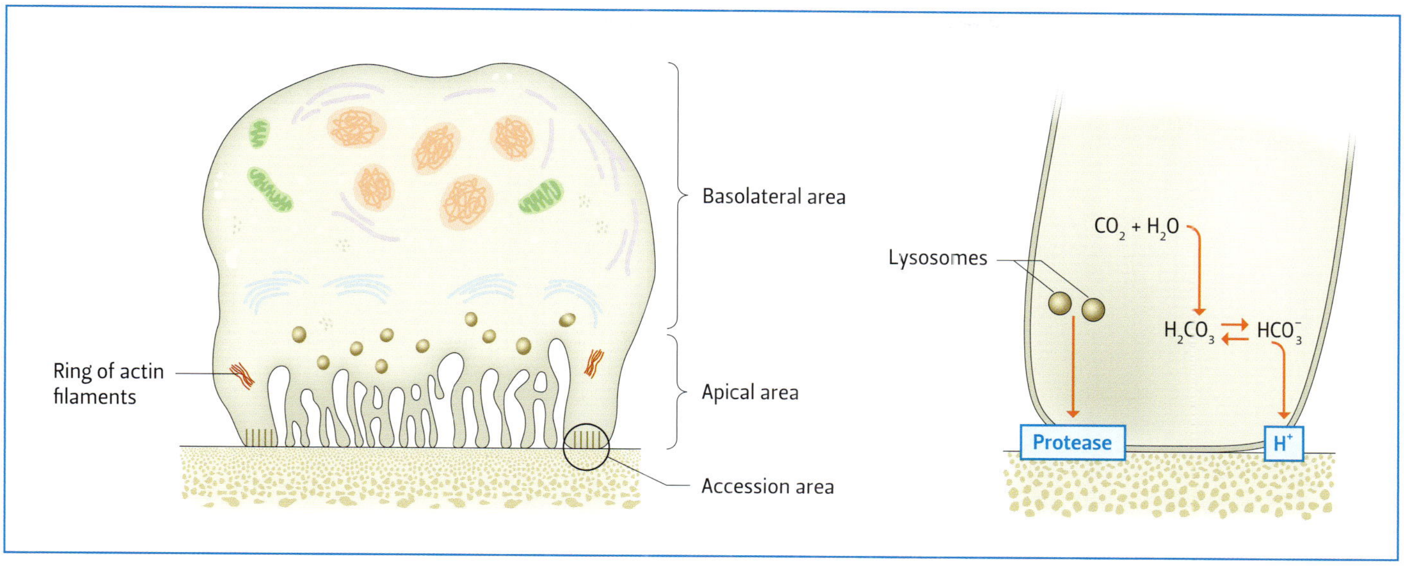

3.7 Osteoclast in business.

Intramembranous bone formation

Intramembranous ossification is the direct formation of bone within highly vascularized layers of primitive mesenchymal condensate. This process occurs in the skull bones, the jaw and collarbones. It begins approximately towards the end of the second month of gestation.

A centre of mesenchymal cells begins to aggregate and differentiate into osteoblasts starting the deposition of the organic matrix. The first calcification crystals appear in association with the extracellular vesicles deposited by the osteoblasts. This deposit rapidly extends to all the collagen fibrils.

The first small amount of bone matrix is uneven and disordered. The trabeculae extend radially creating the characteristic cancellous bone appearance. This bone is called immature bone (*woven bone*).

The cell line deposits a bone matrix and repeats several times the process called appositional growth.

Each generation of osteoblasts produces its own canaliculi so that, when they remain embedded in the bone tissue, the communication and the exchange channels will already be present. As this remodeling process continues, the tissue converts from immature bone to lamellar bone. The central part of the bone will remain as medullary without increasing its size.

This ossification mechanism requires BMP proteins, which activate the *cbfa1* gene in mesenchymal cells by transforming them into osteoblasts.

The difference between immature bone and lamellar bone lays in the arrangement of collagen fibers which in immature bone are intertwined and oriented in all dimensions, while in lamellar bone they are ordered as result of the repeated addition of uniform lamellae during the growth (3.3). Osteocytes appear spherical in immature bone and compressed and flattened in the lamellar bone.

Formation of the endochondral bone

This type of ossification allows the remodeling starting from a cartilage model and occurs in the long bones, vertebrae, ribs and the joint lines of the mandible. This topic, since it is beyond the scope of this textbook, will not be discussed.

Resorption of bone

Beyond its structural role, bone also represents the main storehouse of calcium.[9] In most of the physiological circumstances, bone formation is regulated by functional loads and mediators (growth factors). The control of resorption is carried out by biochemical mediators that control the metabolism of calcium (para-thyroid hormone, estrogen, vitamin D).[10]

The removal of the mineral and organic components goes through three stages:

1. formation of osteoclasts from the hematopoietic line;
2. positioning of osteoclasts on the surface of the mineralized bone;
3. activation of osteoclasts in bone resorption.

3.3 Differences between immature and lamellar bone

Immature bone	Lamellar bone
Intertwined collagen fibers	Organize collagen fibers
Plenty of interfibrillar space	Reduced interfibrillar space
Rapid formation and mineralization	Mineralization and slow formation
Low mineral density	High mineral density
High water content	Low water content
The extra-plasmatic vesicles line an important role in mineralization	Mineralization is mediated by collagen
Osteoclasts can remove all of the immature bone	Osteoclasts can remove a portion towards the lamellar bone

Immediately before the resorption phase, osteoclasts assume a polarity of structure. The margin becomes pleated and the outer part becomes thin, allowing it to seal with the bone. These changes occur only on the part of the cell in contact with the bone.

The initial phase consists in the dissolution of the mineral due to the action of hydrochloric acid (HCl). The pH goes down to about 2.5-3.0 and the organic parts of the bone remain after dissolution by the acid. Proteolytic enzymes (cathepsin-K and MMP-9) degrade collagen and release proteins. All the residues are then packed into gaps on the pleated edge, giving rise to vesicles that are released by exocytosis.

Guided Bone Regeneration (GBR)

The GBR surgical technique with the use of barrier membranes was introduced in 1988.[11]

In the mid-1980s, the principles of GTR (Guided Tissue Regeneration) were introduced.[12]

Considering that bone is a slow-growing tissue, while the epithelium is fast-growing, the GBR technique consists of using a membrane that retains space and seals on the edges of the bone tissue, thus creating an environment in which the osteoprogenitor cells, under the stimulation of growth factors, will transform into osteoblasts and they will begin producing bone tissue by repair, without any interference from fibroblasts.[13]

Two forms of regeneration can be distinguished: a physiological one (natural bone remodeling) and a reparative one, if the tissues have been lost due to an illness or an injury (3.4). GBR takes advantage of the mechanisms of reparative regeneration. Any bone lesion activates the release and the local production of growth factors and other signalling molecules.[14]

Osteoprogenitor cells localize in the bone marrow and periosteum and differentiate directly into osteoblasts. It is clear that one of the focal aspects of the GBR technique concerns the shape of the defect. The more the bone walls are, the greater the supply of mesenchymal and vascular support is. For this reason, there are many classification systems of bone defects suitable for creating predictable protocols for regenerative techniques.

Cells of hematopoietic origin always begin the activity to create space for cells of mesenchymal origin that are committed to reconstruct (3.5).

Bone healing of a GBR occurs in three stages, as indicated below.

3.4 Cell lines involved in bone remodeling

Mesenchymal cells (bone formation)	Hematopoietic cells (bone resorption)
· Fibroblasts · Endothelial cells · Pericytes (pre-osteoblasts) · Adipocytes · Osteoblasts-osteocytes · Chondroblasts	· Erythrocytes · Neutrophils, eosinophils, basophils · Lymphocytes · Monocytes (macrophages-osteoclasts) · Mast cells

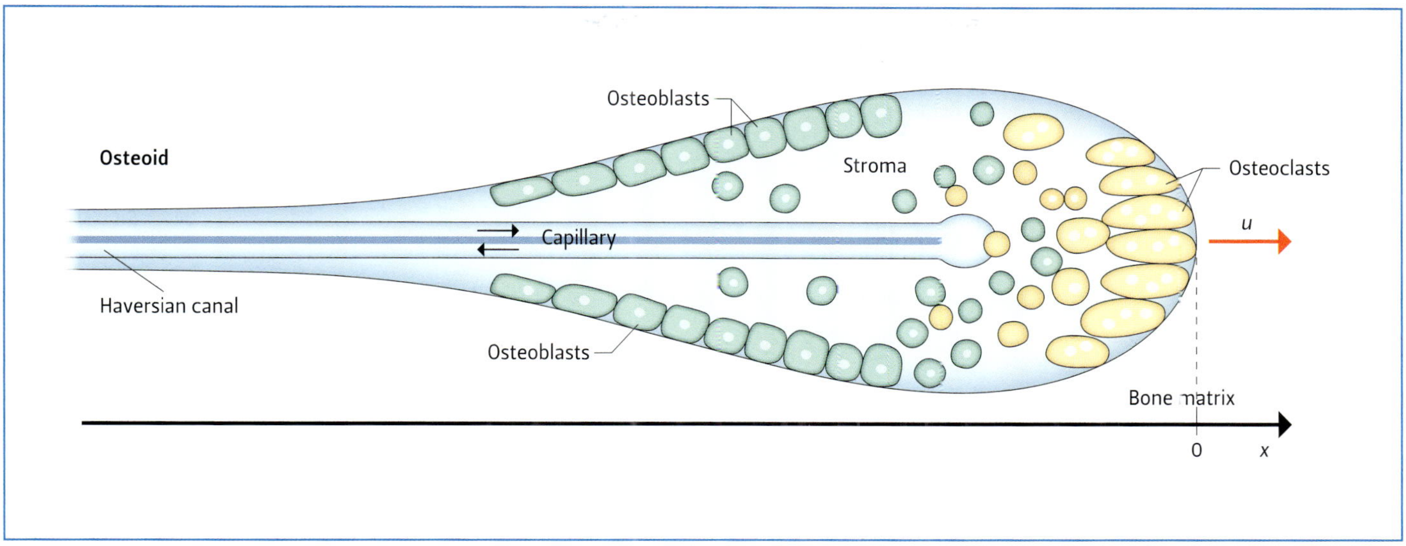

3.8 Bone Multicellular Unit (BMU). This unit is made up of numerous osteoclasts that invade the area in the direction of movement of the unit and eliminate the fibrous bone while the osteoblasts follow by depositing the lamellar bone. The red arrow indicates the direction and the passing time.

Phase 1. **Clot formation and migration of vascular structures from the defect walls (4-6 weeks).** Deposition of osteoid bone starts. The cellular and molecular cascade includes the migration of different cells from the bone walls. This process originates from the edges of the four-walled defect towards its center, following the texture of newly formed vessels, with the osteoblasts performing their function only in the proximity of the vascular framework. Cells produce key factors for bone formation and remodeling. The development of mature bone and bone remodeling are promoted by the stimulation of the osteoblasts and osteoclasts. The central part of the defect, not yet filled with regenerated tissue, is composed of loose connective tissue with orientation-free collagen fibers, fibroblasts, macrophages and vessels.

Phase 2. **Osteoid bone maturation and start of corticalization (2-3 months).** The medullary bone will be mineralized by osteoblasts and new cortical bone will begin to form on its periphery.

Phase 3. **Cortical bone maturation and start of bone remodeling (3-4 months).** New cortex can be seen near the membrane. In this phase, numerous osteoclasts invade the area and eliminate the fibrous bone, while the osteoblasts continue to deposit lamellar bone. This phase creates the osteons.

In the centre, the remodeling process leads to the formation of cancellous bone with trabeculae that follow the orientation of the applied load (3.8).[15]

Membranes

Numerous types of membranes have been proposed. The desirable characteristics for a membrane that can be used in GBR therapy include biocompatibility, barrier prop-

3.5 Conditions for bone regeneration

- Presence of an adequate clot guaranteed by correct vascular supply
- Presence of vital bone as cell lines migrate from it
- Release of growth factors to increase the number of osteoblasts
- Presence of a membrane that protects mechanically and prevents fibrous infiltration
- Membrane stabilization to maintain the biological space and the clot stability
- Membrane resorption time appropriate to the type of defect
- Waiting for an appropriate time to the type of defect

erties, integration into host tissues, clinical handling, maintenance of space and adequate mechanical and physical characteristics.[15,16]

Membranes can be:

- **non-resorbable**, represented by titanium sheet and expanded polytetrafluoroethylene (e-PTFE) with or without titanium reinforcement. One of the disadvantages of non-resorbable membranes is the need for further surgical intervention for their removal. Another negative aspect of e-PTFE membranes is linked to the unfavorable results in case of premature exposure with limited regeneration or infections;[17]
- **resorbable**, consisting of polyglycolic acid (PGA), polylactic acid (PLA) and tissue-derived collagen.[18]

But, if membranes are so effective and useful, why are grafting materials used under the membrane?

In 1990 Buser reported that a frequently observed complication was membrane collapse, resulting in a reduction in the regenerated volume.[19]

In 1992 Nevins added another indication: the use of graft material is recommended not only to prevent membrane collapse but also to promote the formation of new bone.[20]

The grafting materials proposed for this purpose are several. The biological rationale for the use of grafting materials is based on their ability to maintain space and stabilize the clot.[21]

Healing of a defect with GBR requires the presence of the following factors:

- **cells** to produce tissue and support structures from the defect walls and periosteum;
- **growth factors** to promote and guide cellular activities;
- **scaffold** to maintain space and structure for the deposit of the extracellular matrix.

Bone growth factors

The bone induction process is a process of cascade signals, where the differentiation of mesenchymal cells into osteoblasts determines the formation of new bone.

These signals are able to activate receptors on mesenchymal cells and they can be divided into three main families:

- insulin-like growth factors (IGFs);
- transforming growth factor β (TGFβ);
- bone morphogenetic proteins (BMPs).[22]

Insulin-like growth factors (IGFs)

IGF-1 and IGF-2 are the most abundant growth factors stored in bone. They are promoted by GH (Growth Hormone) and they stimulate cell proliferation and differentiate functions such as the expression of type I collagen.

IGF-1 is GH-dependent and peaks in puberty.

IGF-2 has its peak in fetal life and is less sensitive to GH.[23]

They are produced by the bone cells and are, in part, deposited in the new bone in such a way that they can be released during the resorption phases. This activity will increase the number of osteoblasts on the bone surface during the remodeling cycle. A model has been proposed according to which the concentration of bone growth factors incorporated in the bone varies with age and site. For example, cortical bone samples from calvaria had higher concentrations than the iliac crest or vertebral bodies. Some diseases, such as osteoarthritis, are correlated with a high concentration of IGF-1, IGF-2 and TGFβ.[24]

IGFs are small proteins, whose half-life is shorter but they can survive longer when bound together to form IGFBP (Insulin-like Growth Factor Binding Protein).

Transforming growth factors β (TGFβ)

TGFβ-1 and TGFβ-2 are produced by osteoblasts and incorporated into the bone matrix. They are expressed in high levels in mature osteoblasts on bone surfaces and in the healing callus.[25]

TGFβ-1 and 2 are synthesized as precursors and stored as inactive complexes (inactive TGFβ) which will be activated by extreme pH levels or proteases. The bone matrix contains large amounts of inactive TGFβ, which will be activated by the pH conditions present under the pleated edge of the osteoclasts. Their quantity decreases with age.

The activity of TGFβ is stimulated by vitamin D_3, estrogen, testosterone and PTH. Deficiency of D_3 and estrogen reduces the content of TGFβ present in cortical bone.

Their action targets two distinct type 1 and type 2 receptors and enhances the activity of BMPs.[26]

Bone morphogenetic proteins (BPMs)

BMPs are a family of thirteen different proteins (■ 3.6).

These proteins are able to initiate the whole process of bone neoformation both in heterotopic sites (sites other than normal, in this case different from bone) and in orthotopic sites (natural sites) (3.9). The first phase of BMPs' action determines a replication of mesenchymal cells from the neighboring tissues to the area affected by bone remodeling. BMPs repress the WNT signal which keeps the stem cell population stable.

BMP-2s bind to a Bone Morphogenetic Protein Receptor type 1A (BMPR1A), which is found on the cell membrane and is part of the serine/threonine kinase group of transmembrane proteins. BMPs activate the mesenchymal cells to turn into osteoblasts to begin the bone formation.

They are highly soluble proteins and require an insoluble carrier to be able to activate the mesenchymal cells. BMP-2s bindsto type 1 collagen. The soluble signal and the insoluble signal, if tested alone, do not induce any bone formation.[27]

There are also other growth factors not specific for bone but necessary for the regeneration process (3.7).

3.6 Main BMPs and their functions

BMP-2	It induces the formation of bone and cartilage. It determines the differentiation of mesenchymal cells into osteoblasts
BMP-3	It induces the formation of bone
BMP-4	It regulates the formation of the teeth
BMP-7	It induces differentiation into osteoblasts

Scaffold

Scaffolds are materials capable of maintaining space, stabilizing the clot and eventually releasing proteins or cells contained within them.

They must be safe and biocompatible, they must create spaces between the granules where the initial formation of vessels will be possible, they must have surface micropores (100-500 µm) to favour wettability, they must

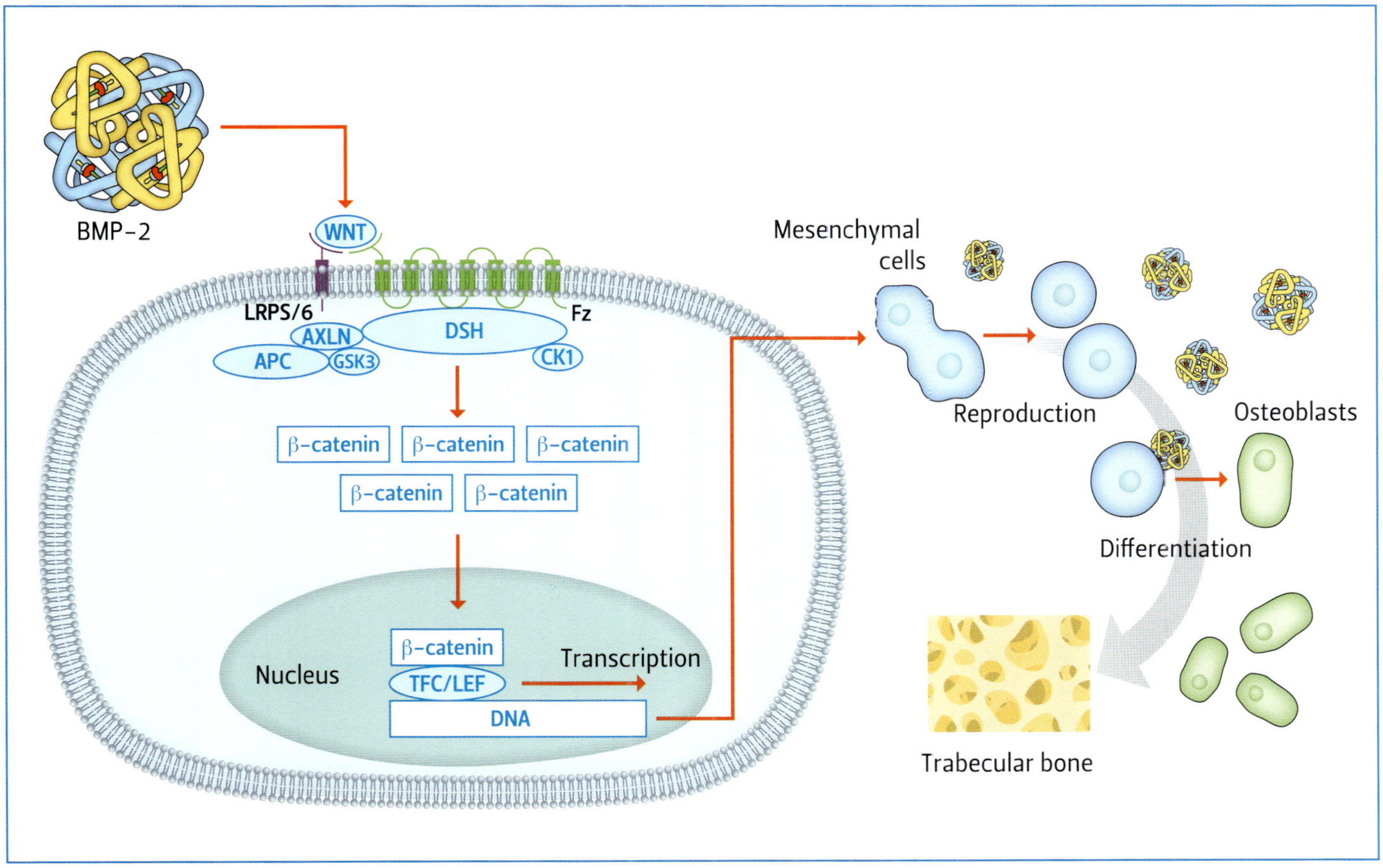

3.9 Mechanism of action of BMPs. From left: BMP-2, action on the transmembrane receptor BMPR1A and reproduction of mesenchymal cells with their differentiation into osteoblasts. WNT, transmembrane signaling gate.

3.7 Growth factors that are not specific to bone but are necessary for regeneration

Osteopontin (OPN)	It is used to maintain bone homeostasis. It binds to hydroxyapatite and provides the basic bone structure
Bone Sialoprotein (BSP)	It stimulates angiogenesis
Osteocalcin	It stimulates endocrine activity and is an indicator of bone activity
Type 1 collagen	Organic bone matrix, connects the mineral parts
Cbfa Run X2	It is essential for the differentiation of osteoblasts

3.8 Classification of scaffolds based on their properties

Osteoconduction	It provides a scaffold for bone regeneration and, during its dissolution, the mineral substrate
Osteoinduction	It produces neoformation of bone tissue even in a heterotopic situation. BMPs are able to initiate this process but must be carried by a specific carrier, in general by type 1 collagen
Osteoproliferation	Starting from the live cells contained in the graft material, it induces bone regeneration

have a correct crystallinity and crystal size and further, they must be easily handled during the surgical phase. All these characteristics are important for the initial stages, the adhesion of osteoblasts and osteoclasts and the deposition of the osteoid.[28]

Scaffolds are classified according to their properties and origin (3.8 and 3.9).

Autologous bone

It is the reference material due to its properties (osteoconduction, osteoinduction, osteoproliferation). Its remodeling capabilities vary depending on whether it is a cortical or a cancellous bone.

Cancellous bone tissue is rapidly vascularized, replaced and quickly resorbed.

The cortical bone, thanks to the greater density and the different structure, determines a high mechanical support but is vascularized more slowly.

All the growth factors are released only when the graft is reabsorbed. So, in this case, a particulate graft is preferable vs a block graft. In the same way, however, the number of the existing cells will be reduced due to the treatment undergone, therefore, if our target is to have the cells, a block will be preferrable, unless it would include only cortical bone.[29]

The disadvantage of using this grafted material consists in its limited availability, in difficult to reach sampling areas and, finally, in creating a second surgical site for the patient. In addition, the number of cells and the concen-

3.9 Classification of scaffolds based on their origin

Origin	Advantages	Disadvantages
Autologous bone	Promotes osteogenesis, osteoinduction, osteoconduction, osteoproliferation and rapid healing	The collection volume is limited, resorption is rapid and a second surgical donor area is required
Human bone Allotransplants, freeze-dried, demineralized bone	Promotes osteogenesis, osteoinduction, osteoconduction	It can induce immune reactions and diseases or infections, lack of quick healing
Xenografts Animal bone or coral	Excellent scaffold, osteoconduction	It shows only osteoconduction, rapid resorption or no resorption, religion risks, BSE risk and infection
Alloplast Synthetic ceramics for biological use β-tricalcium phosphate [β-TCP] and hydroxyapatite	Excellent scaffold, osteoconduction	Fast or no resorption, lack of osteoproliferation
Dentin	Promotes osteogenesis, osteoinduction, osteoconduction and rapid healing	Limited collection volume, requires treatment

tration of growth factors vary considerably according to the age, systemic diseases and the collection site.[30]

Allografted human bone

Allografted human tissue can be taken from cadavers or living donors (for example, the femoral head during orthopedic replacement operations). The structure of the material is similar to the autologous bone, but the cellular component is missing. One of the encountered problems is the immune reactions triggering. There are different types of allografted human bone (■ 3.10).

It is a biocompatible material and contains osteoinductive molecules such as BMPs. Obviously the osteoinductive capacities are related to the physical characteristics (age, diseases) of the donor and the site of the bone sampling.[31]

It resorbs quickly like autografts and can have conflicting interactions with blood type, cross-infection, and it is expensive. The high cost derives from the need for a complicated (■ 3.11) and long procedure to guarantee the final user.[32]

Xenografts

The scaffolds of xenograft origin are made of animal-derived material or bone-like minerals produced by animals.

CORAL

Different species of calcified corals have a calcium carbonate skeleton with a three-dimensional structure similar to the human cancellous bone with macropores of 200-600 μm, but they show an osteoconductive potential lower than that of other bone substitutes.[33]

They have rather long resorption times (24 months).

ANIMAL BONE

The origin can be bovine, equine or porcine. The organic component is removed with a heat treatment or chemical extraction in order to eliminate the risk of immunological reactions and disease transmission.

These are biocompatible and osteoconductive materials, although two bone substitutes treated with different procedures show very different osteoconductive and resorptive properties in vivo and in vitro.[34]

The treatment of bovine material with temperatures above 1000° C causes sintering of the natural hydroxyapatite (HA) by increasing the size of the crystals and decreasing the space between them.

There are many doubts regarding the real reabsorption of DBBMs (Deproteinized Bovine Bone Minerals) as human biopsies carried out after 10 years still showed the presence of the bone substitute in place.

Consequently, they must be considered as non-resorbable.

The enzymatic treatment, carried out with enzymes at 37° C to eliminate the organic parts of bovine bone, allows the resorption after 12 months.

The materials of equine origin undergo enzymatic antigen free processes and resemble natural hydroxyapatite, presenting a temporal resorption compatible with the normal human bone turnover (approximately 12 months).

The materials of porcine origin, always antigen free to be biocompatible, have an average resorption of 12-24 months.

Alloplastic

The alloplastic origin scaffolds consist of bioglasses, bioceramics, polyglycolic and polylactic acid derivatives, hydroxyapatite and calcium sulfate and phosphate

■ **3.10** Types of allographic human bone

FFB (Fresh Frozen Bone)	It is almost never used as it presents a high risk of immunological rejection and disease transmission
FDBA (Freeze-Dried Bone Allograft)	It is degreased with ethanol, dried and frozen and finally crushed into particles of 250-750 μm
DFDBA (Demineralized Freeze-Dried Bone Allograft)	The FDBA process is expanded by soaking the tissue in citric acid for 6-16 hours to remove the mineral part

3.11 Procedure for the use of allographic human bone

Human bone allograft preprocurement steps		
Step 1	Notification of prospective donor's death	Hospitals or morgues notify tissue recovery agencies of human deaths
Step 2	Determination of initial donor eligibility	The tissue recovery agency determines donor eligibility on the basis of readily available information (for example, age, cause of death, evidence of infection, history of systemic disease, evidence of drug use)
Step 3	Consent	If a potential donor is deemed acceptable, the tissue recovery agency obtains and documents consent according to U.S. Food and Drug Administration regulations and state anatomical gift laws.
Step 4	Dispatch of recovery team	Most tissue recovery agencies use their own recovery teams to evaluate and procure potential donor tissues
Step 5	Assignment of a tracking number to prospective donor	The dispatched tissue recovery team assigns a unique tracking number to the potential donor
Step 6	Determination of additional donor eligibility	The tissue recovery team confirms donor identity, reviews medical records, performs a full-body physical assessment, reviews critical time limits and verifies the temperature of the cadaver's storage
Step 7	Tissue procurement	The tissue recovery team must procure the tissue within 12 hours of death for nonrefrigerated cadavers or within 24 hours for refrigerated cadavers
Step 8	Autopsy	Some tissue procurement agencies perform autopsies on potential donors as an additional screening procedure
Step 9	Transport	The tissue recovery team transports harvested donor tissue, blood samples and relevant medical records to the tissue processing center

Human bone allograft pre-processing microbiological and serological testing	
Bacterial test	Detects and identifies contamination with various bacteria
Fungal test	Detects and identifies contamination with various fungi
HIV-1/2Ab test	Detects HIV-1, HIV-2 antibody
HIV/HCV NAT	Detects HIV and hepatitis C virus
HTLV-1/2Ab test	Detects HTLV-1 antibody and HTLV-2 antibody
HBsAg test	Detects hepatitis B surface antigen
HBcAb test	Detects hepatitis B core antibody
HCVAb test	Detects hepatitis C antibody
RPR/STS	Detects syphilis antibody

Steps in the processing of freeze-dried bone allograft		
Processing step 1	Soft-tissue stripping	The technician removes residual muscle, tendon, ligament and so forth
Processing step 2	Initial size reduction	The technician reduces the bone to pieces of approximately 5-millimeter diameter for easier processing
Processing step 3	Initial cleansing and decontamination	The technician flushes, agitates, centrifugates or does all of these to the bone particles, using various solutions such as saline, acetone, ethanol or hydrogen peroxide to remove residual bioburden and reduce antigenicity
Processing step 4	Microbiological treatment	The technician treats the bone particles with antimicrobial, antimycotic and antifungal solutions
Processing step 5	Freezing	The technician freezes the bone particles in liquid nitrogen of a temperature as low as -80° C
Processing step 6	Dehydration	The technician lyophilizes or treats the bone particles with repetitive solvent washes to eliminate moisture content and reduce antigenicity
Processing step 7	Secondary size reduction	The technician reduces the bone particles to final particulate sizes ranging between approximately 250 and 750 micrometers
Processing step 8	Packaging	The technician packages the bone allograft in sterile containers
Processing step 9	Terminal sterilization	The technician applies low-dose γ irradiation at low temperatures to ensure sterility (sterility assurance level, 10-6)

Human bone allograft post processing procedures	
Visual inspection test	Visual detection for such problems as gross graft contamination, packaging defects and product mislabeling
Residual moisture test	Testing of freeze-dried allografts to ensure residual moisture is 6% or less
Residual calcium test	Testing of demineralized freeze-dried bone allograft to ensure residual calcium content is 8% or less

derivatives. Morphologically they can be porous, crystalline, amorphous or granular.

Due to their purely synthetic nature, they do not present any risk of disease transmission. Theoretically it is possible to reproduce the optimal characteristics of the bone tissue, even if, in reality, it has not been possible to reproduce a microporous material with a surface roughness similar to that of the bone tissue yet.

HYDROXYAPATITE (HA)

It has osteoconductive properties and is non-resorbable. There are various forms of HA depending on the surface porosity and the connection of the pores that favor the colonization of osteogenic cells.

β-TRICALCIUM PHOSPHATE (TCP)

It has osteoconductive properties but, unlike the HA, it is resorbable (6-20 months) and has faster bone healing than HA. The explanation is that Ca and P ions are used as a raw material for the formation of new bone. In addition, resorption creates space for new bone.[35]

BIOGLASSES

Bioglasses, in the form of active and amorphous glass crystals, exploit the osteoconductive capacities of phosphate salts. They are biocompatible materials and do not cause immunological reactions, allergies, inflammatory reactions or side effects. Bioactivity is related to a process of surface hydrolytic degradation of glass phosphosilicate. The bond with the bone is formed thanks to a surface layer which, over time, transforms into hydroxyapatite, establishing a stable bond with the bone tissue. The resorption process begins after 2-16 weeks and resorption occurs after about 12-16 months.

DERIVATIVES OF POLYGLYCOLIC AND POLYLACTIC ACID

They are highly biocompatible, do not induce any immunological or inflammatory reactions and they are endowed with osteoconductive capabilities. Not being radiopaque, they allow you to better evaluate the formation of bone tissue in the months following the application. They exhibit a rapid resorption, which usually occurs within 60-90 days.

Dentin

Dentin and enamel can be considered as the aforementioned grafting materials. The process of using the tooth and its characteristics as a graft material will be covered in Chapter 4.

The percentages relating to the use of the different types of scaffolds are shown below (3.12).

3.12 Percentages of use of materials (Infodent analysis 12-2018)

Typology	Percentage of use
Human	4%
Xenographic	54%
Alloplastic	33%
Other	9%

REFERENCES

1. Cattaneo L. Compendio di anatomia umana (2ª edizione). Parma, Monduzzi ed., 1986.
2. Kumar GS. Orban's Oral histology & embriology (14th ed.). New Delhi, Elsevier, 2015.
3. Tamara A, Odendaal F, Hall B. Buried alive: how osteoblasts become osteocytes. Develop Dynamics 2006;235:176-90.
4. Adamo S, De Felici M, Dolfi A, et al. Istologia di Monesi (7ª edizione). Padova, Piccin, 2018.
5. Buser D, Dahlin C, Schenk RK. Guided bone regeneration in implant dentistry (2nd ed.). Chicago, Quintessence Publishing, 1994.
6. Robey PG. Vertebrate mineralized matrix proteins: structure and function. Connect Tissue Res 1996;35:131-6.
7. Lamoureux F, Baud'huin M. Key partners in bone cells biology. Bioessays 2007;29:758-71.
8. Hay ED. Collagen and other matrix glycoproteins in embryogenesis. In: Hay ED. Cell biology of extracellular matrix. New York, Plenum Press, 1991;437-44.
9. Roberts WE, Gretto LP, Arbuckle GR, et al. What are the risk factors of osteoporosis? J Am Dent Ass 1991;122(2):59-61.
10. Baron R, Vignery A, Horowitz M. Lymphocytes, macrophages and the regulation of the bone remodeling. In: Peck WA. Bone and mineral research annual 2. Amsterdam, Elsevier, 1984; 175-243.
11. Dahlin C, Linde A, Gottlow, J, et al. Healing of bone defects by guided tissue regeneration. Plast Reconstr Surg 1988;81(5):672-6.
12. Nyman S, Lindhe J, Karring T. et al. New attachment following surgical treatment of human periodontal disease. J Clin Periodont 1982;9:290-6.
13. Linde A, Thoren C, Dahlin C, et al. Creation of new bone by an osteopromotive membrane technique: an experimental study in rats. Int J Oral Maxillofac Surg 1993;51:892-7.
14. Reddi AH. Cell neology and chemistry of endochondral bone development. Coll Relate Res 1981;1:209-26.
15. Elgali I, Omar O, Dahlin C, et al. Guided bone regeneration: materials and biological mechanisms revisited, Eur J Oral Sci 2017;125: 315-37.
16. Karring T, Nyman S, Gottlow J, et al. Development of the biological concept of guided tissue regeneration-animal and human studies. Periodontol 2000 1993;1: 26-35.
17. Melcher MC, Thomas V., SchmidtG, et al. Recent advances in the development of GTR/GBR membranes for periodontal regeneration - a materials perspective. Dent Mater 2012; 28(7): 703-21.
18. Laney WR. Glossary of oral and maxillofacial implants. Berlin, Quintessence Publishing, 2007; 1-212.
19. Buser D, Bragger U, Lang NP. Regeneration and enlargement of jaw bone using guided tissue regeneration. Clin Oral Implants Res 1990;1:22-32
20. Nevins M, Melloning JT. Enhancement of the damaged edentulous ridge to receive dental implants. A combination of allograft and gore-tex membrane. J Periodontal Restorative Dent 1992;12:97-111.
21. Piattelli A, Degidi M, Di Stefano DA, et al. Microvessel density in alveolar ridge regeneration with autologous and alloplastic bone. Implant Dent 2002; 11(4):370-5.
22. Linkhart TA, Mohan S, Baylink DJ. Growth factors for bone growth and repair: IGF, TGFβ and BMP. Bone 1996; 19(1 Suppl):1-12.
23. Canalis E, Pash J, Varghese S. Skeletal growth factors. Crit Rev Eukaryotic Gene Expression 1993;3:155-66.
24. Dequeker J, Mohan S, Finkelman RD, et al. Generalized osteoarthritis associated with increased insulin-like growth factor types I and II and transforming growth factor 13 in cortical bone from the iliac crest. Possible mechanism of increased bone density and protection against osteoporosis. Arth Rheumat 1993;36: 1702-8.
25. Dodds RA, Merry K, Littlewood A, et al. Expression of mRNA for ILlp, IL6 and TGF/31 in developing human bone and cartilage. J Histochem Cytochem 1994;42:733-44.
26. Dijke P, Miyazono K Heldin, CH. Signaling via hetero-oligomeric complexes of type I and type II serine/threonine kinase receptors. Cm-r Op Cell Biol 1996;8:139-45.
27. Ripamonti U, Ramoshebi LN, Matsaba T, et al. Bone induction by BMPs/OPs and related family members in primates. J Bone Joint Sur 2001;83A (Suppl. 1):116-27.
28. Yamada S, Heymann D, Bouler JM, et al. Osteoclastic resorption of calcium phosphate ceramics with different hydroxyapatite β-tricalcium phosphate ratios. Biomater 1997;18:1037-41.
29. Pallesen L, Schou S, Aaboe M, et al. Influence of particle size on the early stages of bone regeneration. A histologic and stereologic study in rabbit calvarium. J Oral maxillofac Implants 2002;17:498-506.
30. Burchardt H. The biology of bone graft repair. Clinic Orthop Rel Res 1983;174:28-42.
31. Reddi AH, Wientroub S, Muthukumaran N. Biologic principles of bone induction. Orthop Clin North Am 1987;18:207-12.
32. Holtzclaw D, Toscano N, Eisenlohr L, et al. The safety of bone allografts used in dentistry: a review. J Am Dent Assoc 2008;139:1192-9.
33. Buser D, Hoffman B, Bernard JP, et al. Evaluation of filling materials in membrane-protected bone defects. A comparative histomorphometric study in the mandibles of miniature pigs. Clin Oral implants Res 1998;9:137-50.
34. Jensen SS, Aaboe M, Pinholt EM, et al. Tissue Reaction and Material Characteristics of Four Bone Substitutes. Oral Maxillofac Implants 1996;11(1):55-66.
35. Von Arx T, Cochran DL, Hermann JS, et al. Lateral ridge augmentation and implant placement: an experimental study evaluating implant osseointegration in different augmentation materials in the canine mandible. Int J Oral Maxillofac Implants 2001;16:343-54.

The tooth as a source of bone graft

E. Minetti

Embryogenesis and tooth structure

We all know the structure of the human tooth (4.1). But how is this perfect tool for our nutrition and speech formed?

Around the sixth week of the intra-uterine gestation, some areas of basal cells of the ectoderm proliferate more rapidly than the cells of the adjacent areas. These form the primary epithelial band. A week later, the band divides into two lines: one internally (lingual) called the dental lamina, which will serve as the precursor for the ectodermal portion of the deciduous teeth, and one externally (vestibular) called the vestibular lamina. The dental lamina is arranged in a horseshoe shape, following the future shape of the maxillary bones, from which the sketches of the future teeth will start.

The development of the first permanent tooth begins at around 4 months of the intrauterine life. The second molar begins to develop approximately one year after birth and the third molar around the fourth/fifth year.[1]

We will then have two dental laminae, one upper and one lower (4.2). Along the dental lamina the ectodermic cells thicken creating nodes that grow in the underlying mesenchyme forming the future twenty deciduous teeth (ten mandibular and ten maxillary).

Each of these small thickening of the dental lamina represents the beginning of the enamel organ and the dental bud of the deciduous teeth.

The cells proliferate and represent the beginning of the dental papilla; the tissue appears dense and surrounded by mesenchyme, which shows the initial stage of enamel. A third part of the tooth, called the follicular sac, forms around the two embryonic sketches of the enamel

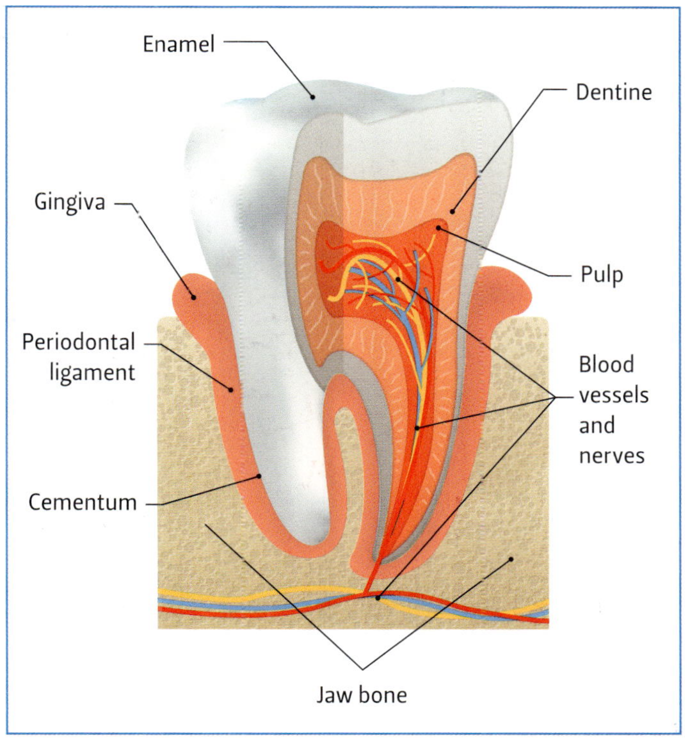

4.1 Structure of the human tooth.

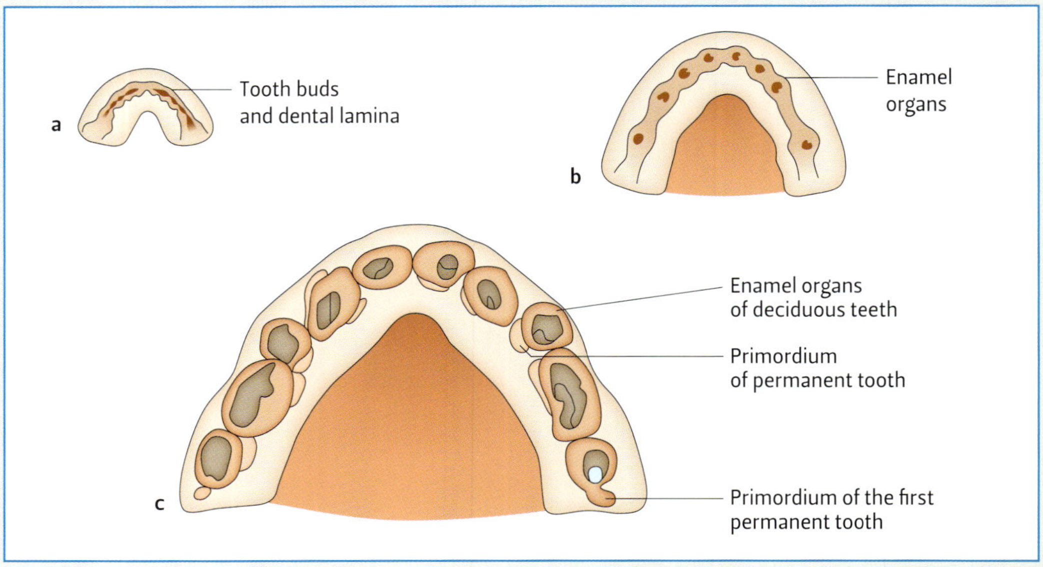

4.2 Stages of cell development of the dental lamina. **(a)** 22 mm embryo, eighth week; **(b)** 43 mm embryo, cap stage, 10th week; **(c)** 163 mm embryo, bell phase, approximately 4 months. The sketches of the permanent teeth are visible as a thickening of the dental lamina on the lingual side of each dental gem.

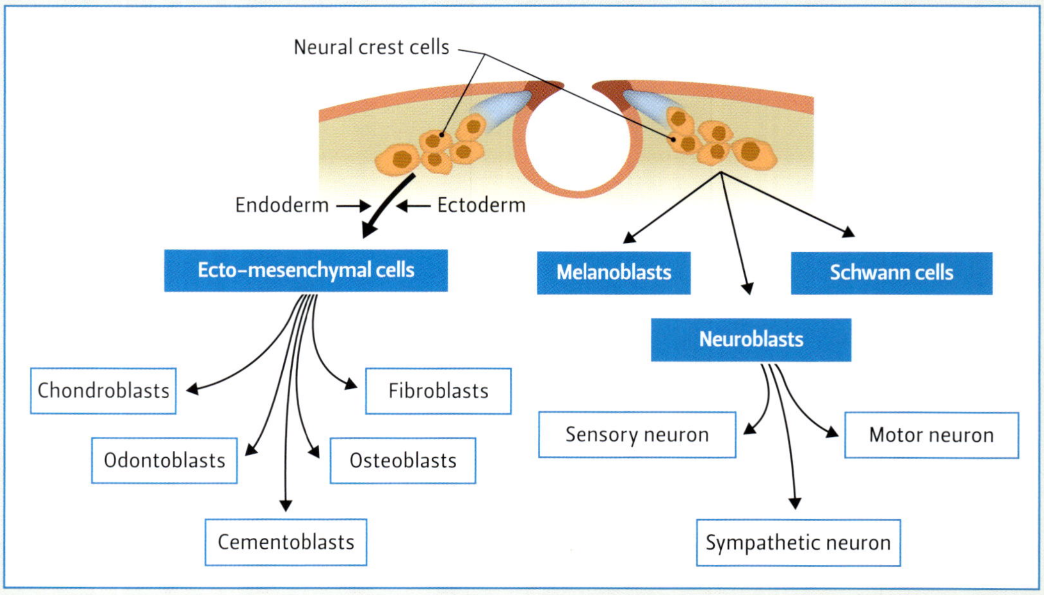

4.3 Differentiation of ecto-mesenchymal and neural cells.

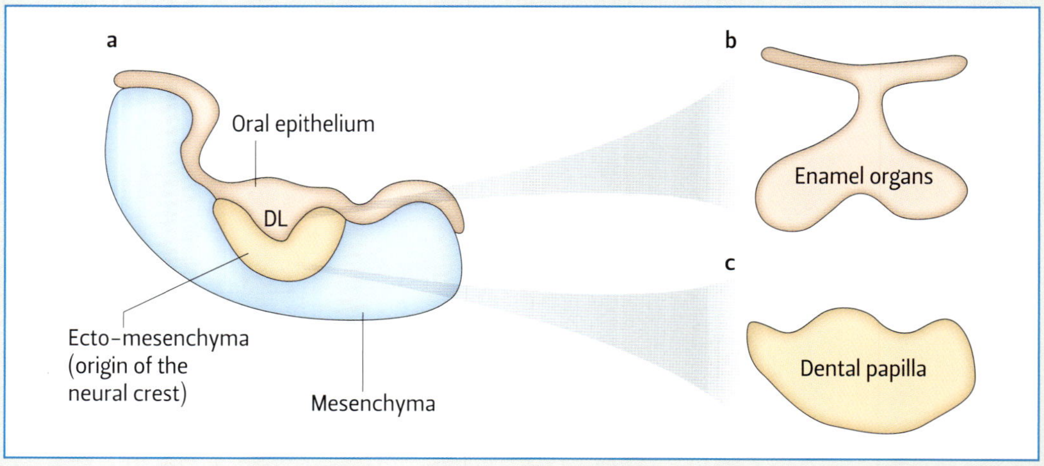

4.4 Stages in the development of the dental bud. **(a)** Development of the dental lamina. **(b)** The enamel organ originates from a specific area of the dental lamina. **(c)** The dental papilla develops from ecto-mesenchymal cells originating from the neural crest. DL: dental lamina.

and the dentin. Therefore, the dental bud is formed by an ectodermal component (dental papilla and the dental follicle) and an ectomesenchymal part (enamel organ) (4.3 and 4.4).

The tooth and its supporting structures will be formed by the dental bud. The enamel will be produced by the enamel organ (4.5). Dentin, dental pulp, cementum, periodontal ligament and alveolar bone will be produced starting from the dental follicle.[2–4]

All the various steps of tooth formation (4.6), such as the coordination of cell proliferation and differentiation, apoptosis, cell matrix synthesis and mineral deposition, are coordinated and controlled by different signaling molecules. The same molecules are repeatedly used during the different phases of dental development and regulate the times precisely.[5,6]

BMPs (Bone Morphogenetic Proteins) regulate epithelium-mesenchymal interactions during the initial stages of the dental development, Wnt and Sonic Hedgehog (Shh) regulate cell proliferation, migration and differentiation, while fibroblast growth factors (FGF) regulate the gene of tooth expression and cell proliferation.[7]

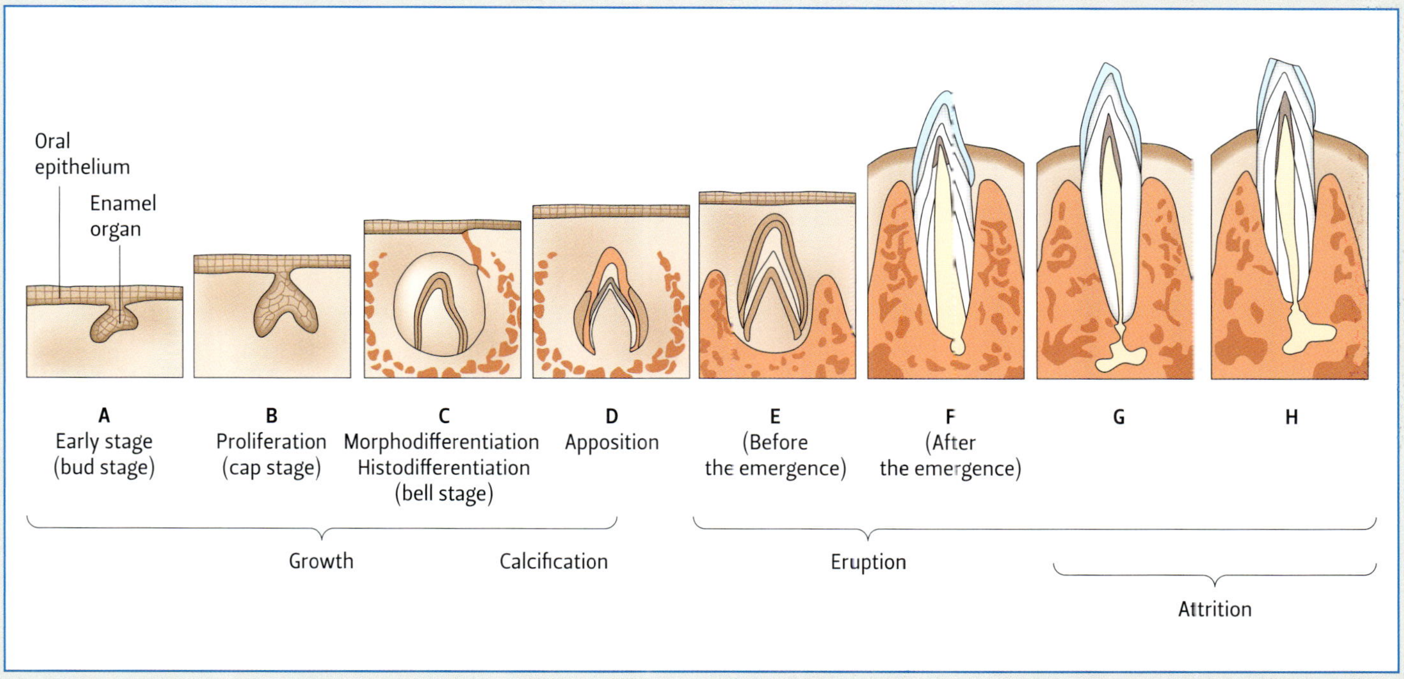

4.5 Tooth life cycle diagram.

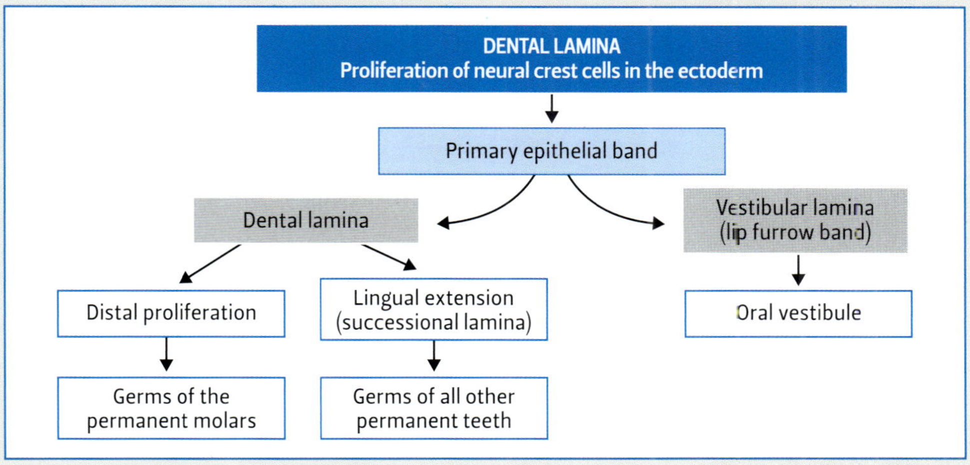

4.6 Development of the dental lamina.[3]

Tooth developmen

Although the development of the teeth is a continuous process (4.7), different morphological "phases" can be recognized in it. Although the size and shape of the teeth are different, they all develop in the same way. The morphological phases are:

- **The bud stage.** The dental bud stage begins between the sixth and seventh week. The proliferation of the ectodermal cells of the lamina gives birth, at regular intervals, to the dental buds which are 10 for each arch (equal to the number of teeth of the deciduous dentition) and invaginates in the underlying mesenchyme. The dental bud first takes the shape of a club, then, due to the invagination of its deeper end, it resembles a bell shape, forming the enamel organ.
- **The cap stage.** The bud stage lasts about a week, in which the spherical shape of the gem moves on the cap shape. The epithelial gem grows in depth and widens, forming the enamel organ. The proliferation of the adjacent mesenchyme gives rise to the dental papilla, which will form the dentin and the pulp. The ectomesenchyme that delimits the dental papilla and encapsulates the enamel organ is called the dental follicle and will form the supporting tissues.
- **The bell stage.** The growth of tooth germs leads to the bell stage. The cells located in the center of the enamel organ secrete acid mucopolysaccharides in the extracellular compartment. Acid mucopolysaccharides are hydrophilic and attract H_2O by increasing the volume of the extracellular compartment. The cells are pushed on both sides, but, being connected by desmosomes, they assume a star-like configuration.[3]

Mineralization of dental tissues

Biological mineralization involves cells that synthesize a protein matrix which the crystals grow on. Mesenchymal cells differentiate, under the stimulation of growth factors, into osteoblasts, odontoblasts and cementoblasts (4.1). Enamel is the only hard tissue of an ectodermal origin.

The main protein structure of hard tissues of mesenchymal origin is collagen. The fibres are intertwined in the classic three-bundle helical shape and are intimately associated with the mineral deposits. Therefore, in these tissues the proteins of the mesenchymal matrix remain trapped in the mineralized tissue.

In the structure derived from the ectoderm, the matrix is similar to a gel and, after it is formed, it is completely replaced by the enamel crystals.

The differences in development between dentin, cementum, bone and enamel are reflected in the size and the arrangement of the crystals (4.8).[8,9]

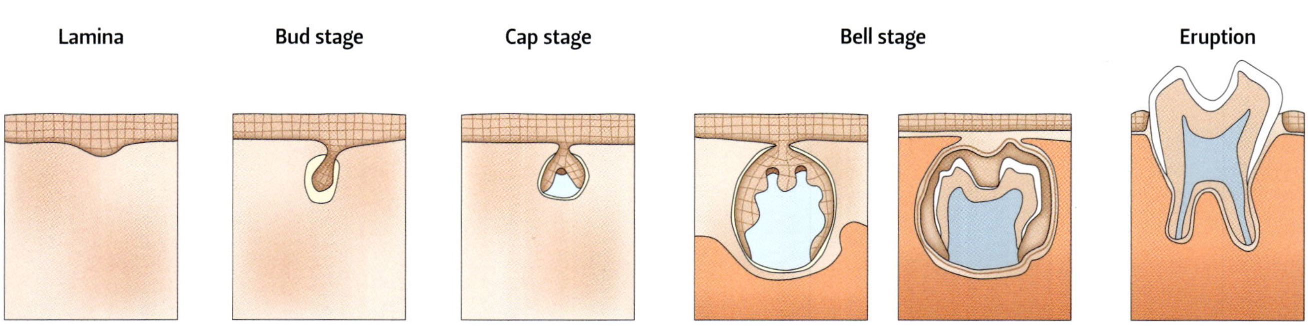

4.7 Stages of tooth development.

4.1 Main cells of mineralized tissues

Cells	Tissue	Function and properties
Chondrocytes	Calcified cartilage	Secretion of the matrix and preparation for calcification
Osteoblasts	Bone	Matrix synthesis and mineral deposit
Osteocytes	Bone	Osteoblasts surrounded by minerals connected to other osteocytes via canaliculi
Osteoclasts	Bone	Multinuclear cells suitable for bone resorption by acids and enzymes
Odontoblasts	Dentin	Cells that produce dentin
Cementoblasts	Cementum	Cells that synthesize cementum
Ameloblasts	Enamel	Cells that produce enamel

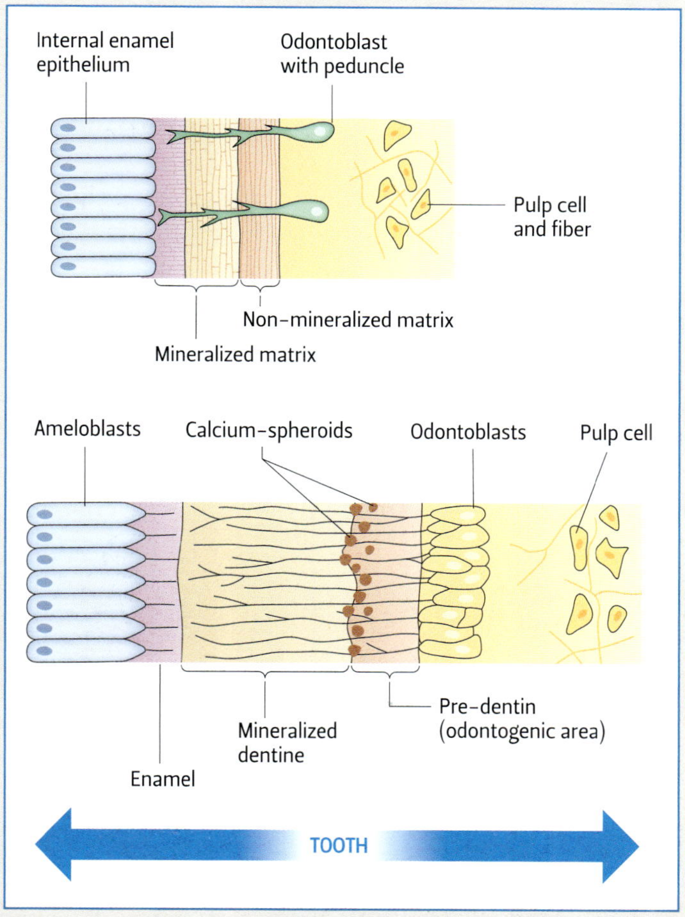

4.8 Deposition of dentin and enamel in section.

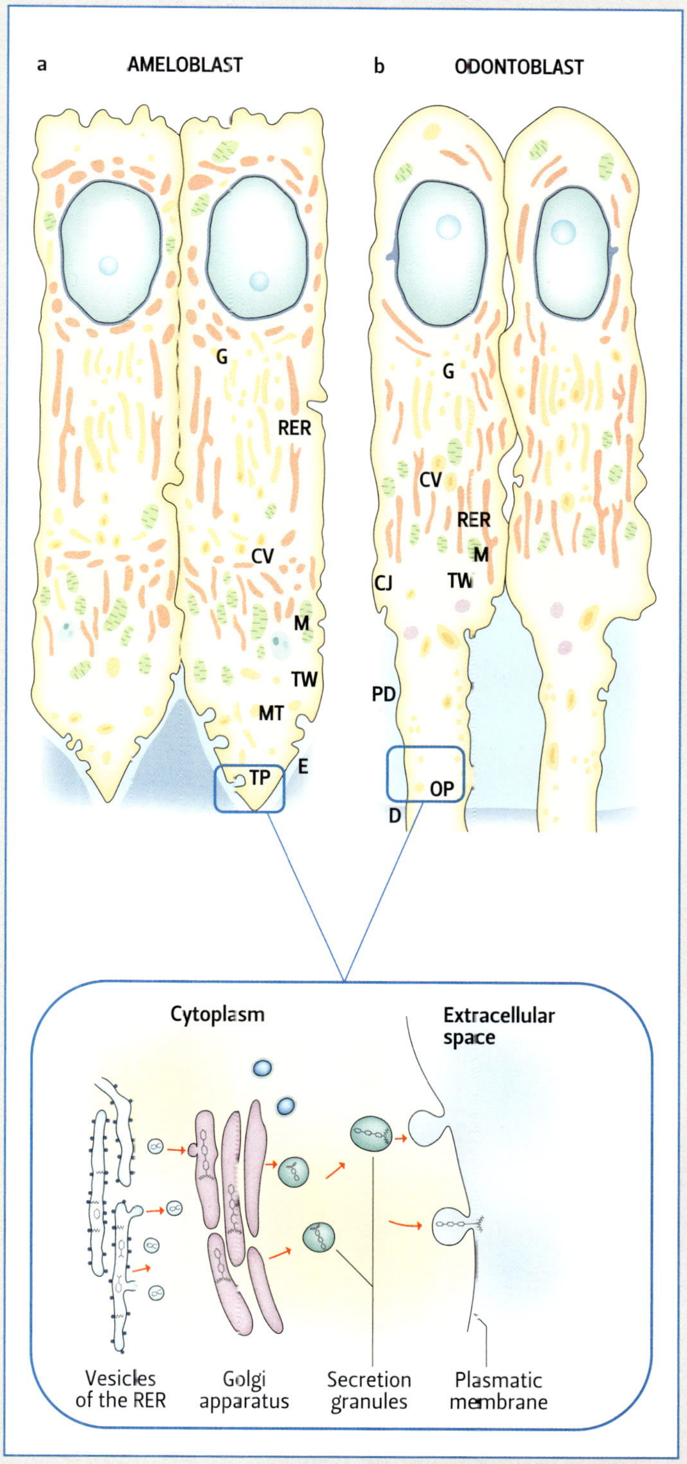

4.9 Ameloblasts **(a)** and odontoblasts **(b)**. Note the different production areas of the secretion granules: the odontoblastic process which will produce the granules for centin and the Tomes process which will produce the granules for the enamel production. In particular (*insert*) production and release of secretion granules. CV: condensation vacuoles; CJ: intercellular junction; D: dentin; E: enamel; G: Golgi apparatus; M: mitochondria; MT: microtubules: OP: odontoblastic process; PD: pre-dentin; RER: rough endoplasmic reticulum; TP: Tomes process; TW, terminal network.

Crystals in mesenchymal tissues (dentin, cementum, bone) measure approximately 5×5×10/50 µm, they are randomly arranged and display a two-dimensional, string-like. Dentin has crystals 10 times larger than bone.[3]

The mature enamel crystals measure approximately 25×25×200 µm and are arranged in a regular three-dimensional manner forming the enamel prisms.[10]

The Golgi apparatus produces vesicles that are conveyed to the apical part of the cell and then released outside. Both the odontoblasts and the ameloblasts have a cytoplasmic extension that protrudes from the cell. The apical portion of the odontoblasts is immersed in the pre-dentine and dentin while the ameloblasts are inserted into the enamel matrix.

The cytoplasmic prolongation of ameloblasts is called the Tomes process while the odontoblasts one is the odontoblastic process (4.9).

Even though the secrets are different, the process is the same. The vesicles contain procollagen which thickens and is then released by exocytosis. These vesicles may contain small crystals which, when the membrane disappears, can thicken and merge to form the mineralized matrix (4.9, detail).

Mineralization can be considered as the result of two distinct processes: the nucleation of the vesicles and the growth of the crystals.

The tooth is made up of three mineralized tissues: enamel, dentin and cementum, which will be analyzed below.

Enamel

The enamel forms a protective covering of varying thickness that covers the entire surface of the crown. The thickness can shift from 2-2.5 mm up to a knife-edged area (amelo-cementum junction).

Due to its high mineral content, enamel is the most densely calcified tissue in mammals. The function of this high calcification is to make the teeth usable for chewing and to protect them from temperature variations.[11]

The colour of the enamel can vary from yellow-white to gray-white.

Translucency can be attributed to the different density of calcification and homogeneity of mineralization.[12]

Enamel mainly consists of inorganic material (96%) and of only a small part of organic substance and water (4%). The organic part is made up of two groups of exclusive enamel proteins, amelogenins (90%) and non-amelogenins (10%). These proteins, unlike those in dentin and bone, have no structural function.

The inorganic part is formed by hydroxyapatite $[Ca_{10}(PO_4)_6(OH_4)_2]$, whose crystals are hexagonal in section and joined together to form the enamel prisms (4.10).

During the secretory phase, the deposition of the enamel matrix is orchestrated by both the pre-ameloblasts and the ameloblasts. Pre-ameloblasts are secretory cells that have not yet developed the Tomes process.

Subsequently the ameloblasts begin the deposition of prismatic enamel by depositing the mineral rapidly on the tip and slowly on the sides. During this phase the ameloblasts also secrete proteins (amelogenins) which are assembled in the form of spheres and occupy the space between the various layers of crystals with the aim of separating and supporting.[13,14]

Enamel prisms are usually oriented perpendicularly to the dentin surface.

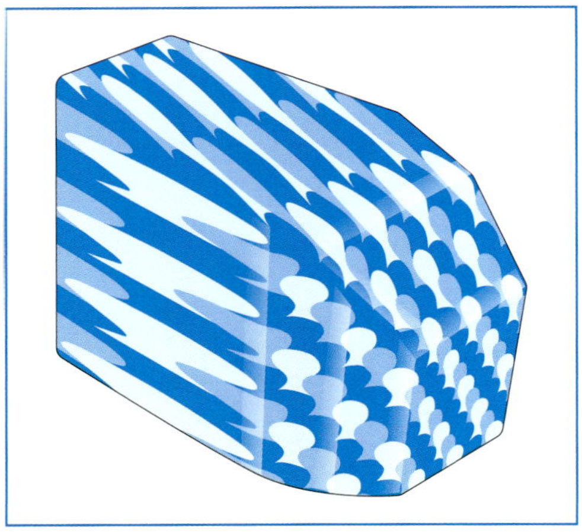

4.10 Enamel prism in section.

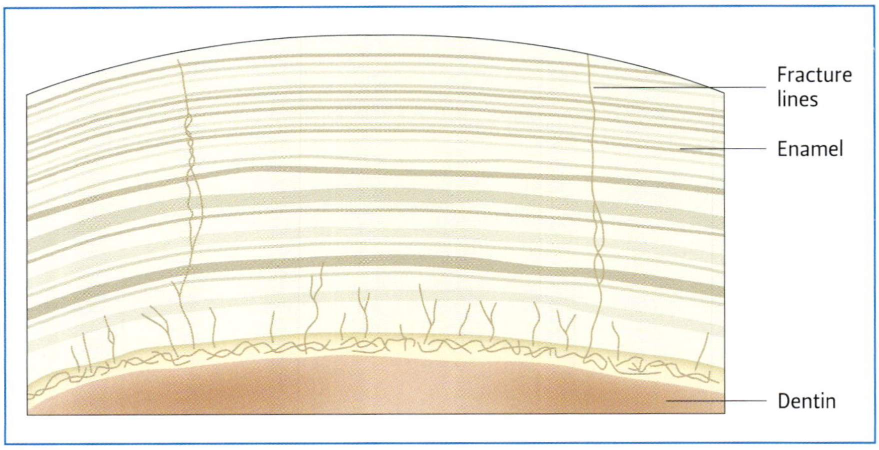

4.11 Incremental Retzius lines.

The Retzius incremental lines

At the microscopic view each prism of the enamel appears to be streaked (transverse striae) by dark lines placed at regular intervals of about 4 µm. These striae are formed following the daily diurnal production rhythm. The Retzius incremental lines (4.11) are spaced 20-80 µm apart and can correspond to a growth period of about 5-20 days. These growth lines can be assimilated to tree rings and can be observed in all the teeth from the same person, representing a characteristic of the individual. They are most noticeable in permanent enamel, but can also be found in deciduous teeth. These lines are more pronounced in prenatal enamel than in the enamel that forms after birth.[10]

Daily growth was demonstrated using ^{3}H-Proline tracers that labeled the developing collagen.[15]

4.2 Components of the extracellular matrix of dentin

Collagen	Type I, III, V
Non-collagenous proteins	Proteoglycans, chondroitin sulfate (biglycan, decorin) heparan sulfate (entactin, perlecan) keratan sulfate, dermatan sulfate
Phosphorylated matrix proteins (SIBLINGs)	DSPP (DSP, DPP), DMP-1, OPN, MEPE, IBSP
Non-phosphorylated matrix proteins	Matrix GLA1 protein, OC (BGLAP2), osteonectin (SPARC3)
Growth factors	TGF-B (TGF-B1, TGF-B2, TGF-B3), BMP (BMP-2, BMP-4, BMP-7), FGF (FGF-2), IGF (IGF-1, IGF-2), PDGF, VEGF-4, NGF-5
Others	MMP6S (MMP-1, MMP-3, MMP-9, MMP-20), TIMP7S (TIMP-1, TIMP-2, TIMP-3)

Dentin

It is the second hardest tissue, even if it is elastic as it has the function of protecting the tooth from fractures. It is produced by the odontoblasts which remain associated with dentin for life and are located on the periphery of the dental pulp. Physically and chemically, dentin resembles bone. The major difference between bone and dentin consists in the fact that osteocytes are found in the bone as included in the bone matrix. On the other hand, the odontoblasts, the dentin cells, always remain external to it, even if their cytoplasmic processes enter the dentinal tubules. The shape of the dentinal canaliculi is similar to the osteocyte processes in the bone.

Young odontoblasts are columnar cells that secrete predentine, rich in type 1 collagen and matrix vesicles.[16]

The continuous secretion of pre-dentine is associated with the progressive elongation of osteoblastic cells in the dentinal canals and the progressive retraction of the cells in the dental pulp.

Dentin is composed of 65% inorganic material and 35% of organic material similar to bone.

- Inorganic component. It consists of $3Ca_3(PO_4)_2Ca(OH)_2$ hydroxyapatite with crystals about 10 times larger than bone and 300 times smaller than enamel. The dentine crystals are similar to bone and cementum ones.
- Organic component. 90% of the organic component is made up of collagen: 94% is type 1, 3% type 3 and 3% type 5. The remaining 10% is made up of non-collagen proteins (4.2).[17]

Odontoblasts (*see* 4.9) originate and differentiate from the dental papillae cells which arise from the neural crest.[18] BMPs are the growth factors most involved in the differentiation of osteoblasts and odontoblasts. Although it is clear that BMPs are strong inducers of the mineralization process, they cannot determine the direction of differentiation of the odontoblast alone. Therefore, all the other factors serve to modulate the differences and modifications necessary for the creation of these structures.[19]

The dentin (4.12-4.14) which forms before the eruption of the tooth is called primary dentin and it is formed in quantities of about 4-8 µm/day, while the dentin which forms after the eruption of the tooth, named as secondary dentin, develops in quantities of about 0.5 µm/day. There is also a tertiary dentin which is a reactive response to an insult or a trauma.[20]

Even in dentin there are daily apposition lines, called Von Ebner lines, similar to those in enamel, which reflect the circadian rhythmic activity. Approximately 4 µm of dentin is deposited every 24 hours. Like enamel, dentin deposited during neonatal life is of a better quality than that deposited after birth.

If we compare a tooth and the alveolar bone, we will notice that the macroscopic structure will be dissimilar, but the closer we get to the microscopic structure and ultrastructure (µ), the more similar they will appear. The final components of the tooth and bone are the

DENTIN MAGNIFICATION'S

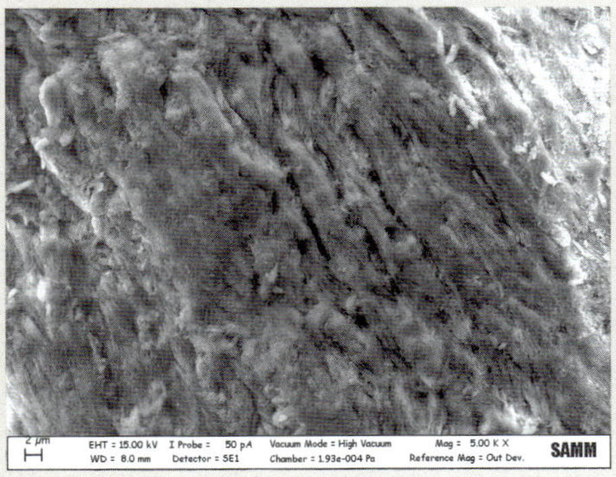

4.12 Collagen fibres of dentin: it is possible to recognize the arrangement of collagen fibres around the dentinal tubules.

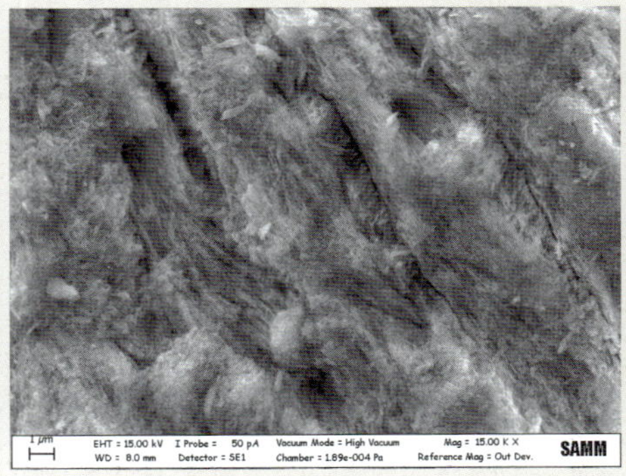

4.13 At a higher magnification, the tubules can be seen.

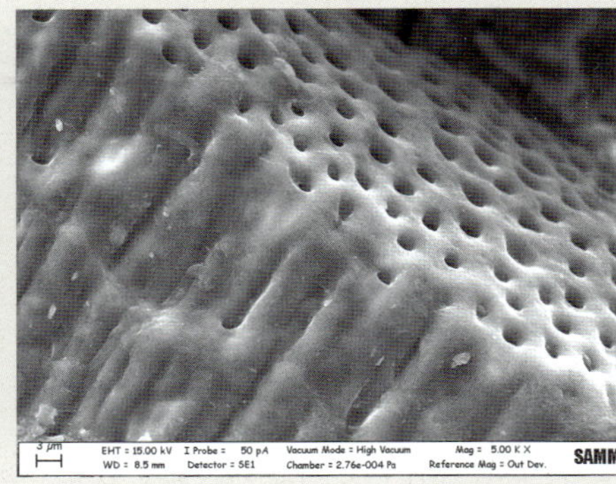

4.14 Dentinal tubules.

same: collagen, hydroxyapatite, non-collagenic proteins and amelogenins.[21]

Cementum

The cementum is circumscribed at the root and is composed of approximately 50% hydroxyapatite and 50% organic material. The cells that produce it are the cementoblasts that differentiate later into cementocytes.

It has a structure similar to the bone, it completely covers the root of the tooth and it is placed between the dentin and the periodontal ligament. The thickness of the cementum varies: it is thinner at the CEJ (20-50 µm) and thicker (4.15) in the apical area (150-200 µm).[22]

Embryologically, two types of cementum can be highlighted: a primary (acellulated) one, which develops slowly when the tooth erupts, and a secondary one, which develops when the tooth is in occlusion. When the cementum develops rapidly, the cementoblasts can become trapped in the structure and, similarly to the osteocytes, they transform into cementocytes. Proteins are represented, as in bone tissue, by collagenic (type 1, 3, 5, 6, 12) and non-collagenic ones.[16,22-24]

The cementum has a concentric laminate structure which, like the enamel and the dentin, represent the expression of cyclical growth.

Sharpey fibres are radially oriented to the tooth and penetrate the cementum, connecting it with the alveolar bone. These fibres are produced by periodontal fibroblasts.

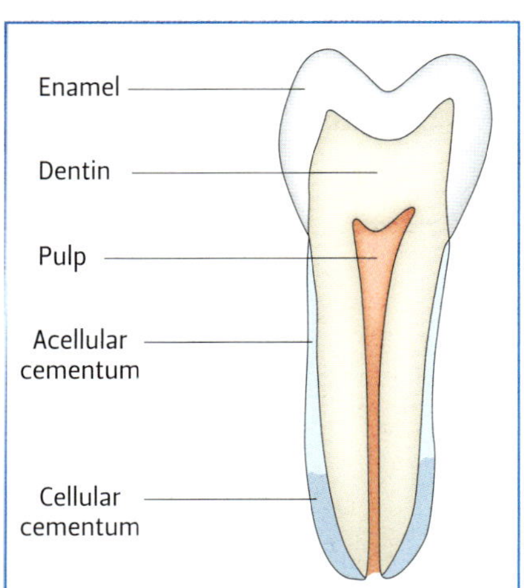

4.15 Section of the cementum with thickening in the apical area.

History and literature review

What is meant by history? Is the tooth as a graft material new? Why can it be used? Are there any advantages?

Leafing through the main histology books, it is immediately clear that the tooth has a significant similarity with another graft material: the bone (4.3).[25,26]

The reasons that led us to think of using the tooth as a graft material arose from the observations of Yeomans and Urist in 1967 (4.4).[27]

The authors performed tests using tendons, muscles, decalcified cortical bone and decalcified dentin in three different sites: rectus abdominis, mandibular bone defect created with a bur and post-extraction sockets using New Zealand rabbits. All samples were decalcified using 0.6 M HCl, then washed and sterilized in 70%

4.3 The tooth in the books of Histology

Histology by Monesi[25]	*Histology and Microscopic Anatomy by Wheater*[26]
Chapter 18 – Bone tissue ***18.4 Dentin and tooth cementum*** Dentin and tooth cementum are two specialized forms of bone tissue. Dentin is a special form of bone tissue, harder than compact bone. The substance of the dentin consists of an organic matrix (28%) and an inorganic matrix (72%).	***Chapter 13 – Oral cavity*** ***13.3 Lip and tooth*** Dentin is a mineralized tissue that has a chemical composition similar to that of bone. ***13.4 Structure of the tooth*** Dentin forms most of the crown and roots and is composed of a calcified organic matrix similar to that of bone. The inorganic component is more abundant in dentin than in bone.

4.4 Representation of bone production in tests carried out by Yeomans and Urist in 1967[27]

	Incidence of induction in various sites		
Tissue	**Muscle**	**Drill-hole in mandible**	**Extracted tooth socket**
Decalcified dentine	+	+	+
Undecalcified dentine*	+	+	+
Decalcified bone	+	+	+
Tendon	0	0	0
Muscle	0	0	0
Control	0	0	0

+ = presence of newly formed bone; 0 = lack of newly formed bone.
* Induces bone in 75% of cases, but only after a period of 8-12 weeks.

alcohol before grafting. The grafts were analyzed at 4, 8 and 12 weeks.

In defects filled with decalcified bone, the matrix was resorbed within 4 weeks. Decalcified dentin was better tolerated, but reabsorbed and replaced more slowly than bone. Dentin didn't induce dentinogenesis but osteogenesis. Decalcified tendons and muscles were resorbed and replaced with fibrous tissue and delayed the repair processes of the defect.

Microscopically, dentin was resorbed thanks to the increased number of mesenchymal cells, macrophages and osteoclasts that carry collagenolytic enzymes. The resorption of the undecalcified dentin was incomplete or delayed. Minerals seemed to make the matrix inaccessible to the action of collagenolytic enzymes. For this reason, undecalcified dentin was not resorbed for 8-12 weeks, much later than the decalcified dentin.

But how did they come to these surprising conclusions? In 1965 Urist wrote an article in which he analyzed numerous liquids (4.5 and 4.6) suitable for decalcification using demineralized cortical bone and the results of the graft.[28]

The bone was demineralized in 0.6 M HCl for 5 days and then removed with a prolonged washing in sterile 0.15 M NaCl. They were then grafted into a pocket of the rectus abdominis, quadriceps or erector spinal muscle of 250 rabbits, 20 rats, 10 mice and 5 guinea pigs. A defect was created on the ulna in 10 rabbits and a defect on the lumbar vertebrae in 3 dogs. In an attempt to find out

4.5 Alternatives to HCl tested for demineralization

Preparation	Result
Calcium chloride	It delays the reabsorption and hinders the ostoegenetic reaction
EDTA (ethylenediaminetetraacetic acid) + formic acid + citric acid	It produces bone as with HCl but in a reduced percentage of positive cases
EDTA (ethylenediaminetetraacetic acid) + formic acid + acetic acid	It produces bone as with HCl but in a reduced percentage of positive cases
Lactic acid	Failed to remove all the mineral and a diffuse deposit which remained seemed to increase inflammation and prevent osteogenesis
Heat 70° C	Did not induce bone formation
Nitrous acid + HCl + β-propiolactone	Did not induce bone formation
Nitric acid + HCl + β-propiolactone	Did not induce bone formation
FDNB (dinitrofluorobenzene)	Did not induce bone formation
IAA (iodoacetamide) + HCl	Did not induce bone formation

which decalcifing solution was best, numerous alternatives were tested (*see* 4.6).

The implant, using HCl, after about 3 weeks began to produce bone tissue. The first deposits of mineralized material were evident after 4-6 weeks.

In 1974 Linden[29] reproduced the Urist experiment using 68 3-10 week old gray rats. Decalcified bone, allogenic bone, decalcified dentin, non-decalcified bone dipped in alcohol were used. The enamel was removed from the dentin with a scalpel. This was then decalcified in 0.6 M HCl for 72 hours at 4° C, then soaked in several 70% alcohol baths and rinsed in distilled water.

Dentin grafts were able to produce bone more easily and to form it more quickly.

The inflammatory response was short and after 5 days the fibroblasts surrounded the grafts.

The decalcified bone and dentin exhibited a brief inflammatory reaction, then they were permeated by mesenchymal cells. Some of the mesenchymal cells transformed into multinucleated giant cells which proceeded by the erosion of tunnels in the matrix enlarging pre-existing cavities. The matrix was immediately recalculated, probably thanks to the diffusion of the ionic residues of the resorption. Then the osteoblasts replaced the multi-

4.6 Summary of the results obtained with heterotopic grafting by various procedures

Giver	Preparation	Site	Host	Positive results %
Mouse	HCl 0.6 N	Rectus abdominus	Mouse	95
			Rat	60
Rat	HCl 0.6 N	Rectus abdominus	Rat	90
			Rabbit	70
Guinea pig	HCl 0.6 N	Rectus abdominus	Guinea pig	95
			Rat	50
Rabbit	HCl 0.6 N	Rectus abdominus and quadriceps	Rabbit	98
			Rat	60
Calf	HCl 0.6 N	Rectus abdominus	Rabbit	50
			Rat	60
Rabbit	EDTA 1 N	Rectus abdominus	Rabbit	80
Rabbit	1 M formic citric acid	Rectus abdominus	Rabbit	85
Rabbit	0.6 M lactic acid	Rectus abdominus	Rabbit	10
Rabbit	Acetic acid 0.6 N	Rectus abdominus	Rabbit	50
Rabbit	Nitric acid 0.6 N	Rectus abdominus	Rabbit	0
Rabbit	Nitrous acid 0.6 N	Rectus abdominus	Rabbit	0
Rabbit	β-propiolactone 10%	Rectus abdominus	Rabbit	0
Rabbit	0.6 M HCl + 0.1% toluidine blue	Rectus abdominus	Rabbit	80
Rabbit	0.6 M HCl + 70° C heat	Rectus abdominus	Rabbit	20
Rabbit	0.6 M HCl + 70% alcohol	Rectus abdominus	Rabbit	85
Rabbit	0.6 M HCl + freeze-drying	Rectus abdominus	Rabbit	80
Rabbit	0.6 M HCl + 0.1% 1.2 fluorodynitrobenzene	Rectus abdominus	Rabbit	0
Rabbit	0.6 M HCl + 0.1% iodoacetamide	Rectus abdominus	Rabbit	10
Rabbit	$CaCl_2$ 25 mmol/L	Rectus abdominus	Rabbit	50
Rabbit	HCl 0.6 N	Ulna	Rabbit	95
Human	HCl 0.6 N	Various bone defects	Human	90
Calf	HCl 0.6 N	Lumbar spinal fusion	Dog	50

Note: the percentages are always high if HCl is used on autologous. With the addition of heat, the percentages dropped to 20%.

nucleated cells and formed new bone starting from the cementing line.

But why did the tooth induce bone production in these experiments? The bone is considered the gold standard, but the tooth, according to the experiences of these authors, was not different, indeed perhaps it showed some more advantages.

The BMP-mediated mechanism of bone induction was analyzed and proposed by Urist in 1971[30] indicating BMPs as possible determinants.

«These observations suggest that the hypothetical BMPs (Bone Morphogenetic Proteins) are structurally linked both to the telopeptides of the collagen molecules and to the proteoglycans of bone and may be linked to both.» Different systems have been analyzed to demineralize bone and teeth, but it seems that some procedures may affect the results in the bone tissue production.

In the same article Urist looked at tests by Huggins and colleagues,[31] which demineralized using 0.5 M HCl at room temperature and created a powder treated with ethanol and water saturated with phenol for 30 minutes which was then rinsed in 70% ethanol and water, frozen in liquid nitrogen and dehydrated with ethanol and ether overnight at 37° C and then implanted in mice. The results produced bone in a significant number of grafts.

Nade[32] tests on rabbit bone demineralized using HCl or EDTA were also evaluated, observing that some procedures reduced the yield of new bone. In particular, it was noted that the fine particles used by Huggins and colleagues[31] treated as such, could have lost their morphogenetic capabilities. Grafts with EDTA did not result in any morphogenetic activity in guinea pigs. Instead, the use of EDTA at low concentrations for a short time and at low temperatures resulted in a certain morphogenetic activity. Instead, optimal results were obtained if the EDTA was replaced with HCl or H_3PO_4 (phosphoric acid) at 2° C.

In 1972, Bang,[33] analyzing 168 samples of dentin, soaked in different solutions and grafted into 43 Guinea pigs, found the high osteoconductive properties of dentin.

The tests were carried out by the dentin demineralization in different HCl solutions: 0.2 M, 0.4 M, 0.6 M, 0.8 M, 1.0 M, 2.0 M.

While for the concentrations between 0.2 and 0.6 the success rates were high (75-85%), with higher concentrations the number of positive outcomes (cases in which bone was generated) was drastically reduced. This seems to indicate that high concentrations of HCl cause changes in the matrix responsible for negative effects on the induction mechanism. Any of the lyophilization or cryogenization processes using liquid nitrogen have no influence on the results.

Proteins have a pile-like structure. If an alteration of the structure occurs by chemical, thermal or mechanical denaturation, the functionality of the proteins is lost. A denatured protein (4.16), even if quite similar to the original one, as far as the coarse structure is concerned, is no longer able to perform its biological functions.

In 1985, Sato and Urist[34] showed that when BMPs were used without any vector, a large amount was needed for an adequate bone induction.

Bessho[35] has then shown that the BMPs are very soluble in vivo and, if used without a carrier, they are rapidly washed out, invalidating their action. Based on these observations, the use of an appropriate carrier (collagen) for clinical use was suggested.

For Kuboki and colleagues,[36] BMP carriers can be considered of three types: bone-inducing, cartilage-inducing and bone-cartilage-inducing. The geometry of the carrier is of crucial importance for bone formation (4.17). Closed tubules induced chondrogenesis while open tubules induced osteogenesis and the granule sizes of demineralized bone, ranging from 420 to 850 µm, induced more bone using as a carrier vs a powder of about 44-74 µm thinner.

Koga and colleagues[37] demonstrated that demineralized dentin can be used as a grafting material. They carried out an analysis on cleaned human teeth, pulverized with a percussion mill and separated accordingly, to obtain particles (180 µm, 212 µm, 425 µm, 600 µm, 800 µm and 1200 µm) divided, according to the size, into three groups:

- group 1: 180-212 µm;
- group 2: 425-600 µm;
- group 3: 800-1200 µm.

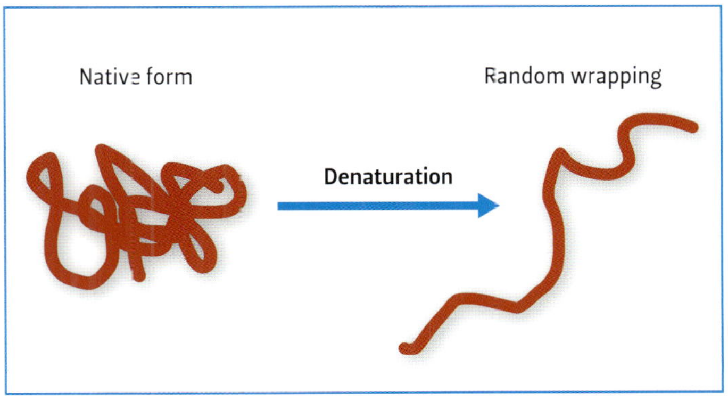

4.16 Appearance of a protein after denaturation.

They were also separated according to the degree of demineralization, by the use of nitric acid (HNO_3) in UDD (UnDemineralized Dentin), PDDM (Partially Demineralized Dentin) and CDDM (Completely Demineralized Dentin).

The granules treated in this way were then grafted into the rat calvaria. Confirming Bang's observations,[33] complete demineralization and the untreated tooth did not result in a greater amount of bone produced. The tooth with partial demineralization and with a particle size between 800 and 1200 µm (as analyzed by Kuboki and colleagues)[36] had the best results at both 4 and 8 weeks (4.18).

Another aspect analyzed by Koga[37]concerned the in vitro observation of the different reactions of osteoblasts to the untreated surface compared to the demineralized one. In fact, the osteoblasts adhered only to the demineralized surface. Osteoblasts were deposited on the UDD (non-demineralized) and DDM (demineralized) surface. The SEM images showed that the mor-

Categories by geometry	Fundamental shapes		Examples
Convex	Fibre	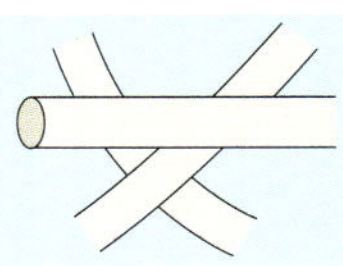	Fibres of collagen membranes, fibrous glass membrane, titanium mesh (50 µm fibres), CPSA glass fibres
	Particles	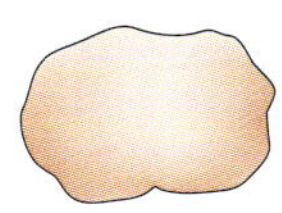	Insoluble bone matrix, porous particles of hydroxyapatite (PPHAP, particles with pores)
Plane	Planes		Conventional culture dishes
	Sheets (membrane)	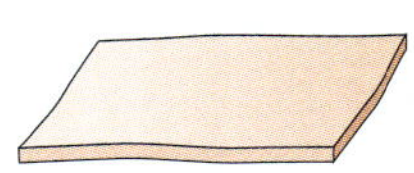	Laser perforated membrane (LPM, sheet with pores)
	Blocks	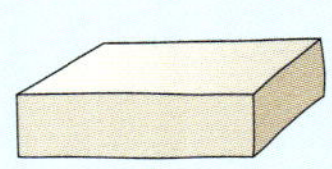	Porous block of hydroxyapatite (PBHAP, blocks with pores)
Concave	Pores	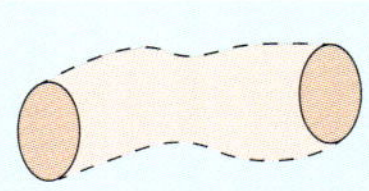	Hydroxyapatite BMP carrier
	Tunnel	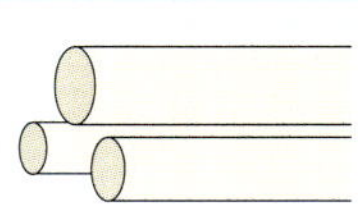	Honeycomb shaped hydroxyapatite
	Concavities	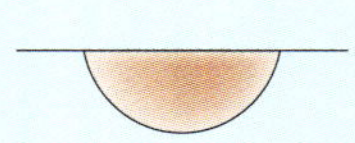	Concavity of monolithic hydroxyapatite
	Micropits	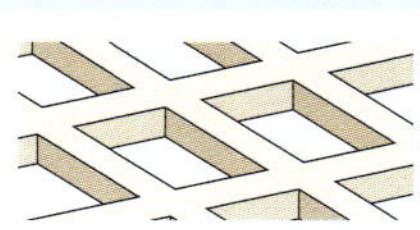	Micropits on silicon tip
	Groove	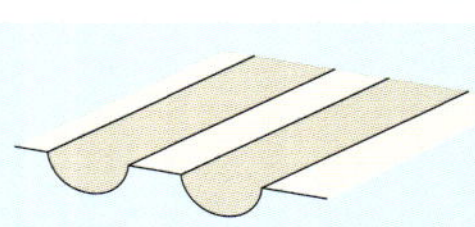	Micro grooves

4.17 Classification of surfaces that can be used as carrier of BMP.

phology of the cells was reacting to the nanosurface, with dentinal tubules clearly visible in the DDM image, but not observable on the UDD surface, and only in the DDM the attachment of osteoblast cells to the surface was noticed (4.19).

His conclusions were that demineralized dentin can be used as a grafting material, demonstrating a high cellular compatibility and rapid bone regeneration by an optimal balance between the resorption and the production of new bone (4.20).

Therefore, the demineralization process turns out to be a key factor in cell adhesion and in promoting regeneration. Blum,[38] based on an animal model, claimed that, by reducing the mineral part, demineralization facilitates the release of GFs from the bone matrix. Similarly, Kim,[39] analyzing 100 different sources and proposing a process to obtain a graft material from demineralized dentin, stated that demineralization is a necessary process to release various growth factors and proteins, as this is blocked by the presence of hy-

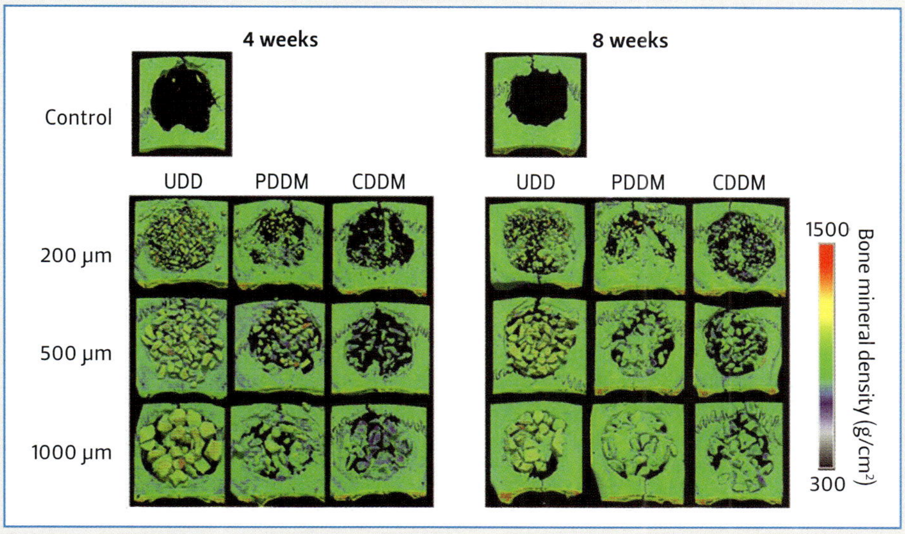

4.18 Result of the bone production of defect bone filled with non-demineralized (UDD), partially demineralized (PDDM) and fully demineralized (CDDM) dentin. (From Koga et al.)[37]

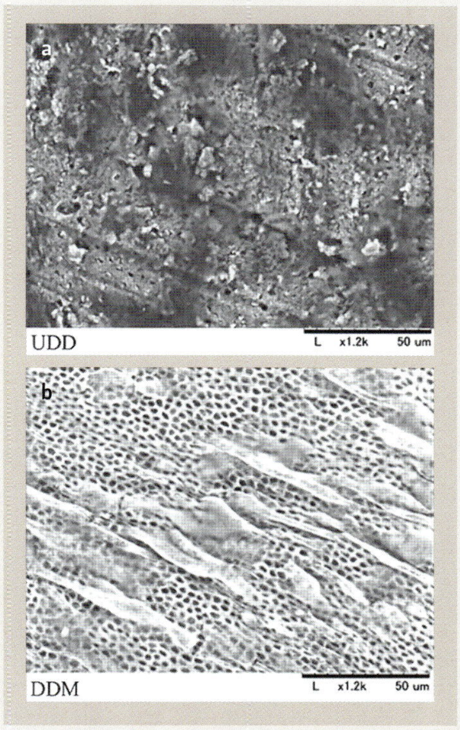

4.19 Osteoblasts grown on the surface of UDD and DDM. The cells are sensitive to the surface nanostructure. Dentinal tubules can be seen on the DDM surface but not on the UDD surface. (From Koga et al.)[37]

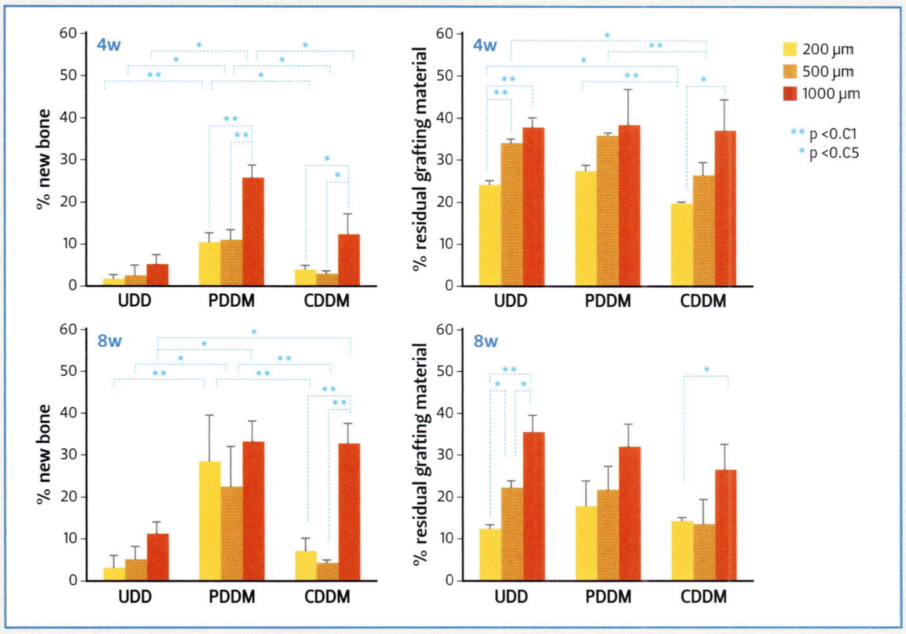

4.20 Percentages of bone formed according to size and healing time. (From Koga et al.)[37]

droxyapatite crystals. Bone production is induced when demineralized dentin is grafted into rabbit, pig and rat muscle. The decalcification of the dentin induces the release of BMPs thus causing osteoinduction.

The highly soluble BMPs (as claimed by Bessho),[35] have no osteoinductive effect when used alone. The graft material must be used as a carrier for the BMP proteins. Indeed, numerous graft materials have been proposed as carriers for BMP, collagen, TCP[40] and polyesters.[41,42]

Demineralized dentin naturally contains proteins, it has a type 1 collagen structure and therefore can be considered an optimal carrier of an osteoinductive graft material.

Human demineralized dentin, according to Kim's protocol,[43] placed under the skin in some in vivo tests on 15 mice, showed at a histological level at 2, 5 and 8 weeks (4.21-4.23), the formation of new bone.

In the same publication, considered as a milestone in the use of the tooth as grafting material, the surfaces, the dissolution of ions and the X-ray diffraction analysis of dentin, dental crown, cortical bone, Bio-Oss, phosphate synthetic biphasic calcium and allograft human bone were also analyzed and compared (4.24).

According to these analyses, it can be considered that the tissue from dental origin has the same physiochemical characteristics of the human bone. To all intents and purposes, the tooth has already been considered as mineralized bone.[25]

The presence of BMPs in the demineralized human tooth (4.25) was demonstrated by Bessho[44] who extracted them and then determined their amino acid sequence.

Approximately 2 kg of freshly extracted vital human teeth were used to achieve this. Enamel, cementum, pulp and caries were removed mechanically and rinsed with cold distilled water. The dentin thus treated was placed in liquid nitrogen and then crushed using the Wiley Milling machine, giving 1 to 3 mm granules then treated with 4 mol/L guanidine HCl. Following an extraction procedure for chromatography, all the samples were subjected to SDS-PAGE test and an isoelectric focusing (IEF). The thin line in the SDS-PAGE and IEF tests indicated the molecular weight of the sample under analysis.

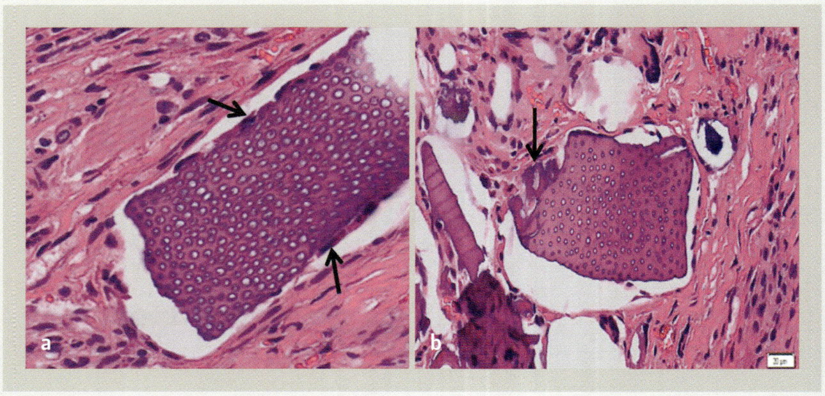

4.21 (**a, b**) Two-week histological analysis. Cells can be seen enveloping the treated dentin granules and attaching to them. (From Kim et al.)[39]

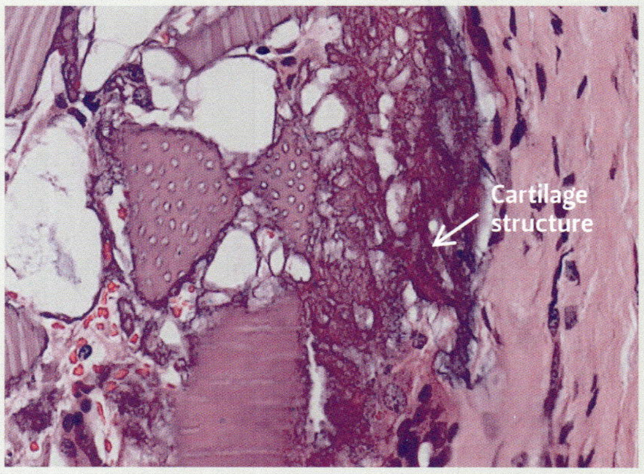

4.22 Cartilage tissue forming around dentin granules at five weeks. (From Kim et al.)[39]

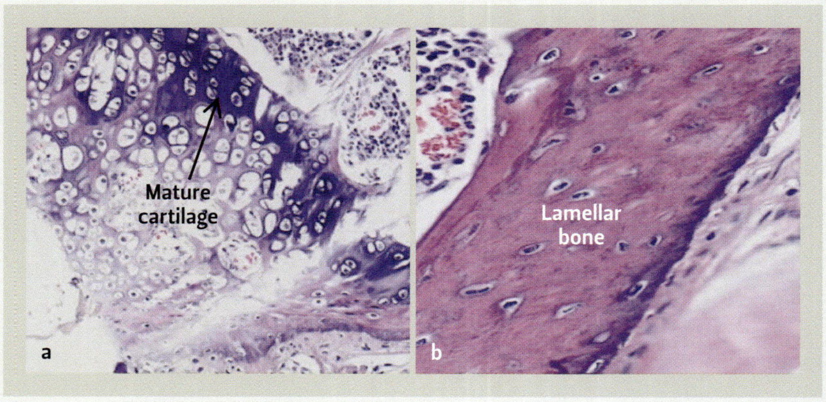

4.23 (**a**) Endochondral ossification and (**b**) lamellar bone at eight weeks. (From Kim et al.)[39]

Kim,[43] using his own protocol for the use of dentin for regeneration, has also demonstrated the presence of proteins in dentin after a treatment (4.26).

It is possible to explain the presence of all these proteins in the tooth structure as growth factors (GFs), such as the transforming factor crescin-β and bone morphogenetic proteins (BMPs) are involved in the dental repair and play a role during embryonic tooth development by stimulating pulp and bone development and the osteo-differentiation.[45-48]

Demineralized dentin stimulates bone formation in vivo. The specific mechanisms by which the dentinal tubules influence bone formation have been investigated by means of a three-dimensional reconstruction using the SEM and the FIB/SEM technique.[49]

Using this technique, it was discovered that the osteocytes from the new bone surrounding the DDM (demineralized dentin), built a network connected by cellular processes and formed bone tissue, and that the cellular processes of the osteocytes extended into the dentinal tubules.

The size of mesenchymal cells, as well as of the osteoblasts and the other bone cells, varied from 10 to 20 µm, and the size of osteoclasts varied from 20 to 100 µm or more.

Therefore, it is natural to assume that the penetration of cells into the dentinal tubules is impossible. However, it is interesting that the current analysis was able to demonstrate the invasion of the dentinal tubules by the osteocyte processes and their cytoplasm. Under these

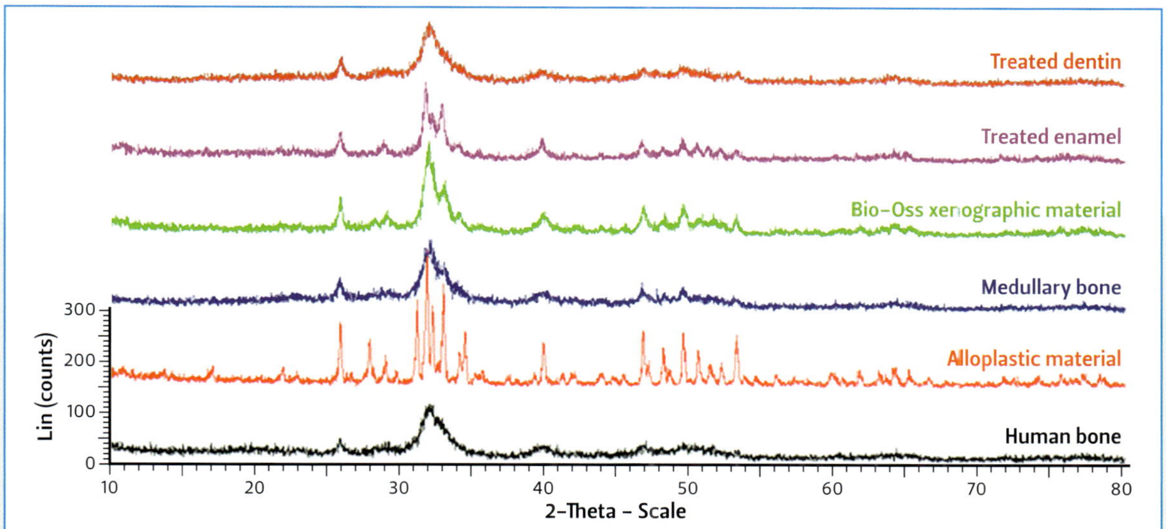

4.24 Results of the X-ray diffraction analysis of different materials; from top to bottom, dentin, enamel, Bio-Oss, medullary bone, alloplastic, human bone. (From Kim et al.)[43]

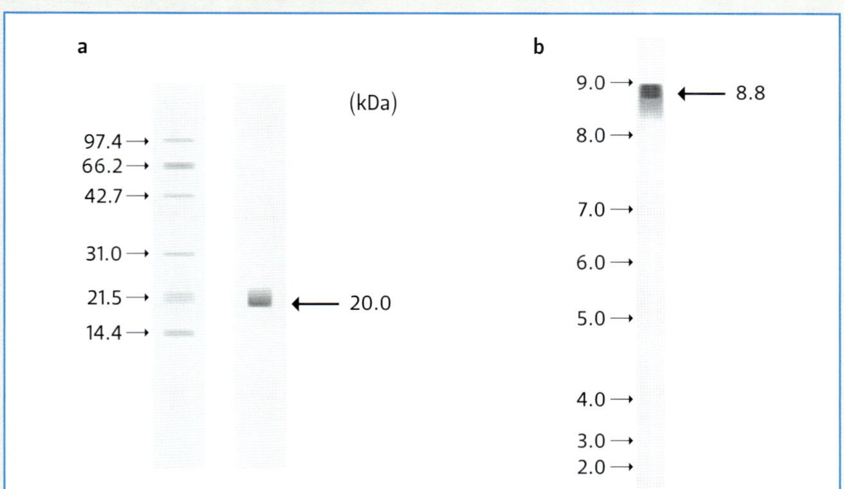

4.25 **(a)** SDS-PAGE test for the presence of BMP in dentin. **(b)** IEF test for the presence of BMP in dentin.

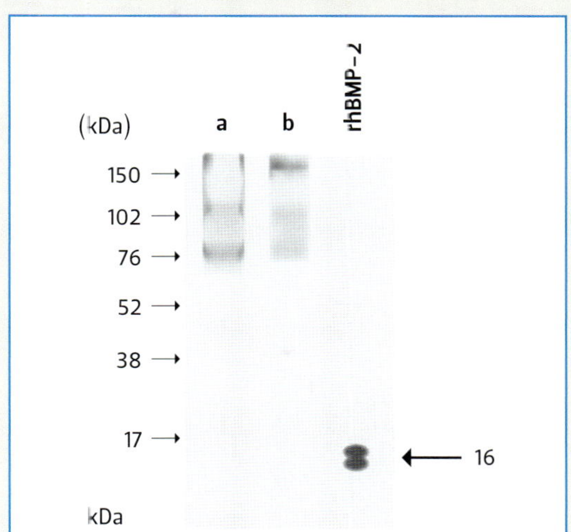

4.26 SDS-PAGE test to evaluate the presence of proteins in the treated dentin.

conditions, the degree of invasion was approximately 5 µm from the new DDM bone interface. Later the cellular processes of the osteocytes extended into the dentinal tubules and the bone tissue formed and filled the DDM surface (4.27-4.31).

Therefore demineralization, by increasing the size of the dentinal tubules, supports the adhesion and the activity of the osteoblasts and their total number (4.30 and 4.32).

Numerous **tests** have been carried out **on animals** (*see* 4.18) using different methods of demineralization, with the aim of understanding whether the grafting material from dental origin might have characteristics that could be used in regeneration and all of them were positive. Herein are listed some test examples.

- Sixty rats, divided into three groups of twenty, were histologically analyzed at 6 and 8 weeks:[50] group 1 tooth, group 2 iliac bone, group 3 control; tissue reabsorption in group 2 was very high, despite the rapid initial regeneration. The reaction to dentin produced greater amounts of bone at both 6 and 8 weeks.
- Muscle pockets were prepared in 24 mice[51] where demineralized human dentin induced bone formation at 2, 4 and 8 weeks.
- In 20 laboratory mice[52] two defects were formed in the central part of the skull bones. In one defect the demineralized *deciduous dental graft material* was placed, while the other was the control. Physio-chemical analyzes, SEM, plasma spectrometry, X-ray analysis, X-ray diffraction and histological and histomorphometric analyses were performed, discovering that deciduous dentin induced bone formation. This research was innovative and interesting, as the deciduous tooth as a graft material was proposed and analysed for the very first time.
- Also 6 foxhounds[53] were treated bilaterally with extractions and alveolar preservation, where one side

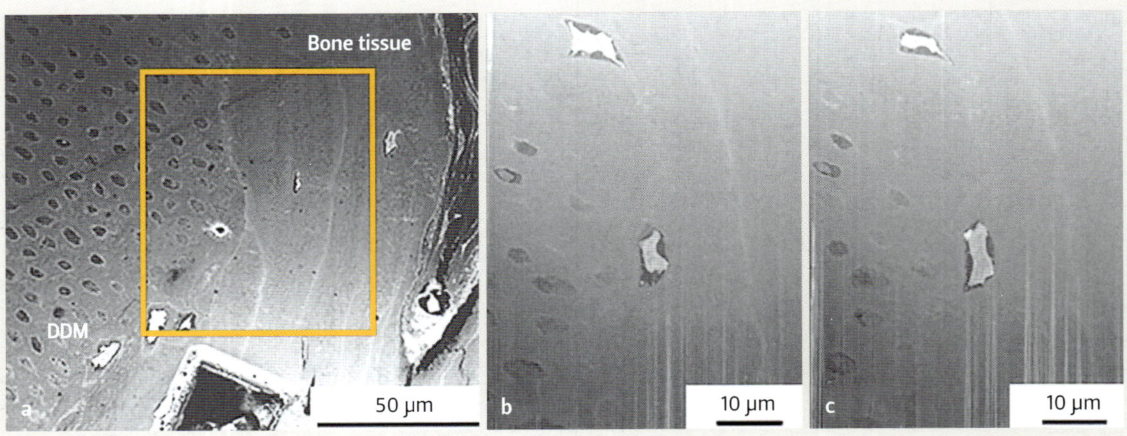

4.27 Enlargement of the DDM yellow box with osteocytes, consecutive sections. These sections demonstrate penetration into the tubules. (From Tanoue et al.)[49]

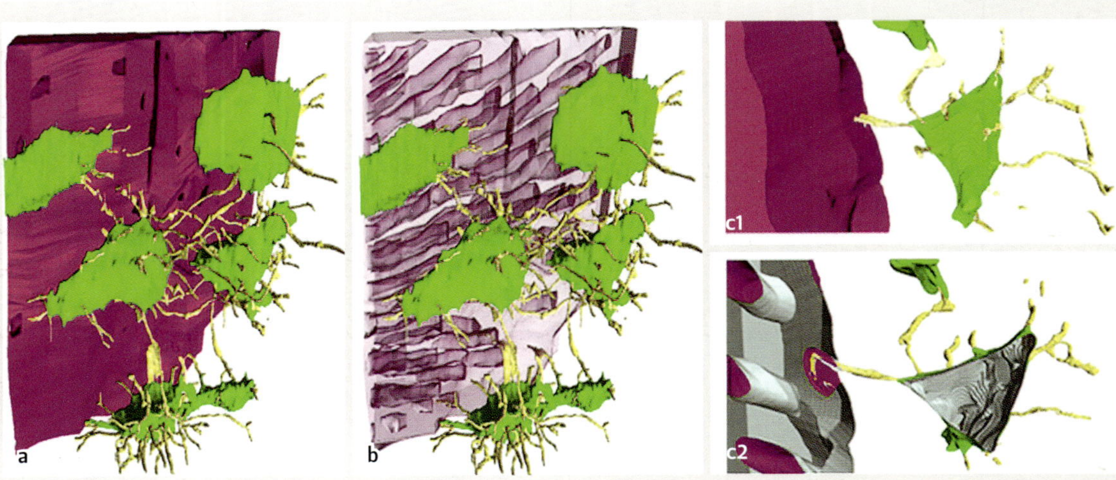

4.28 Digital reconstruction of the images of Figure 4.27, where it can be observed how the osteocytes create a network with the tooth by penetrating into the dentinal tubules. (From Tanoue et al.)[49]

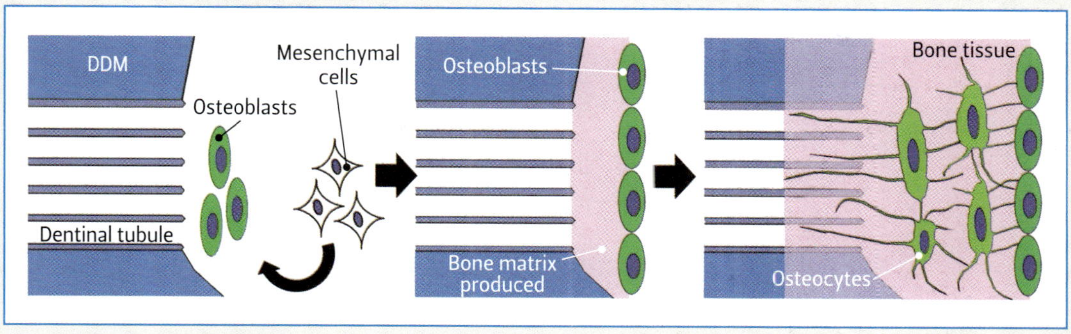

4.29 Schematic example of the penetration. (From Tanoue et al.)[49]

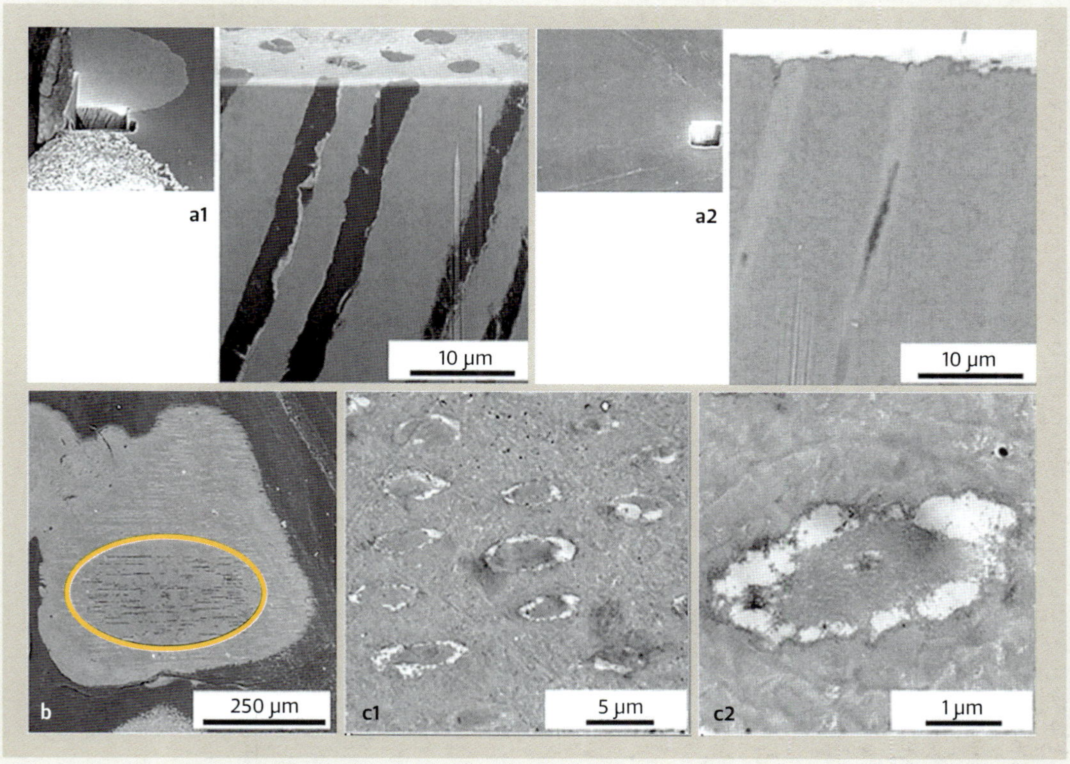

4.30 SEM images of bone penetration into the granules. (From Tanoue et al.)[49]

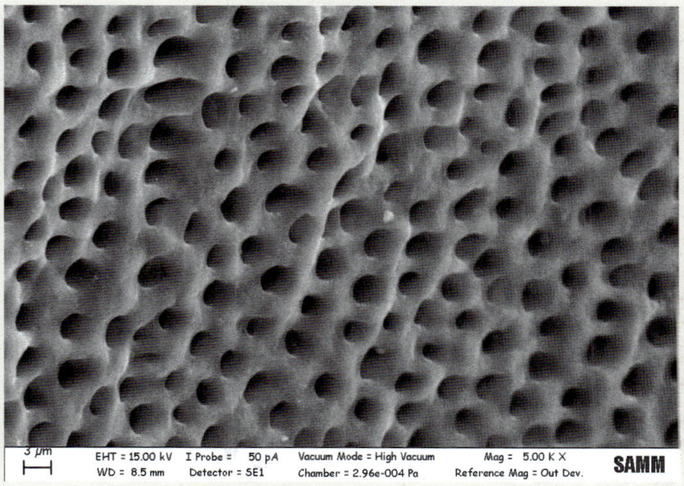

4.31 Dentinal tubules after treatment with Tooth Transformer.

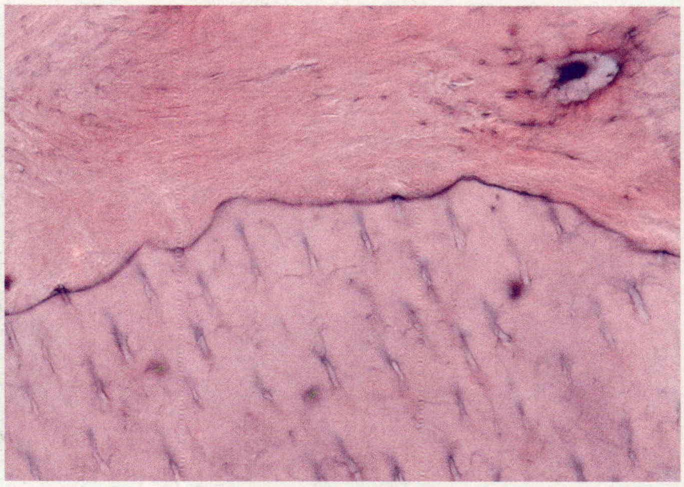

4.32 Granule in intimate contact with bone tissue that appears to penetrate the tubules.

represented the control and, on the other, the sockets were filled with treated tooth graft and the evaluation was set at 60 and 90 days. At 60 days there was a significant statistical difference between the two groups as there was new bone on the treated side with values of 82.22 ± 1.7% and on the untreated side 57.29 ± 0.11%. At 90 days the statistical difference was maintaining values of 91.32 ± 0.8% in the test group and 65.89 ± 0.6% in the control group.

- Molars were extracted from 6 mini pigs[54], creating vertical defects to place implants. Two groups were set: one in which the defects were filled with the extracted, after treating and demineralizing them and then checked after 4, 8 and 12 weeks (4.7) and another control without any grafting material. It is interesting to note in Kim's results how at 12 weeks the test continued to grow in an inversely proportional rate compared to the control.

These data were also confirmed by a study carried out on sheep[55] in which untreated tooth granules and tooth granules treated using the Tooth Transformer machine (4.33-4.37), were placed in artificially created cavities and then analyzed after 2 months by histological and histomorphometric sampling (4.38). The cavities filled with treated tooth had a mean vital bone value of 31.68%, while the control cavities only had 1.77%.

Many trials on humans have been reported and some examples are given below.

- Six patients with GBR (Guided Bone Regeneration) and concomitantly placed implants,[43] who underwent histological analysis on biopsies at three months, showed bone formation in 46-87% of the grafted areas. The same study presented 37 patients in whom 54 implants were placed in regenerated areas using autologous dentin between October 2008 and December 2009 with a follow-up at 31 months. The marginal bone loss around the implants was found to be 0.33 ± 0.63 mm.
- Two hundred and fifty patients[56] were divided into GBR + implants, GBR, alveolar preservation and sinus lift using both the granules and the blocks from dental perforated and treated. The recorded crestal bone loss was 0.29 ± 0.30 mm and the histological examinations showed the formation of new bone, thickening of the lamellar bone, osteoblasts and some parts of enamel that appeared to be in the resorption phase. Only 9% of the implants were unsuccessful.
- One hundred patients[57] with a 24-month follow-up were treated with maxillary sinus lifts and alveolar preservation and they showed dense composite bone in which dentin granules were embedded on histological examinations.
- Clinical cases of comparison with other biomaterials (4.8)[58] were also presented as in one study where 24 patients were divided into the following three groups: group 1, demineralized dentin; group 2, biocera; group 3, Bio-Oss.

In the context of the comparison studies, Wu's[59] was particularly interesting: 30 patients (12 women and 18 men) were divided into two groups with 30 implants, 15 per group, in which also endodontically treated teeth were used. The aim was to compare the autologous tooth with xenografts in the management of immediate implants with bone defect. The tooth was crushed using a hammer, and the pulp, or the endodontic filling material, was removed. The size of the fragments was selected using a sieve. All implants were successful during the observation period. None of the implants had biological, infective or mechanical complications. Patients were asked to complete a satisfaction and quality questionnaire (4.39) which indicated how healing perception was better with the use of the autologous tooth. The percentages of ridge reabsorption after 12 months were approximately the same in the two groups.

Up to this point, all human clinical studies have been performed with healthy extracted elements. However, a prospective multicenter clinical study was carried out

4.7 Comparison histomorphometric evaluations of the newly formed bone

	Control (no graft)	Test (tooth graft)
4 weeks	37.00 ± 11.53	48.15 ± 18.02
8 weeks	32.25 ± 26.99	45.50 ± 28.37
12 weeks	1.33 ± 2.31	77.13 ± 15.30

4.8 Percentage of mineralization after 4 months of the dentin, biocera and Bio-Oss tests

Group	% mineralized after 4 months
Dentin	52.5 ± 10.7%
Biocera	52.0 ± 23.4%
Bio-Oss	51.0 ± 18.3%

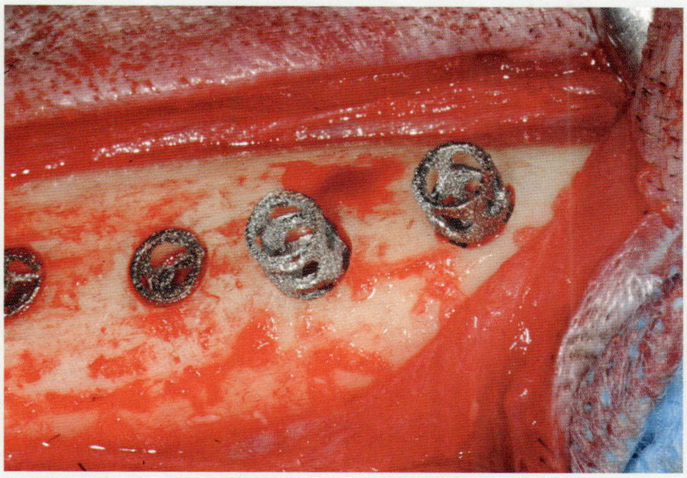

4.33 Placement of titanium cages in sheep bones.

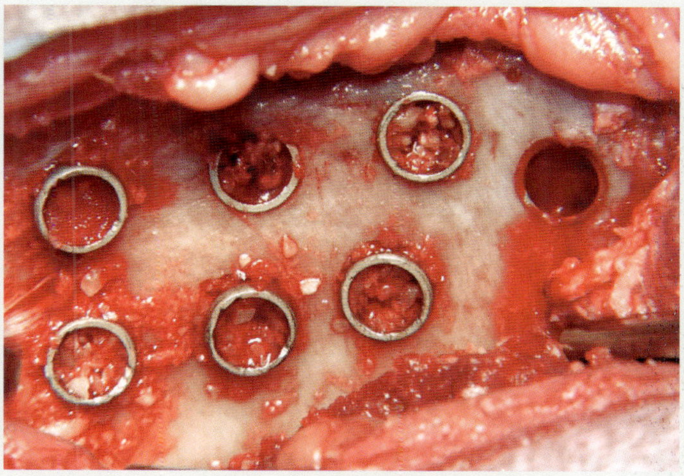

4.34 Filling of the cages placed in sheep bone with the granulate of dental origin.

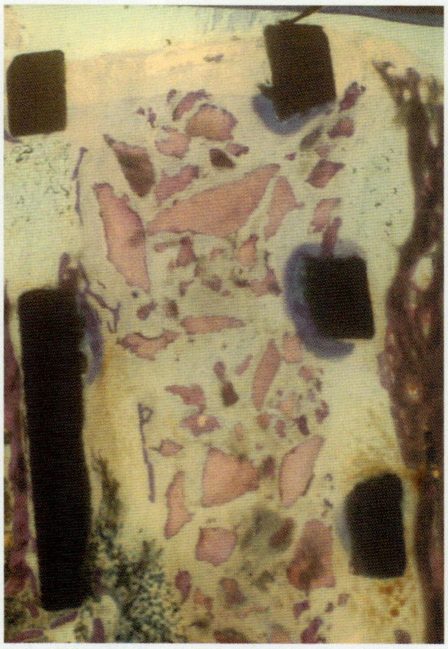

4.35 Particulate without treatment after 2 months from implantation.

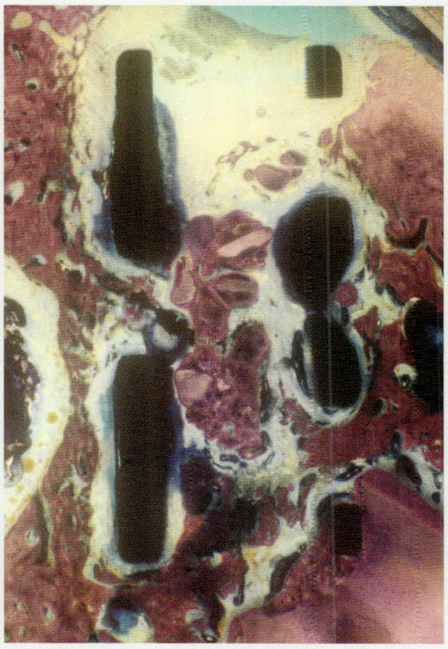

4.36 Particulate matter with treatment 2 months after implantation.

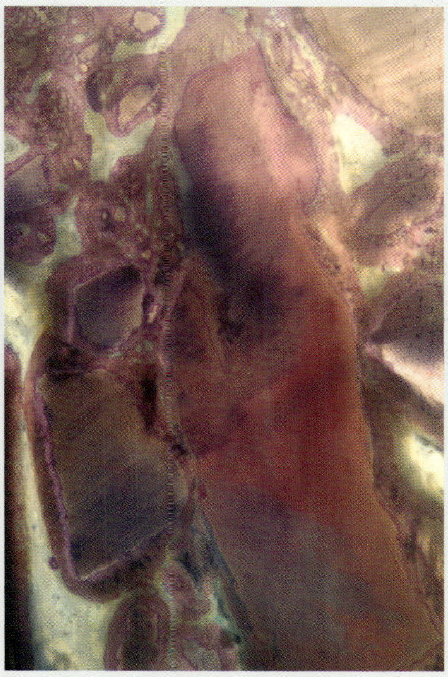

4.37 Particulate enlargement with treatment 2 months after implantation.

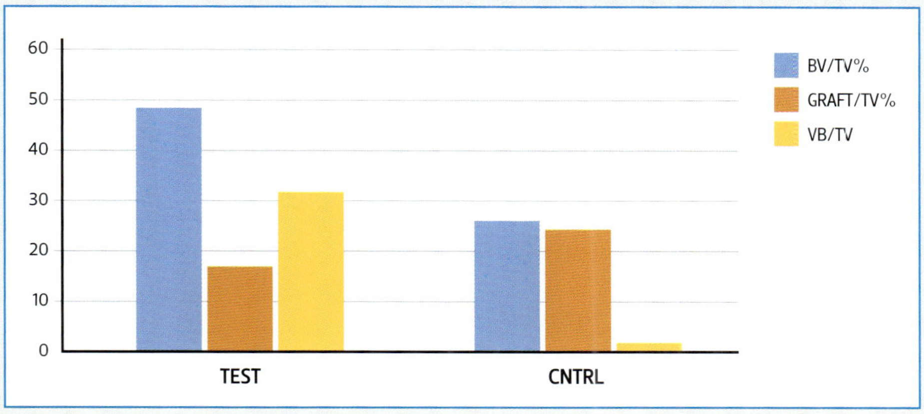

4.38 Histomorphometric evaluations in animal tests.

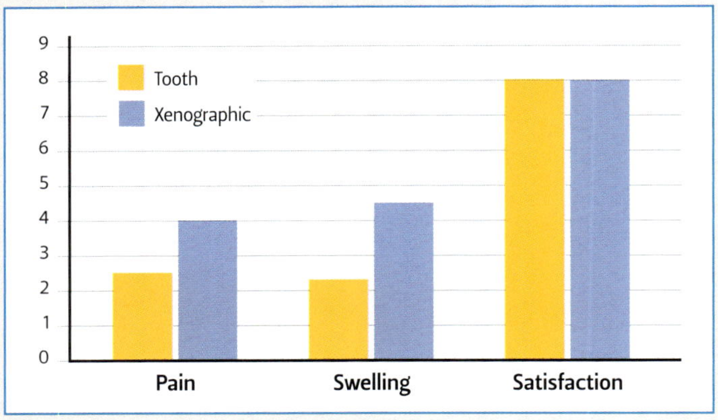

4.39 Result of the evaluation questionnaires of patients undergoing regeneration surgery using various types of grafting material.

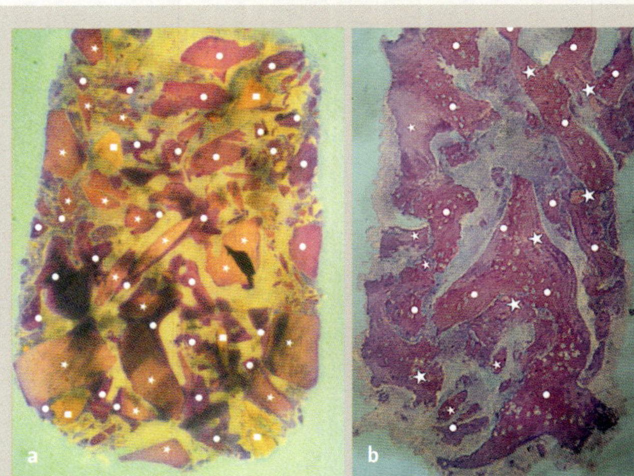

	Group 1	Group 2
Number of histologies performed	28	
Bone volume/Total volume	40.48% (±8.90)	40.28% (±11.51)
Residual graft/Total volume	19.70% (±13.75)	17.39% (±7.09)
Vital bone/Total bone	20.78% (±13.29)	22.89% (±9.72)

4.40 Histological and histomorphometric images of the two groups.

4.9 Results of the histomorphometries performed

Number of histologies performed	13
Bone volume/Total volume	41.47 ± 11.51
Residual graft/Total volume	16.60 ± 7.09
Vital bone/Total bone	24.87 ± 9.72

4.10 Statistical data and comparison with the p value

	Bone volume		Residual graft		Vital bone	
Dataset	1	2	1	2	1	2
Sample size	19	13	19	13	19	13
Average	40.4800	40.2801	19.7017	17.3983	20.7800	22.8900
Standard deviation	8.9032	11.5104	13.7533	7.0935	13.2970	9.7245
T	0.6871		0.5536		0.4887	
Degree of freedom	30		30		30	
P value (level of significance)	0.4973		0.5840		0.6286	

Analysis: $p > 0.05$ value not statistically significant; $p < 0.05$ wrong hypothesis.

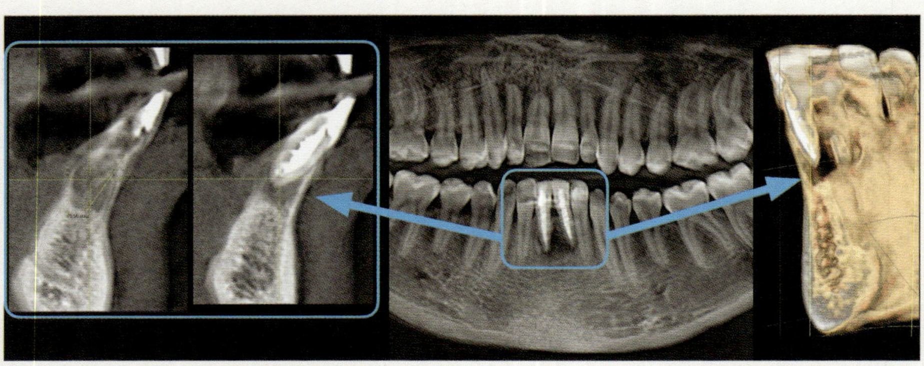

4.41 Initial situation.

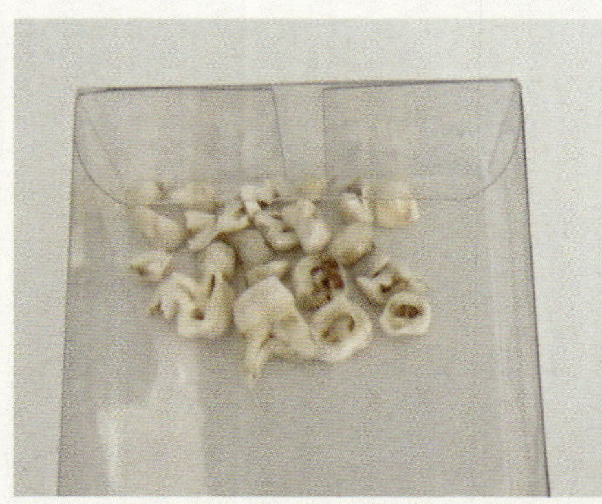

4.42 Plastic box in which the patient's deciduous teeth were stored for 20 years.

in which only the elements treated endodontically[60] were considered. A group of 98 patients were treated with crest preservation and 13 out of them got a biopsy to perform a histomorphometrical evaluation (4.9).

Statistical differences were also analyzed by a prospective histological clinical multicenter study[61] for ridge preservation between healthy (group 1) and RCT teeth (group 2) (4.40) using histological and histomorphometric examinations. There was no statistical difference between the two groups (4.10).

Tooth performance in sinus lift was evaluated in other studies.[62] Twenty-three patients received sinus lift via vestibular access with a 24-month success rate of 97.5%. Five histologies performed at 4 months (4.11) were analyzed with values comparable to the other multicenter tests presented.

In 2020, Minetti presented[63] a case report using deciduous teeth in a 26-year-old patient. The patient had a cyst in area 4.1-3.1 (4.41) which had caused the extraction of the two teeth which, due to root canal treatments and prostheses, could not be used as grafting material. The patient denied consent to the use of the wisdom tooth 4.8 but came to the dental office after a few days with a plastic box (4.42) containing her deciduous teeth kept by her mother. Only some of the deciduous teeth extracted and stored for 15-20 years were selected to be transformed into grafting material.

About 5 months after the surgical procedure, two implants were inserted, and a biopsy was taken.

The results were comparable to those achieved with the use of permanent teeth from a histomorphometric (47.22% of BV, 18.68% of graft volume and 28.55% of VB) and a clinical point of view with a follow-up at 24 months. This finding opens up the scenario to a possible routine use of the deciduous teeth.

The list of studies reported in the literature is very long and in the recent years has undergone a strong quantitative and qualitative increase. It is possible then to compare the data as placing them on the same scale (4.43-4.45), up to 2015 and from 2015 onwards, looking at the articles in the literature and noting their numerical increase.

From these data it is understood how the number of human cases in the literature has increased by 2.5 times in just 5 years, while the animal studies have decreased by about 10 times. The availability of some devices has undoubtedly increased the number of cases but it has also raised the predictability and effectiveness of the treatment.

REVIEW OF THE LITERATURE ON THE TOOTH AS GRAFT MATERIAL

In recent years, some literature reviews about dental grafting material have been carried out.

In one case, the conclusions pointed out the absence of an adequate uniformity and standardization in the process, which results in the impossibility of comparing the various materials and, moreover, it damages the clinical usefulness of this grafting material.[64]

This systematic review clearly demonstrated the diversity of treatment methods used to produce tooth-derived graft material.

4.11 Histomorphometric data of the mean values obtained from the histologies in the sinus lift

Number of histologies performed	5
Bone volume/Total volume	36.284 ± 9.77
Residual graft/Total volume	14.61 ± 14.61
Vital bone/Total bone	21.5 ± 8.61

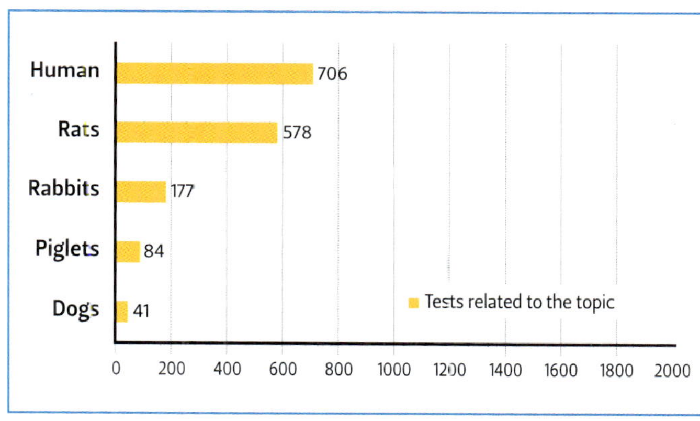

4.43 Clinical cases carried out from 1967 to 2015 using a tooth.

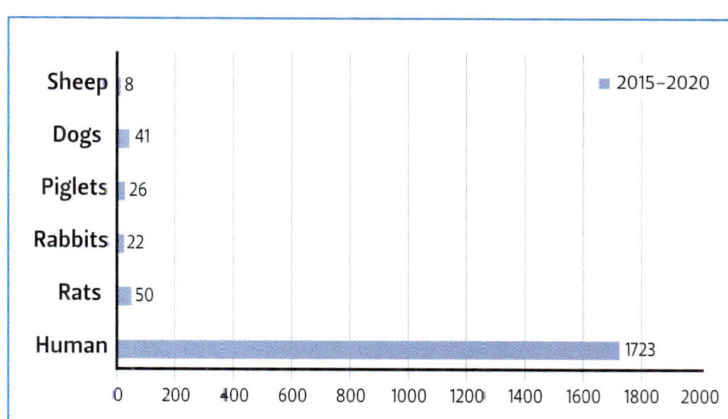

4.44 Clinical cases carried out from 2015 to 2020 using a tooth.

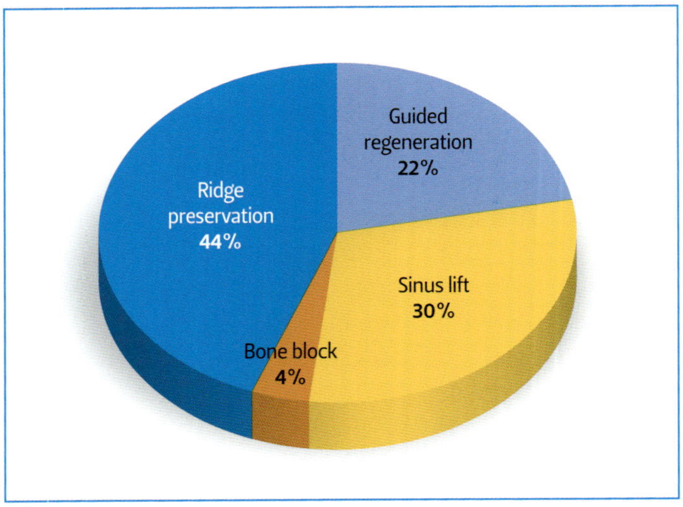

4.45 Percentages of studies on surgical modalities.

The other reviews concluded that the preparation, size and shape of the granules play an important role in the properties of the graft material. A standardization of these methods is recommended, but future studies and technologies will make it accessible and usable with success, given its undoubted qualities, similar to the autologous bone.[65,66]

RESEARCH ON TOOTH PRESERVATION

One of the researches carried out on the particularities of the tooth as a carrier and as a potential graft material is the Schmidt-Schultz et al.[67]

For the first time, GFs were extracted, solubilized and identified as IGF-II (Insulin Growth Factor II), BMP-2 (Bone Morphogenetic Protein-2) and TGFβ (Transforming Growth Factor β) from teeth dated in the late pre-ceramic Neo-lithic period (about 8000 years ago) and from teeth dated in the early Middle Ages and they were compared with recent extracted teeth. These molecules are an integral part of dental structures throughout life. Tests for protein quantification and recognition were performed using electrophoresis (SDS-PAGE).

The incredible results were that the proteins were still present (4.46) and active (that is not denatured) even after 8000 years and the quantity was similar in all the three groups.

The conclusions were that the ECM (Extra Cellular Matrix) proteins of the bone and tooth are very well protected. The apatite in which the proteins are embedded, ensures considerable protection from chemical and physical agents even after death (4.47). These structures are therefore preserved for thousands of years.

We must therefore imagine that the tooth could be considered as similar to a structure where the building blocks of HA support, protect and enclose the delicate proteins over time.

This also indicates that, while the alloplastic mineralized material is known to be only osteoconductive, the osteoinductive factors (that is proteins) contained in the mineralized structure may be usable when the mineralized structure is resorbed during the regeneration process.[68]

Some Polish researchers[69] extracted mouse incisor teeth and stored them for 30 months, then they implanted the grafts intra-muscularly in order to evaluate in vivo the maintenance of their osteoinductive potential. They were then analyzed at different time intervals ranging from 10 to 450 days and it was seen that, in 87% of cases, there was an induced intramuscular ossification

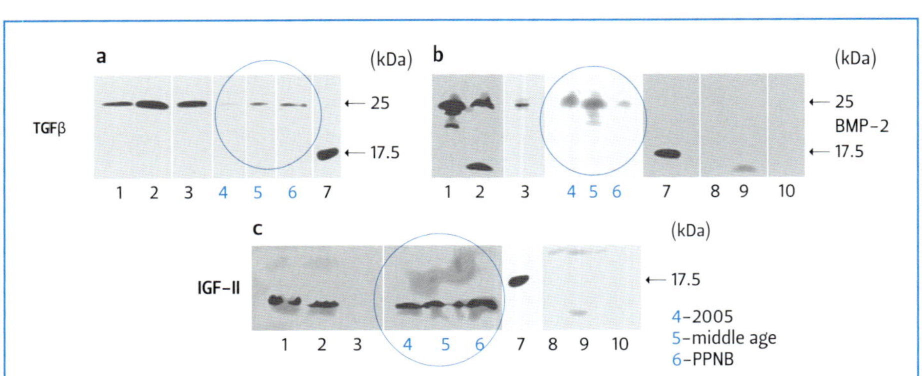

4.46 TSDS-PAGE comparison test between teeth extracted at different times. **(a)** TGFβ; **(b)** BMP-2; **(c)** IGF-II.

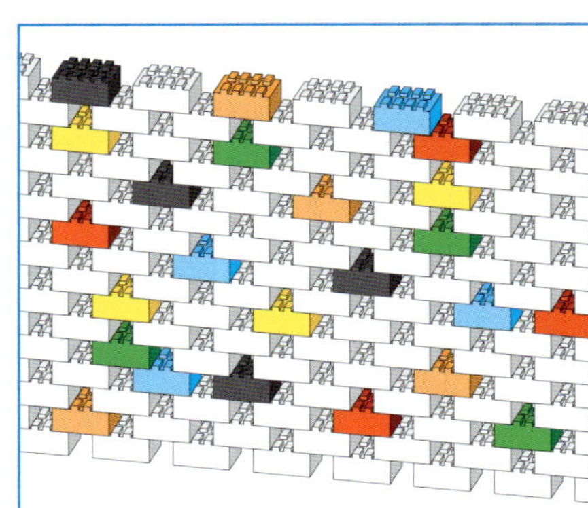

4.47 The image provides an idea of how proteins are protected by the presence of a mineralized structure that surrounds, supports and protects them.

process. In conclusion, the results actually agree with those obtained by Schmidt-Shultz on the maintenance of proteins over time that cause osteinduction, indicating that the storage of teeth for 30 months seems not to have any effect on the osteoinductive properties of the teeth.

DIFFERENT PROCESSING METHODS PROPOSED BY LITERATURE

The table below (4.12) lists all the treatment methods for demineralization proposed so far in the literature. The differences in treatment are evident.

The tooth, which is an autologous structure of type 1 mineralized collagen with autologous HA, can be considered as an excellent grafting material with osteoconductive properties. The presence of internal proteins transforms it into an osteoinductive grafting material. However, these proteins are numerically reduced (3.5-4%) and each treatment can reduce their numerical presence or their effectiveness.

The proposed treatments are many and all extremely different. From these considerations we started to understand which could be the best procedure to maintain intact all the qualities of the tooth.

4.12 Overview of the procedures proposed in the literature for the treatment of tooth demineralization

Procedures	Literature
Cleaned in 4% hydrogen peroxide, 70% ethanol for 10 min, stored at -20° C, reduced to 800-1000 µm powder, demineralized in 0.6 M HCl for 10 min, then washed in saline solution and sterilized with a peracetic acid-ethanol solution and then washed in saline	Park M, Mah YJ, Kim DH, et al. Demineralized deciduous tooth as a source of bone graft material: its biological and physicochemical characteristics. Oral Surg Oral Med Oral Pathol Oral Radiol 2015;120:307-14
Cleaned in 4% hydrogen peroxide, 70% ethanol for 10 min, stored at -20° C, reduced to 800-1000 µm powder, demineralized in 0.6 M HCl for 15 min, then washed in saline solution and sterilized with a peracetic acid-ethanol solution and then washed in saline	Park M, Mah YJ, Kim DH, et al. Demineralized deciduous tooth as a source of bone graft material: its biological and physicochemical characteristics. Oral Surg Oral Med Oral Pathol Oral Radiol 2015;120:307-14
Cleaned in 4% hydrogen peroxide, 70% ethanol for 10 min, stored at -20° C, reduced to 800-1000 µm powder, demineralized in 0.6 M HCl for 20 min, then washed in saline solution and sterilized with a peracetic acid-ethanol solution and then washed in saline	Park M, Mah YJ, Kim DH, et al. Demineralized deciduous tooth as a source of bone graft material: its biological and physicochemical characteristics. Oral Surg Oral Med Oral Pathol Oral Radiol 2015;120:307-14
Cleaned in 4% hydrogen peroxide, 70% ethanol for 10 min, stored at -20° C, reduced to 800-1000 µm powder, demineralized in 0.6 M HCl for 25 min, then washed in saline solution and sterilized with a peracetic acid-ethanol solution and then washed in saline	Park M, Mah YJ, Kim DH, et al. Demineralized deciduous tooth as a source of bone graft material: its biological and physicochemical characteristics. Oral Surg Oral Med Oral Pathol Oral Radiol 2015;120:307-14
Cleaned in 4% hydrogen peroxide, 70% ethanol for 10 min, stored at -20° C, reduced to 800-1000 µm powder, demineralized in 0.6 M HCl for 30 min, then washed in saline solution and sterilized with a peracetic acid-ethanol solution and then washed in saline	Park M, Mah YJ, Kim DH, et al. Demineralized deciduous tooth as a source of bone graft material: its biological and physicochemical characteristics. Oral Surg Oral Med Oral Pathol Oral Radiol 2015;120:307-14
Cleaned in 4% hydrogen peroxide, 70% ethanol for 10 min, stored at -20° C, reduced to 800-1000 µm powder, demineralized in 0.6 M HCl for 60 min, then washed in saline solution and sterilized with a peracetic acid-ethanol solution and then washed in saline	Park M, Mah YJ, Kim DH et al Demineralized deciduous tooth as a source of bone graft material: its biological and physicochemical characteristics. Oral Surg Oral Med Oral Pathol Oral Radiol 2015;120:307-14
Cleaned in 4% hydrogen peroxide, 70% ethanol for 10 min, stored at -20° C, reduced to 800-1000 µm powder, demineralized in 0.6 M HCl for 90 min, then washed in saline solution and sterilized with a peracetic acid-ethanol solution and then washed in saline	Park M, Mah YJ, Kim DH, et al. Demineralized deciduous tooth as a source of bone graft material: its biological and physicochemical characteristics. Oral Surg Oral Med Oral Pathol Oral Radiol 2015;120:307-14
Demineralized in 0.6 m HCl for 5 days and then removed with prolonged washing in sterile 0.15 M NaCl	Yeomans JD, Urist MR. Bone induction by decalcified dentine implanted into oral, osseous and muscle tissues. Arch Oral Biol 1967;12:999-1008
Descaled in 0.6M HCl for 72 hours at 4° C, then immersed in many 70% alcohol baths and rinsed in distilled water	Urist MR. Bone formation by autoinduction. Science 1965; 150(3698):893-9
Demineralized by 0.5 M HCl at room temperature, created a powder treated with ethyl alcohol and water saturated with phenol for 30 min. Then rinsed in 70% ethanol and water, frozen in liquid nitrogen dehydrated with ethanol and ether overnight at 37° C	Huggins C, Wiseman S, Reddi AH. Transformation of Fibroblasts by allogeneic and xenogeneic transplants of demineralized tooth and bone. J Exp Med 1970;132:1250-8

(Continued on the next page)

4.12 *(Continued from the previous page)*

Procedures	Literature
HCl 0.6 M	Nade N. Bone graft surgery reappraised: the contribution of the cell to ultimate success. Brit J Surg 1970;57:752-6
EDTA	Nade N. Bone graft surgery reappraised: the contribution of the cell to ultimate success. Brit J Surg 1970;57:752-6
Different HCl solutions: 48 hours at 0.2 M	Bang G. Induction of heterotopic bone formation by demineralized dentin: an experimental model in Guinea pigs. Scand J Dent Res 1973;81:240-50
Different HCl solutions: 48 hours at 0.4 M	Bang G. Induction of heterotopic bone formation by demineralized dentin: an experimental model in Guinea pigs. Scand J Dent Res 1973;81:240-50
Different HCl solutions: 48 hours at 0.8 M	Bang G. Induction of heterotopic bone formation by demineralized dentin: an experimental model in Guinea pigs. Scand J Dent Res 1973;81:240-50
Different HCl solutions: 48 hours at 1.0 M	Bang G. Induction of heterotopic bone formation by demineralized dentin: an experimental model in Guinea pigs. Scand J Dent Res 1973;81:240-50
Different HCl solutions: 48 hours at 2.0 M	Bang G. Induction of heterotopic bone formation by demineralized dentin: an experimental model in Guinea pigs. Scand J Dent Res 1973;81:240-50
Demineralization by HNO_3 (nitric acid)	Koga T, Minamizato T, Kawai Y, et al. Bone regeneration using dentin matrix depends on the degree of demineralization and particle size. PLoS One 2016;11(1):e0147235
Dimensions 500 µm in ice + B-TCB	Nampo T, Watahiki J, Enomoto A, et al. A new method for alveolar bone repair using extracted teeth for the graft material. J Periodontol 2010;81:1264-72
70% ethyl alcohol and then to Korea Tooth Bank	Kim KW. Bone Induction by demineralized dentin matrix in nude mouse muscles. Maxillofac Plast Reconstr Surg 2014;36(2):50-6
Crushed with high speed Kometabio - alcohol to remove bacteria and physiological solution to remove alcohol[52]	Calvo-Guirado JL, Cegarra del Pino P, Sapoznikov L, et al. A new procedure for processing extracted teeth for immediate grafting in post-extraction sockets. An experimental study in American Foxhounds. Ann Anat 2018;217:14-23
Immersed in 70% ethyl alcohol and sent to Korea Tooth Bank where they dehydrated with ethyl alcohol and a solution of ethyl ether, lyophilized and disinfected with oxide of ethylene and packaged and shipped to the surgeon	Kim SK, Kim SW, Kim KW. Effect on bone formation of the autogenous tooth graft in the treatment of peri-implant vertical bone defects in the minipigs. Maxillofac Plast Reconstr Surg 2015;37:2
Crushed for 3 s with Kometabio 300-1200 µm. 10 min in 0.5 M NaOH + 30% alcohol (called basic alcohol) rinsed twice with saline sulphate solution. If necessary, store for the future, place at 140° C for 5 min	Bindermann I, Hallel G, Nardy C, et al. A novel procedure to process extracted teeth for immediate grafting of autogenous dentin. J Interdiscipl Med Dent Sci 2014;2:154
10% EDTA calcium hydroxide MTA for 14 days	Tomson PL, Grover LM, Lumley PJ, et al. Dissolution of bio-active dentine matrix components by mineral trioxide aggregate. J Dent 2007;35:636-42
10% EDTA calcium hydroxide MTA for 14 days	Graham L, Cooper PR, Cassidy N, et al. The effect of calcium hydroxide on solubilisation of bio-active dentine matrix components. Biomaterials 2006;27(14):2865-73
Stored in sodium chloride solution then immersed in ethanol for 20 hours, pulp removed, minced in ice immersion, 10% EDTA and 5 M PMSF for 14 days	Kim HS, Lee DS, Lee JH, et al. The effect of odontoblast conditioned media and dentin non-collagenous proteins on the differentiation and mineralization of cementoblasts in vitro. Arch Oral Biol 2009;54:71-9
37% phosphoric acid for 15 s 3 weeks in 0.5 M EDTA at 4° C	Vennat E, Bogicevic C, Fleureau J-M, et al. Demineralized dentin 3D porosity and pore size distribution using mercury porosimetry. Dent Mater 2009;25:729-35

(Continued on the next page)

4.12 *(Continued from the previous page)*

Procedures	Literature
Placed at -80° C for 24 hours 0.6 M HCl 1 week + chloroform and methanol for 24 hours and then granulated with a Spex Industries shredder	Yagihashi K, Miyazawa K, Togari K, et al. Demineralized dentin matrix acts as a scaffold for repair of articular cartilage defects. Calcif Tissue Int 2009;84:210-20
17% EDTA pH 7.5 15 min 17% EDTA pH 9 15 min 10% EDTA pH 7.5 15 min 10% EDTA pH 9 15 min	Parmar G, Chhatariya A. Demineralising effect of EDTA at different concentration and pH - A spectrophotometer study. Endodont 2004;16:54-7
Boiling in water for 2 hours, 2 hours in isopropranol and dried at 100 degrees and sterilized with gamma rays	Moharamzadeh K, Freeman C, Blackwood K. Processed bovine dentine as a bone substitute. Br J Oral Maxillofac Surg 2008;46: 110-3
Boiling water 30 minutes, 735° C calcination and sintering at 1150° C for 1 hour	Elkayar A, Elshazly Y, Assaad M. Properties of hydroxyapatite from bovine teeth. Bone Tissue Regen Insights 2009;2:31-6
3 s of grinding, alcohol 0.5 M NaOH (sodium hydroxide) + 30% alcohol (alcohol solution) for 10 minutes rinse in saline solution	Cardaropoli D, Nevins M, Schupbach P. New bone formation using an extracted tooth as a biomaterial: a case report with histologic evidence. Int J Periodontics Restorative Dent 2019;39(2):156-63
Bon Maker- (simple formulation) HCl 0.45 M-H_2O_2 130 volumes-ethanol 62.6% chloroform 31.3% water 6.1%; (aggressive formulation) HCl 0.56 M-H_2O_2 120 volumes-ethanol 47.2% chloroform 47.2% water 5.6%	Tests carried out at POLIMI, 2016
Tooth Transformer - 01 M HCl + H_2O_2 10% (34 volumes)	
0.6 m HCl at 2° C + 70% ethyl alcohol and gentamicin	Pinheiro Carvalho VA, de Oliveira Tosello D, de Castillo Salgado MA, et al. Histomorphometric analysis of homogenous demineralized dentin matrix as osteopromotive material in rabbit mandibles. Int J Oral Maxillofac Implants 2004;19:679-86 Gomes MF, Banzi EC, Destro MF, et al. Homogenous demineralized dentin matrix for application in cranioplasty of rabbits with alloxan-induced diabetes: histomorphometric analysis. Int J Oral Maxillofac Implants 2007;22:939-47 Gomes MF, Destro MF, Banzi EC, et al. Optical density of bone repair after implantation of homogenous demineralized dentin matrix in diabetic rabbits. Braz Oral Res 2008;22:275-80
Liquid nitrogen -169° C for 2 weeks then in 70% ethyl alcohol 30-60 min	Al-Namnam NM, Shanmuhasuntharam P, Ha KC, et al. Processed allogenic dentine as a scaffold for bone healing: an in vivo study. Aust J Basic Appl Sci 2010;4:5932-40
10 EDTA at 25° C for 3 months	Reis-Filho CR, da Silva ER, Martins AB, et al. Demineralised human dentine matrix stimulates the expression of VEGF and accelerates the bone repair in tooth sockets of rats. Arch Oral Biol 2012;57:469-76
10% EDTA for 3 minutes	de Oliveira GS, Miziara MN, Silva ER, et al. Enhanced bone formation during healing process of tooth sockets filled with demineralized human dentine matrix. Aust Dent J 2013;58:326-32
Cleansed 10% H_2O_2 + pulverized + decalcified 1 group 2% H_2SO_4 20 min/ 2 group 2% HCl 20 min/ 3 group 2% HNO_3 20 min/ 4 group 2% EDTA 20 min All rinsed with physiological solution 3 times 10 minutes and disinfected with ethylene oxide	Jang HS, Kim SG, Lim SC et al. Osteogenic ability according to the decalcified modality of auto-tooth bone grafts in peri-implant defects in dogs. Implant Dent 2014;23:482-8
Washed 10% H_2O_2 - dehydrated ethyl alcohol - degreased ether ethyl-freeze-dried and disinfected with ethylene oxide	Kim SK, Kim SW, Kim KW. Effect on bone formation of the autogenous tooth graft in the treatment of peri-implant vertical bone defects in the minipigs. Maxillofac Plast Reconstr Surg 2015;37:2

(Continued on the next page)

4.12 *(Continued from the previous page)*

Procedures	Literature
In ultrasonic tank with 75% alcohol then sintered at 800° C and gamma rays	Huang YC, Lew WZ, Feng SW, et al. Histomorphometric and transcriptome evaluation of early healing bone treated with a novel human particulate dentin powder. Biomed Mater 2016;12:015004
0.2 HCl for 144 hours, lyophilized and sterilized with ethyl alcohol	Movin S, Borring-Møller G. Regeneration of infrabony periodontal defects in humans after implantation of allogenic demineralized dentin. J Clin Periodontol 1982;9:141-7
Ground with a coffee grinder> 700 rpm. Demineralized with 1 M lactic acid for 15-20 min, rinsed with saline for 60 seconds	Joshi CP, Dani NH, Khedkar SU. Alveolar ridge preservation using autogenous tooth graft versus beta-tricalcium phosphate alloplast: a randomized, controlled, prospective, clinical pilot study. J Indian Soc Periodontol 2016;20:429-34
Immersed in a gentamicin solution + 70% ethyl alcohol at 2° C	Gomes MF, de Abreu PP, Morosolli AR, et al. Densitometric analysis of the autogenous demineralized dentin matrix on the dental socket wound healing process in humans. Braz Oral Res 2006; 20:324-30
Calcium chloride	Urist MR. Bone formation by autoinduction. Science 1965;150:893-9
EDTA + formic acid + citric acid	Urist MR. Bone formation by autoinduction. Science 1965;150:893-9
EDTA + formic acid + citric acid	Urist MR. Bone formation by autoinduction. Science 1965;150:893-9
Lactic acid	Urist MR. Bone formation by autoinduction. Science 1965;150:893-9
Heat 70° C	Urist MR. Bone formation by autoinduction. Science 1965;150:893-9
Nitric acid + HCl + β-propiolactone	Urist MR. Bone formation by autoinduction. Science 1965;150:893-9
Nitric acid + HCl + β-propiolactone	Urist MR. Bone formation by autoinduction. Science 1965;150:893-9
DNFB (dinitrofluorobenzene)	Urist MR. Bone formation by autoinduction. Science 1965;150:893-9
IAA (iodoacetamide) + HCl	Urist MR. Bone formation by autoinduction. Science 1965;150:893-9

REFERENCES

1. Sharpe PT. Neural crest and tooth morphogenesis. Adv Dent Res 2001;15:4.
2. Berkovitz BKB, Holland GR, Moxham BJ. Oral Anatomy, histology and embriology. (3rd edition). St. Louis, Mosby, 2005;290-303.
3. Kumar GS. Orban's Oral histology & embryology (14th edition). New Delhi, Elsevier, 2015.
4. Papagerakis P, Mitsiadis T. Development and structure of teeth and periodontal tissues. In: Rosen CJ. Primer on the metabolic bone diseases and disorders of mineral metabolism (8th edition). Ames, John Wiley & Sons, 2013;904-13.
5. Vainio S, Karavanova I, Jowett A, et al. Identification of BMP-4 as a signal mediating secondary induction between epithelial and mesenchymal tissues during early tooth development. Cell 1993;75:45-58.
6. Dassule HR, McMahon AP. Analysis of epithelial mesenchymal interactions in the initial morphogenesis of the mammalian tooth. Dev Biol 1998;202:215-27.
7. Bei M. Molecular genetics of ameloblast cell lineage. J Exp Zool B Mol Dev Evol 2009;312B:437-44.
8. Caruso S, Bernardi S, Pasini M, et al. The process of mineralisation in the development of human tooth. Eur J Paediatr Dent 2016;17(4):322-6.
9. Reith EJ. The early stage of amelogenesis as observed in molar teeth of young rats. J Ultrastruct Res 1967;17:503-26.
10. Mjor IA, Fejerskov O. La struttura del dente umano. Milano, Edi-ermes, 1981.
11. Daculsi G, Menanteau J, Kerebel LM, et al. Length and shape of enamel crystals. Calcif Tissue Int 1984;36:550-5.
12. Helmcke J-G. Ultrastructure of enamel. In: Miles AEW. Structural and chemical organization of teeth, vol II. New York, Academic Press Inc., 1967.
13. Robinson C, Brookes SJ, Shore RC, et al. The developing enamel matrix: Nature and function. Eur J Oral Sci 1998;106(Suppl 1):282-91.
14. Simmer JP, Papagerakis P, Smith CE, et al. Regulation of dental enamel shape and hardness. J Dent Res 2010;89:1024-38.
15. Ohtsuka M, Saeki S, Igarashi K, et al. Circadian rhythms in the incorporation and secretion of 3H-proline by odontoblasts in relation to incremental lines in rat dentin. J Dent Res 1998;77:1889-95.
16. Reith EJ. The early stage of amelogenesis as observed in molar teeth of young rats. J Ultrastruct Res 1967;17:503-26.
17. Goldberg M, Kulkarni AB, Young M, et al. Dentin: structure, composition and mineralization. Front Biosci (Elite Ed) 2011;3:711-35
18. Ruch JV, Lesot H, Begue-Kirn C. Odontoblast differentiation. Int J Dev Biol 1995;39:51-68.
19. Wang HG, Kawashima N, Iwata T, et al.. Differentiation of odontoblasts is negatively regulated by MEPE via its C-ter-

minal fragment. Biochem Biophys Res Commun 2010;398:406-12.

20. Bleicher F. Odontoblast physiology. Exp Cell Res 2014;325:65-71.

21. Boskey AL. Mineralization of bone and teeth. Elements 2007;3:387-93.

22. Yamamoto T, Domon T, Takahashi S, et al. The structure and function of the cemento-dentinal junction in human teeth. Periodontal Res 1999;34(5):261.

23. McCulloch CA, Lekic P, McKee MD. Role of physical forces in regulating the form and function of the periodontal ligament. Periodontol 2000;24:56-72.

24. MacNeil RL, Somerman MJ. 1993. Molecular factors regulating development and regeneration of cementum. J Periodontal Res 28:550-9.

25. Adamo S, De Felici M, Dolfi A, et al. Istologia di Monesi (7ª edizione). Padova, Piccin, 2018.

26. Young B, O'Dowd G, Woodford P. Wheater - Istologia e anatomia microscopica (6ª edizione). Milano, Edra, 2014.

27. Yeomans JD, Urist MR. Bone induction by decalcified dentine implanted into oral, osseous and muscle tissues. Arch Oral Biol 1967;12:999-1008.

28. Urist MR. Bone formation by autoinduction. Science 1965;150:893-9.

29. Linden GJ. Bone induction in implants of decalcified bone and dentine. J Anat 1975;119:359-67.

30. Urist MR, Strates BS. Bone morphogenetic proteins. J Dent Res 1971;50(6): 1392-406.

31. Huggins C, Wiseman S, Reddi AH. Transformation of fibroblasts by allogeneic and xenogeneic transplants of demineralized tooth and bone. J Exp Med 1970;132:1250-8.

32. Nade S. Bone graft surgery reappraised: the contribution of the cell to ultimate success. Brit J Surg 1970; 57:752-6.

33. Bang G. Induction of heterotopic bone formation by demineralized dentin: an experimental model in Guinea pigs. Scand J Dent Res 1973;81:240-250.

34. Sato K, Urist MR. Induced regeneration of calvaria by bone morphogenetic protein (BMP) in dogs. Clin Orthop 1985;197:301-11.

35. Bessho K, Tagawa T, Murata M. Purification of bone morphogenetic protein derived from bovine bone matrix. Biochem Biophys Res Commun 1989;165:595-601.

36. Kuboki Y, Jin Q, Takita H. Geometry of carriers controlling phenotypic expression in BMP-induced osteogenesis and chondrogenesis. J Bone Joint Surg Am 2001;83-A Suppl 1(Pt 2):105-15.

37. Koga T, Minamizato T, Kawai Y, et al. Bone regeneration using dentin matrix depends on the degree of demineralization and particle size. PLoS One 2016;11(1):e0147235.

38. Blum B, Moseley J, Miller L, et al. Measurement of bone morphogenetic proteins and other growth factors in demineralized bone matrix. Orthopedics 2004;27(1 Suppl):161-5.

39. Kim YK, Lee J. Tooth derived bone graft material. J Korean Assoc Oral Maxillofac Surg 2013:39:103-11.

40. Urist MR. Experimental delivery systems for bone morphogenetic protein. In: Wise DL, Altobelli DE, Schwartz ER, et al. Handbook of biomaterials and applications. Section 3: Orthopaedic biomaterials applications. Boston, Marcel Dekker, 1995;1093-133.

41. Herford AS, Boyne PJ. Reconstruction of mandibular continuity defects with bone morphogenetic protein-2 (rhBMP-2). J Oral Maxillofac Surg 2008;66:616-24.

42. Boerckel JD, Kolambkar YM, Dupont KM, et al. Effects of protein dose and delivery system on BMP-mediated bone regeneration. Biomaterials 2011;32:5241-51.

43. Kim YK, Lee JK, Kim KW, et al. Healing mechanism and clinical application of autogenous tooth bone graft material. In: Pignatello R. Advances in Biomaterials Science and Biomedical Applications. Rijeka, InTech, 2013; pp. 405-435.

44. Bessho K, Tanaka N, Matsumoto J, et al. Human dentin-matrix-derived bone morphogenetic protein. J Dent Res 1991;70(3):171-5.

45. Young CS, Terada S, Vacanti JP, et al. Tissue engineering of complex tooth structures on biodegradable polymer scaffolds. J Dent Res 2002;81:695-700.

46. Duailibi MT, Duailibi SE, Young CS, et al. Bioengineered teeth from cultured rat tooth bud cells. J Dent R 2004;83:523-8.

47. Nakashima M. Bone morphogenetic proteins in dentin regeneration for potential use in endodontic therapy. Cytokine Growth Factor Rev 2005; 16(3):369-76.

48. Yang W, Harris MA, Cui Y, et al. MP is required for odontoblast differentiation and pulp vasculogenesis. J Dent Res 2012;91(1):58-64.

49. Tanoue R, Ohta K, Miyazono Y, et al. Three-dimensional ultrastructural analysis of the interface between an implanted demineralised dentin matrix and the surrounding newly formed bone. Sci Rep 2018; 8:2858.

50. Nampo T, Watahiki J, Enomoto A. A new method for alveolar bone repair using extracted teeth for the graft material. J Periodontol 2010;81:1264-72.

51. Kim KW. Bone induction by demineralized dentin matrix in nude mouse muscles. Maxillofac Plast Reconstr Surg 2014;36(2):50-6.

52. Park M, Mah YJ, Kim DH, et al. Demineralized deciduous tooth as a source of bone graft material: its biological and physicochemical characteristics. Oral Surg Oral Med Oral Pathol Oral Radiol 2015;120:307-14.

53. Calvo-Guirado JL, Cegarra del Pino P, Sapoznikov L, et al. A new procedure for processing extracted teeth for immediate grafting in post-extraction sockets. An experimental study in American Fox Hound dogs. Ann Anat 2018;217:14-23.

54. Kim SK, Kim SW, Kim KW. Effect on bone formation of the autogenous tooth graft in the treatment of peri-implant vertical bone defects in the minipigs. Maxillofac Plast Surg 2015:37:2.

55. Minetti E, Palermo A. Comparison between the bone regeneration using tooth graft with or without tooth transformer in sheep. BAOJ Dentistry 2019;5(1):54-7.

56. Park SM, Um IW, Kim YK, et al. Clinical application of auto-tooth bone graft material. J Korean Assoc Oral Maxillofac Surg 2012;38:2-8.

57. Bindermann I, Hallel G, Nardy C, et al. A novel procedure to process extracted teeth for immediate grafting of autogenous dentin. J Interdisciplinar Med Dent 2014;2:154.

58. Lee JY, Kim YK, Kim SG, et al. Histomorphometric study of sinus bone graft using various graft material. J Dent Rehabil Appl Sci 2011;27:141-7.

59. Wu D, Zhou L, Lin L, et al. Immediate implant placement in anterior teeth

with grafting material of autogenous tooth bone vs xenogenic bone BMC. Oral Health 2019;19:266.

60. Minetti E, Palermo A, Ferrante F, et al. Autologous tooth graft after endodontical treated used for socket preservation: a multicenter clinical study. Appl Sci 2019;9(24):5396.

61. Minetti E, Giacometti E, Gambardella U, et al. Alveolar socket preservation with different autologous graft materials: preliminary results of a multicenter pilot study in human. Materials 2020:13(5):1153.

62. Minetti E, Palermo A, Contessi M, et al. Autologous tooth graft for maxillary sinus augmentation: a multicenter clinical study. Int J Growth Factors Stem Cells Dent 2019;2:45-51.

63. Minetti E, Taschieri S, Corbella S. Autologous deciduous tooth-derived material for alveolar ridge preservation: a clinical and histological case report. Case Rep Dent 2020;6:1-6.

64. Gharpure A, Bhatavadekar NB. Clinical efficacy of tooth-bone graft: a systematic review and risk of bias analysis of randomized control trials and observational studies. Implant Dent 2018;27(1):119-34.

65. Khanijou M, Seriwatanachai D, Boonsiriseth K, et al. Bone graft material derived from extracted tooth: a review literature. J Oral Maxillofac Surg Med Pathol 2019;31(1):1-7.

66. Tabatadei FS, Tatari S, Samadi R, et al. Different methods of dentin processing for application in bone tissue engineering: a systematic review. J Biomed Mater Res A 2016;104(10):2616-27.

67. Schmidt-Schultz TH, Schultz M. Intact growth factors are conserved in the extracellular matrix of ancient human bone and teeth: a storehouse for the study of human evolution in health and disease. Biol Chem 2005;386:767-76.

68. Lohmann CH, Andreacchio D, Kuster G, et al. Tissue response and osteoinduction of human bone grafts in vivo. Arch Orthop Trauma Surg. 2001; 121(10):583-90.

69. Wlodarski KH, Szcesny G, Kuzala B, et al. Longterm preservation of Bone Morphogenetic Activity in stored demineralized murine incisors. Pol Orthop Traumat 2013;78:97-100.

In vitro studies with dental materials

E. Minetti

In order to understand and to be able to develop a protocol that could be the basis for a completely automated device capable of constantly reproducing the same results and maintaining osteo-inductive abilities, a research project was carried out at the Natta Institute of the Polytechnic University of Milan, Italy, with the help of prof. Candiani, Dr. Bono, Dr. Gelosa and Dr. Brunella.

The studies were divided into several phases evaluating:

- type of grinding and granule sizes;
- liquid assessment;
- in vitro tests;
- cytotoxicity tests;
- tooth weight checks.

These tests took place over a wide temporal and fan-shaped spectrum so that only at the end it was possible to go back to reevaluate them and follow other paths; it can therefore be difficult to justify the research timeline in this textbook.

Analysis of the type of grinding

Grinding is the first step toward using the tooth as a graft material.

Some authors analyzed the size of graft material grains to understand which size performed better. Dozza[1] created defects in the sheep's cortical bone by inserting scaffolds of different sizes (Large, 1-2 mm), (Small, <0.5 mm), (Medium, 0.5-1 mm). The best results were obtained with a Medium particle size.

Koga and colleagues[2] also performed an analysis using clean, pulverized human teeth divided according to size into three groups. The best result was obtained for dimensions ranging between 0.5 and 1 mm. Smaller particles are too quickly resorbed to ensure sufficient space retention over time and allow for bone formation.

It is therefore obvious that the best performances are obtained when the dimensions of the granules are homogeneous and they are between 0.5 and 1 mm.

If you think about the surgical use of the tooth, extreme care must be taken not to disperse an unrepeatable sample (the extracted tooth) due to grinding techniques that can create particles that are not homogeneous in size (for example, too small) and that this size is as similar as possible to optimal weights. In fact, if you have 1 gr of tooth it would be absurd to lose 0.5 gr due to the grinding technique.

In the effort of trying to understand which was the system that guaranteed the best performance, two different grinding systems were evaluated, one at high speed, like a coffee grinder, and one at low speed, with concentric conical blades.

A tooth was triturated, then analyzed under a microscope to highlight the shape of the produced granules, filtered through calibrated sieves and, finally, the quantity of granules with a size between 0.5 and 1 mm was weighed.

Comparison by grinding

High-speed grinding results in granules of different sizes and with dissimilar shapes (5.1).

Low speed grinding results in similar granules of size and shape (5.2).

Comparison by grinding product weight

Tests were carried out to understand the percentage dispersion in terms of dry weight of a ground tooth and then filtered through a sieve to keep only the granules with a size between 0.5 and 1 mm. The tooth was weighed (5.3) before grinding and after grinding by the use of two devices.

A sample of 11 natural human teeth was used without restorations, prostheses or root canal treatments. In the case of the low-speed grinder, the teeth were sectioned due to problems of insertion into the space between the blades and this resulted in a weight loss caused by the cuts; in any case, it was decided not to weigh the tooth after sectioning because this is one limitation of this system and therefore must be fully evaluated. In the high-speed grinder, however, the teeth were inserted whole.

This first analysis, with all the limitations due to the number of elements analyzed and the tools used, made it possible to understand that grinding at low speed, resulting in a more homogeneous grinding, is more efficient and therefore allows a greater percentage of tooth to be used (5.1).

The granules thus produced were then inserted into the -Mastersizer 3000 device (5.4) which allows the quantification of both dry and wet granules through laser diffraction. The test indicated that the average particle size varied between 406 and 815 µm with peaks up to 1110 µm (5.2). The dimensions of the granules, therefore, appeared to be in agreement with the literature.[1,3-8]

5.1 Differences between the two types of grinding in weight and in average percentages of the analyzed samples

	Weight before (g)	Weight after (g)	% residual
High speed grinding	1.31 ± 0.56	0.56 ± 0.24	43.09% ± 2.17
Low speed grinding	1.51 ± 0.65	1.36 ± 0.61	93.5% ± 2.18

Liquid evaluation

Treatment of permanent teeth: search for liquids

The first phase of the research was aimed at understanding the chemical composition of the tooth in order to evaluate the possible effects of the demineralization process.

The granules were produced using a low-speed grinder and then filtered by size using metal sieves (Filtra, Seneco Srl, Milan, Italy) in three groups:

- group A: particles from 200 to 700 µm;
- group B: particles <200 µm;
- group C: particles >700 µm.

Only group A granules were used for the tests.

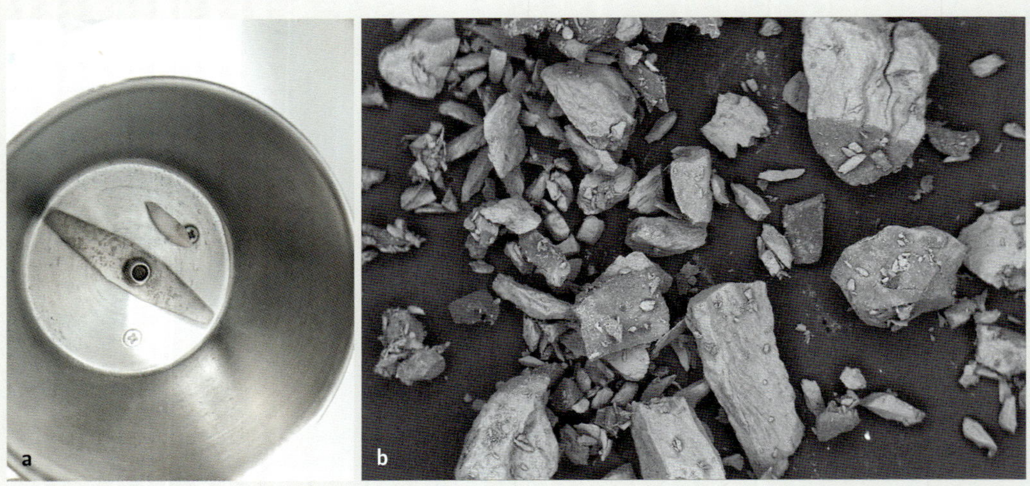

5.1 (a) High speed grinder. (b) Granules produced with the high-speed grinder. Different sized granules can be seen, many of which are very small.

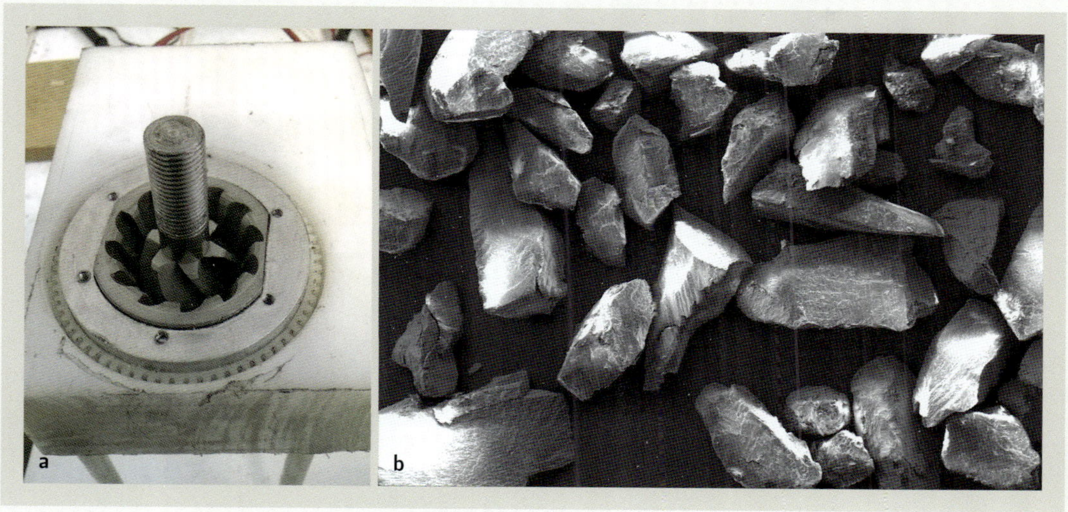

5.2 (a) Low speed grinder. **(b)** Granules produced with a low-speed grinder, similar in size.

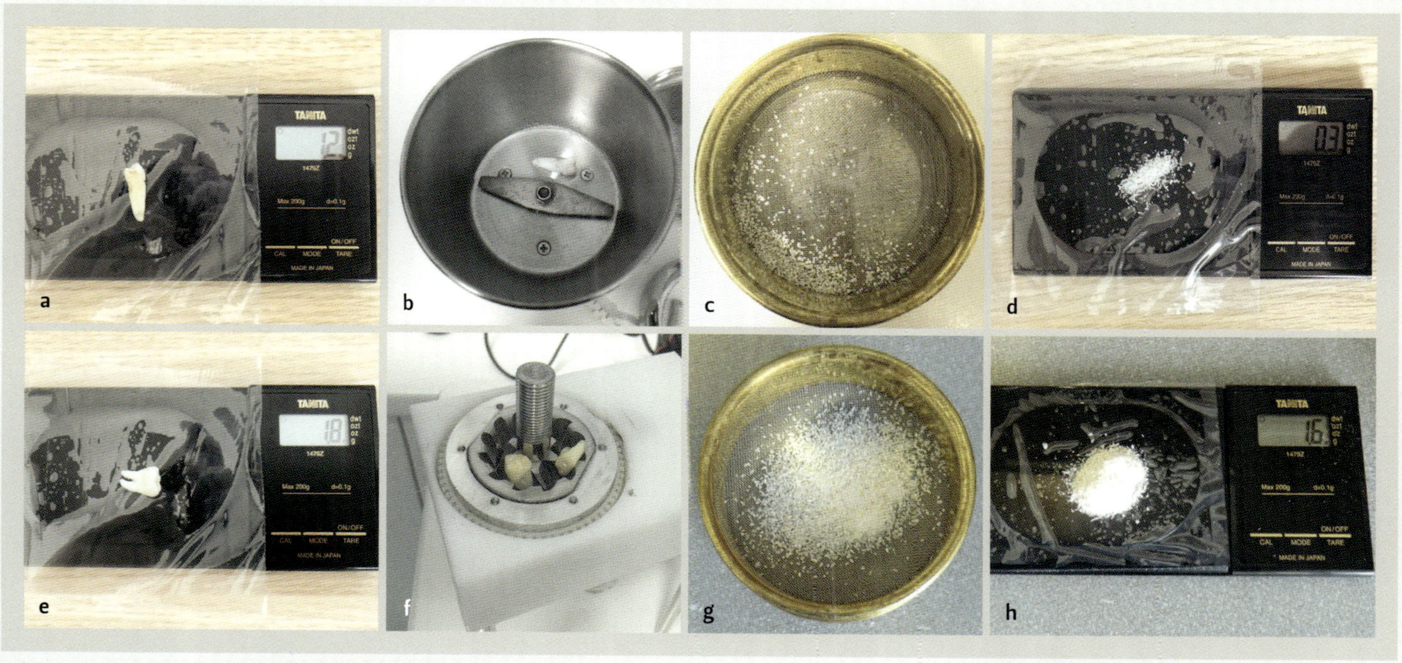

5.3 High speed grinding: **(a)** mini digital scale to measure the initial weight of the tooth; **(b)** the same tooth in the high-speed grinder; **(c)** metal sieve to select the granules of the desired size; **(d)** weight of the dental granulate after being sieved. Low speed grinder: **(e)** mini digital scale to measure the initial weight of the tooth; **(f)** the same tooth in the low-speed grinder; **(g)** metal sieve to select the granules of the desired size; **(h)** weight of the dental granulate after sieving.

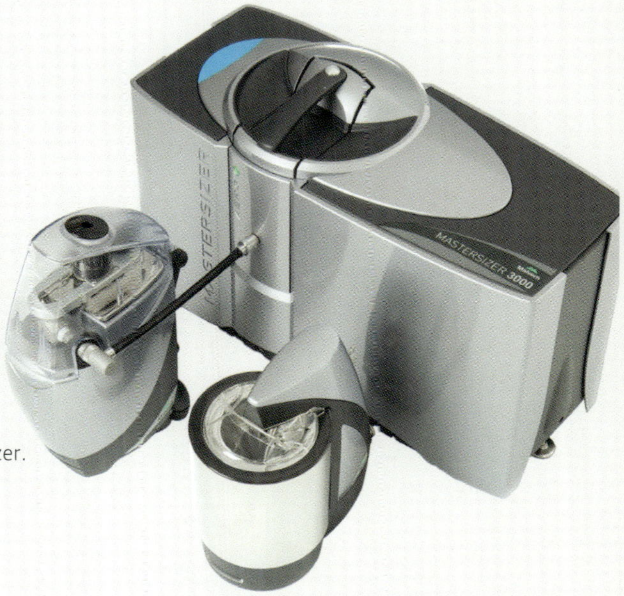

5.4 Laser diffraction particle size analyzer. (Courtesy of Malvern Panalytical Ltd, UK.)

5.2 Dimensions measured after grinding at low speed by Tooth Transformer using master size 3000

Analysis

Measurement Details

Operator Name Ricerca2
Sample Name thooth trasformer
SOP File Name AeroM.cfg

Measurement Details

Analysis Date Time 05/06/2018 14:05:23
Measurement Date Time 05/06/2018 14:05:23
Result Source Measurement

Analysis

Particle Name Tooth
Particle Refractive Index 1,600
Particle Absorption Index 0,100
Dispersant Name
Dispersant Refractive Index
Scattering Model Mie
Analysis Model General Purpose
Weighted Residual 0,93 %
Laser Obscuration 2,96 %

Result

Concentration 0,0429 %
Span 1,864
Uniformity 0,576
Specific Surface Area 52,39 m^2/kg
D [3;2] 115 µm
D [4;3] 422 µm
Dv (10) 59,0 µm
Dv (50) 406 µm
Dv (90) 815 µm

Frequency (compatible)

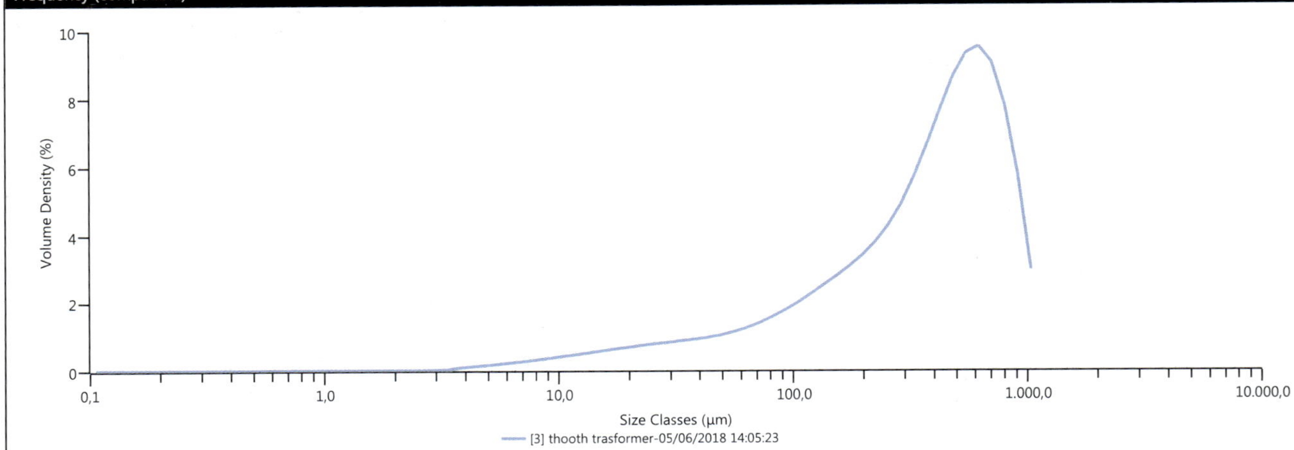

Result

Size (µm)	% Volume Under	Size (µm)	% Volume Under	Size (µm)	% Volume Under	Size (µm)	% Volume Under	Size (µm)	% Volume Under	Size (µm)	% Volume Under	Size (µm)	% Volume Under
0,0995	0,00	0,461	0,00	2,13	0,00	9,86	1,37	45,6	8,21	211	28,25	976	97,52
0,113	0,00	0,523	0,00	2,42	0,00	11,2	1,71	51,8	9,06	240	31,39	1110	100,00
0,128	0,00	0,594	0,00	2,75	0,00	12,7	2,09	58,9	9,98	272	34,93		
0,146	0,00	0,675	0,00	3,12	0,00	14,5	2,51	66,9	11,01	310	39,00		
0,166	0,00	0,767	0,00	3,55	0,00	16,4	2,98	76,0	12,16	352	43,73		
0,188	0,00	0,872	0,00	4,03	0,07	18,7	3,49	86,4	13,46	400	49,26		
0,214	0,00	0,991	0,00	4,58	0,16	21,2	4,05	98,1	14,94	454	55,65		
0,243	0,00	1,13	0,00	5,21	0,28	24,1	4,65	111	16,60	516	62,85		
0,276	0,00	1,28	0,00	5,92	0,43	27,4	5,29	127	18,48	586	70,64		
0,314	0,00	1,45	0,00	6,72	0,61	31,1	5,96	144	20,57	666	78,62		
0,357	0,00	1,65	0,00	7,64	0,82	35,3	6,67	163	22,88	756	86,20		
0,405	0,00	1,88	0,00	8,68	1,08	40,1	7,42	186	25,44	859	92,73		

A scanning electron microscope (SEM ESEM Zeiss EVO50; Carl Zeiss, Milan, Italy) (5.5) was used as an instrument and microanalyses were carried out with an EDX energy dispersion X-ray spectrometer (Bruker model Quantax 200 6/30), with an acceleration voltage of 15 kV, to investigate the surface composition and surface image. The EDS exam consists of an instrumental analytical method that exploits the emission of X-rays generated by an accelerated electron beam incident on the sample, which allows to determine the quantification and identification of the individual elements that compose the analyzed material (5.6).

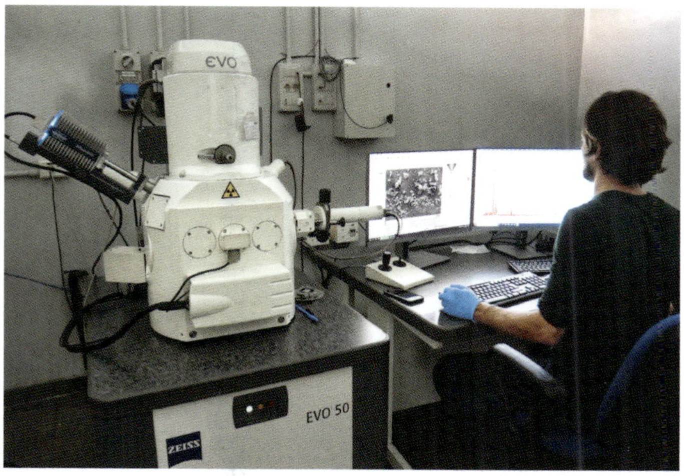

5.5 Microscope SEM Zeiss EVO50.

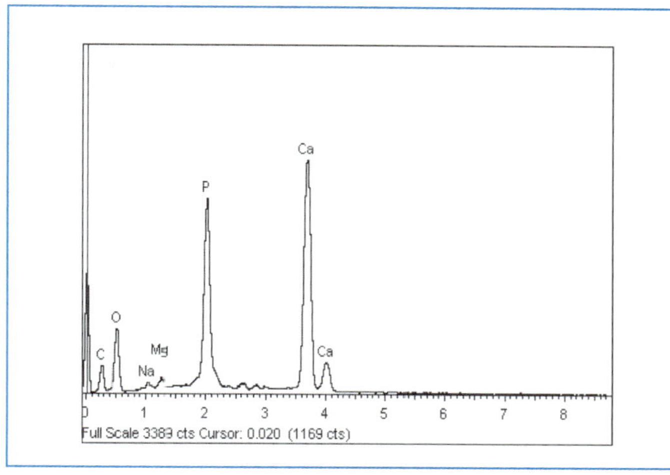

5.6 EDS curve graph.

5.3 Average composition of the analyzed samples

Sample	C %	O %	P %	Ca %
Native dentine	27.79 ± 4.55	47.06 ± 4.85	8.59 ± 1.33	16.56 ± 3.73
Native enamel	12.90 ± 2.68	55.21 ± 5.54	11.04 ± 0.82	20.25 ± 3.16
Native deciduous tooth	22.08 ± 4.88	55.37 ± 2.32	8.54 ± 1.62	12.94 ± 3.06
Xenographic material	15.95 ± 2.46	62.32 ± 2.74	8.62 ± 0.20	12.45 ± 0.41

The EDS spectrum graph confirms the presence of diffuse calcium phosphate deposits over the entire surface of the sample.

The tooth surface was also analyzed at this stage (5.3).

The samples were first fixed in 1.5% (v/v) glutaraldehyde solution for 20 minutes, then dehydrated in subsequent ethanol baths and, finally, sprinkled with gold particles.

The surface of the non-demineralized tooth is characterized by mineral crystals which cover it (5.7).

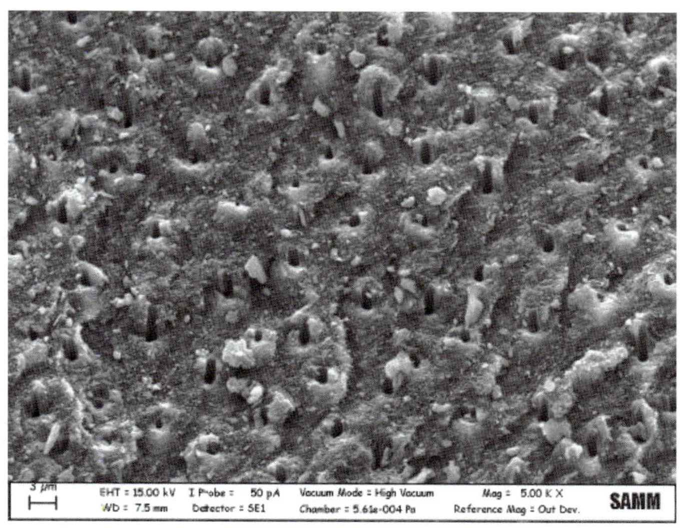

5.7 Untreated dentin surface.

Search for liquids: literature review

Based on the analysis of the literature, various liquids proposed by numerous authors have been identified (5.4).

With regard to their use suggested in the literature, however, a series of factors related to the purpose of the research must be taken into consideration.

The potential of the tooth as a grafting material, given its possible osteoinductive effect, has been evident since 1967. The real challenge is to find a repeatable, simple and short system capable of crushing, detoxifying and demineralising the tooth structure while keeping all its features.

For this purpose, 37 articles (5.5) were evaluated in which various protocols were proposed for the use of the tooth as grafting material or protocols designed to demineralize or detoxify the tooth for an in vitro or an in vivo study.

The number of possible protocols resulting from these articles is 50, as some authors have tested different procedures in each single article.

In order to decide in which direction to orientate the in-depth analyzes, it was decided to take into consideration the most tested liquids, as all the tests reported had positive results, but it was not possible to make any quantitative or qualitative comparison between them.

The most used liquids for demineralization were:

- HCl (hydrochloric acid), within 25 tests;
- ethyl alcohol, within 12 tests;
- EDTA, within 7 tests;
- peracetic acid, within 7 tests (all tests were collected in a single article);

Regarding detoxification, Bhat[9] analyzed seven different systems for disinfecting the teeth:

- 10% formalin;
- 3% H_2O_2 (hydrogen peroxide);
- 5.25% sodium hypochlorite;
- 2% glutaraldehyde;
- 0.1% thymol in distilled water;
- boiling in water;
- 121° C autoclave, 15 psi.

The ones that proved to be the most effective were formalin, sodium hypochlorite, autoclave treatment and H_2O_2.

5.4 Treatment liquids proposed by the literature

Demineralization	Detoxification	Rinsing
· Ethanol · HCl · EDTA · Nitric acid · Sodium hydroxide · Calcium chloride · Lactic acid · FDNB · Calcium hydroxide · Phosphoric acid · Hexamethyldisilazan · Liquid nitrogen · Sulfuric acid	· Hydrogen peroxide · Peracetic acid · Ethanol · Ethyl alcohol · Phenol · Ethyl ether · Ethylene oxide · Temperature · ß-propiolactone · Chloroform · Methanol · Isopropanol · Gamma rays · Gentamicin	Sodium chloride Distilled water

In literature the most used liquids were:

- hydrogen peroxide, 14 tests;
- chloroform, 5 tests.

The most used liquid for washing was a saline sulfate solution (12 tests). It was therefore decided to analyze all these liquids following the indications of the tests already carried out, obviously eliminating the chloroform because it was considered toxic.

HCl has been tested at different concentrations (0.1, 0.2, 0.45, 0.5, 0.6, 0.8, 1.0, 2.0) with usage times ranging from 1 to 5, 10, 15, 20, 25, 30, 60, 90 minutes, 72 hours, 144 hours, 5 days, 1 week.

5.5 Treatment liquids proposed by the literature divided by number of tests performed

Substance	Tests carried out	Bibliographic reference
HCl	25 test	10–23
EDTA	7 tests	13, 21, 24–29
Nitric acid	2 tests	21, 2
Sodium hydroxide	2 tests	32, 33
Lactic acid	1 test	34
Calcium hydroxide	2 tests	25, 34
Phosphoric acid	1 test	29
Liquid nitrogen -168°C	2 tests	20, 35
Sulfuric acid	1 test	21
Hydrogen peroxide	14 works	10, 15, 21, 36
Peracetic acid	7 tests	10
Ethyl alcohol	12 tests	10, 12, 15, 22–24, 31, 35–37
Phenol	1 test	12
Ethyl ether	2 tests	12, 36
Ethylene oxide	2 tests	21, 36
Temperature	4 tests	38–41
Chloroform	5 tests	15, 20, 42
Methanol	1 test	42
Isopropanol	1 test	39
Gamma rays	1 test	39, 41
Gentamicin	1 test	17–19
PBS saline sulfate solution	12 works	10, 11, 31, 32, 37, 43

EDTA was tested at concentrations of 10 and 17%.

Ethyl alcohol was tested at concentrations of 75, 70, 62 and 30%.

H_2O_2 was used at different concentrations: 14, 34, 120 and 130 volumes.

Obviously, for surgical routine purposes, protocols in which the waiting time exceeds 30/40 minutes cannot be used due to the procedure.

Analysis of different demineralization systems

The lines suitable for demineralization and detoxification were analyzed at different concentrations to verify their capability and with different cell lines in order to understand their cytotoxicity.

The granules of group A were then evaluated after treatment at different concentrations. The tables include C, N, O, Na, Mg, P and Ca but, to make it easier for the reader to understand, only the percentage values with the standard deviation are included in the table below (5.6) for P and Ca which both indicate the mineral part of the tooth.

The right column shows the Ca/P ratio values. The native bone has a mineral ratio between Calcium and Ca/P phosphorus = 1.67.[44]

A ratio very similar to the natural human bone indicates that the use does not alter the natural chemistry of

5.6 Values of minerals expressed on the analyzed granules with and without treatment

		P%	Ca%	Ca/P ratio (Control 1.67)
Untreated dentine	Reference values	8.59 ± 1.33	15.56 ± 3.73	1.92
Untreated Deciduous		8.54 ± 1.62	12.94 ± 3.06	1.51
Enamel		11.04 ± 0.82	20.25 ± 3.16	1.83
Xenograft (Bio-Oss)		8.62 ± 0.20	12.45 ± 0.41	1.44
0.001 M HCl	3% H_2O_2	8.56 ± 0.54	13.23 ± 1.68	1.54
0.001 M HCl	10% H_2O_2	10.39 ± 0.66	27.29 ± 27.29	2.62
0.001 M HCl	36% H_2O_2	8.11 ± 0.56	12.10 ± 1.40	1.49
0.01 M HCl	3% H_2O_2	8.02 ± 0.33	12.84 ± 1.00	1.60
0.01 M HCl	10% H_2O_2	8.16 ± 1.79	18.18 ± 4.76	2.23
0.01 M HCl	36% H_2O_2	7.75 ± 1.56	11.56 ± 3.03	1.49
0.1 M HCl	3% H_2O_2	7.14 ± 3.08	14.28 ± 4.31	2.00
0.1 M HCl	10% H_2O_2	5.04 ± 0.60	8.59 ± 1.37	1.70
0.1 M HCl	36% H_2O_2	2.34 ± 0.59	3.56 ± 1.08	1.52
0.6% HCl	3% H_2O_2	-0.23 ± 0.21	0.30 ± 0.15	-1.30
0.6% HCl	10% H_2O_2	0.52 ± 0.12	0.39 ± 0.12	0.75
0.6% HCl	36% H_2O_2	-0.27 ± 0.07	0.14 ± 0.05	-0.51
EDTA 17%		5.48 ± 2.91	13.39 ± 7.37	2.44
EDTA 10%		8.37 ± 0.39	21.55 ± 0.45	2.57
Alcol etilico 70%		9.29 ± 1.64	25.88 ± 1.99	2.78
Alcol etilico 62%		10.03 ± 2.17	27.45 ± 5.70	2.73
EDTA 17%	H_2O_2 10%	9.44 ± 1.63	25.47 ± 2.75	2.69
EDTA 10%	H_2O_2 10%	8.50 ± 1.43	22.50 ± 4.46	2.64
Ethyl alcohol 70%	H_2O_2 10%	11.18 ± 3.27	27.97 ± 5.88	2.50
Ethyl alcohol 62%	H_2O_2 10%	11.74 ± 1.42	30.61 ± 2.72	2.60
Ethyl alcohol 70%	EDTA 17%	10.44 ± 0.8	28.33 ± 0.92	2.70
Ethyl alcohol 62%	EDTA 10%	8.59 ± 1.8	23.17 ± 3.92	2.69

In *aqua green* color: solution that at the end of the tests was considered as more effective in maintaining proteins and detoxifying.

the bone. It can be seen that only few procedures allow to keep the ratio in the proximity of the natural values.

If the percentage values of the two minerals (Ca and P) are higher than the reference ones, it means that the quantities of the other components not present in the table have been reduced as the values are 100% optimized.

If, on the other hand, the values are lower than the reference, it means that the treatment has led to a reduction in the quantity of P or Ca and to an increase in the values of the other components.

Optimal demineralization should result in a similar percentage reduction of both the minerals.

Blum[45] on an animal model stated that, by reducing the mineral part, demineralization facilitates the release of GFs from the bone matrix.

From these data it is understood that, for example, ethyl alcohol increases calcium. This indicates a decrease in C, O, N, Na and Mg, and therefore could interfere or decrease the protein content (made up of carbon, oxygen, hydrogen and nitrogen).

Indeed, Firschein[46] has affirmed that when a segment of rat bone is demineralized in HCl and implanted in rat muscle, new bone is deposited.

However, if the identical test is performed by demineralizing the bone using HCl + 60/70% alcohol before implantation in the muscle, the matrix is resorbed in a similar way but replaced only with fibrous tissue.

This might be the reason why EDTA alone, in terms of the amount of calcium present, gives better results than EDTA + alcohol.

For all intents and purposes, some combinations of liquids seem to be able to completely eliminate the mineral part from the tooth. But the question must be asked whether this is sufficient, or it can lead to a loss of some component of the tooth.

Scanning Electron Microscope (SEM) analysis

As part of the same test, SEM images of treated samples with all possible variations were carried out (■ 5.7).

It is particularly interesting to note how, depending on the liquid or set of liquids used, a different image of the surface was obtained with a greater or lesser opening of the dentinal tubules.

Upon careful evaluation of the surface of the granules subjected to different treatments, two things were evident:

- the surfaces may appear clean or with residues of various origins;
- the shape and size of the dentinal tubules varies.

One of the focal aspects of this surface variation is the increase in wettability, with an increase in the hydrophilicity of the surface.

The hydrophilic surfaces demonstrated an increase in osteoblast maturation, an increase in the production of local factors and a mineralization compared to the hydrophobic surfaces.

Evidently, the maturation of osteoblasts is influenced by microtomography.[47,48]

Hydrophilic surfaces tend to promote more cell adhesion, proliferation, differentiation and bone mineralization compared to hydrophobic surfaces in the initial stages.The size of osteoblasts growing on the hydrophilic surface is greater.

Surface wettability can affect several important aspects of the biological system:

- adhesion of proteins and other macromolecules to the surface (conditioning);
- interaction between soft and hard tissues with pre-conditioned surfaces;
- reduction of bacterial adhesion and subsequent reduction of biofilm formation;
- increased in vivo osseointegration;
- the hydrophilic surface in contact with the blood and biological fluids promotes adsorption in a way that facilitates and improves the cell adhesion;
- the hydrophilic surfaces interact closely with biological liquids allowing the normal adsorption of proteins on the surface and the consequent interaction with cell receptors.[49]

Koga,[2] in 2016, found different sensitivities of osteoblasts to the untreated surface compared to the demineralized one. In fact, the osteoblasts only adhered to the demineralized surface. Osteoblasts were deposited on the UDD (non-demineralized) and DDM (demineralized) surface. The SEM images showed that the morphology of the cells is sensitive to the nanosurface, with dentinal tubules clearly visible in the DDM image but not observable on the UDD surface, and only in DDM the attachment of osteoblasts to the surface can be noted.

It is therefore probable that the mineral residues on the surface (which correspond to higher Ca and P values in the EDS table and therefore to the various levels of demineralization) may interfere with cell adhesion.

5.7 SEM images corresponding to the type of treatment

Untreated dentine		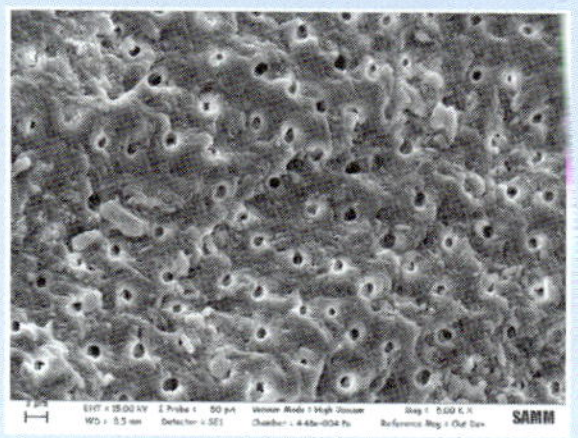
Untreated deciduous		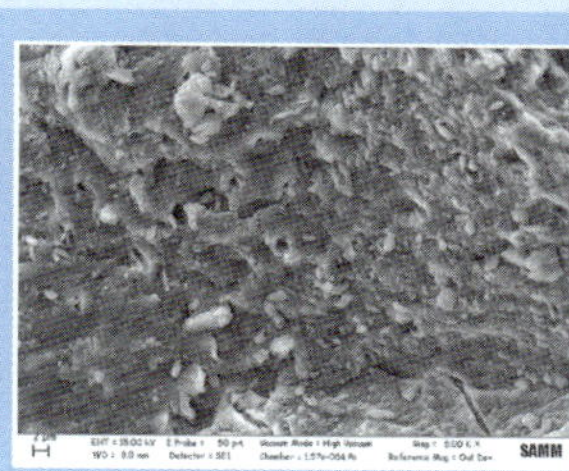
Enamel		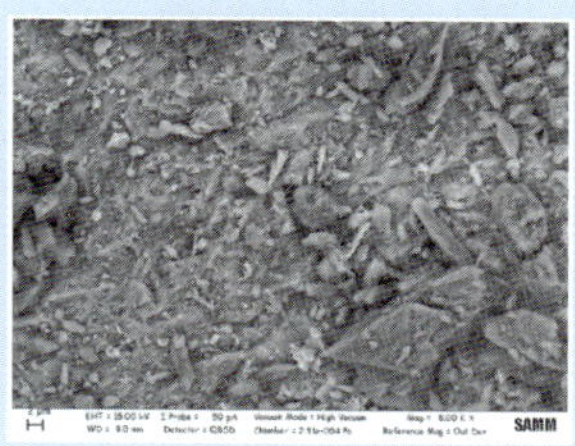
Xenograft		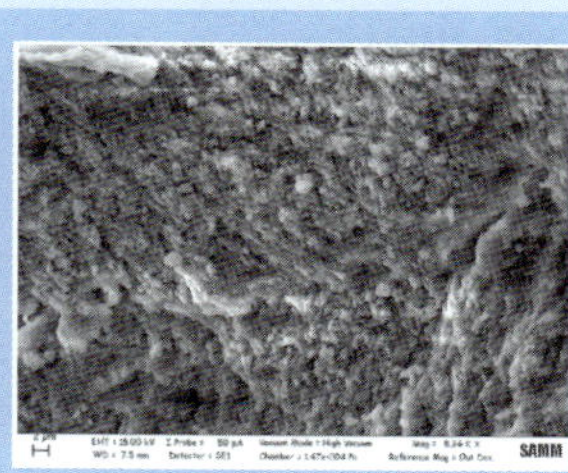
0.001M HCl	3% H_2O_2	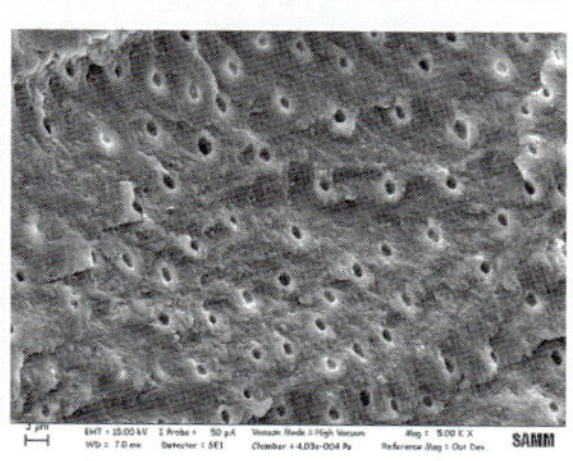
0.001 M HCl	10% H_2O_2	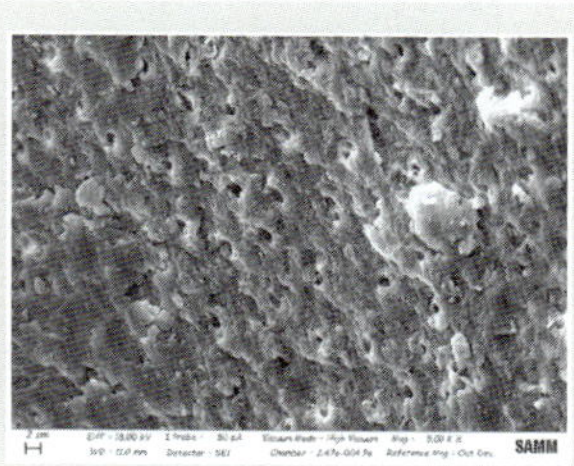
0.001 M HCl	36% H_2O_2	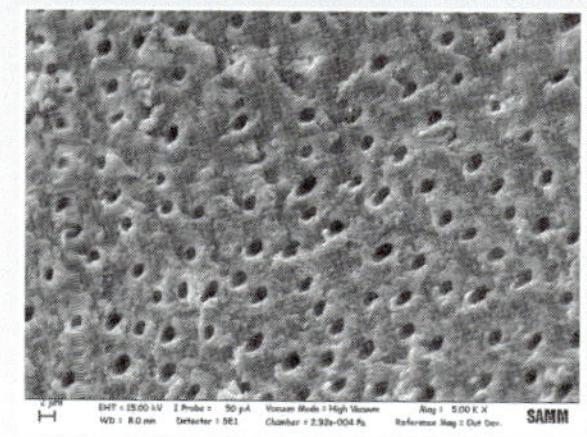
0.01 M HCl	3% H_2O_2	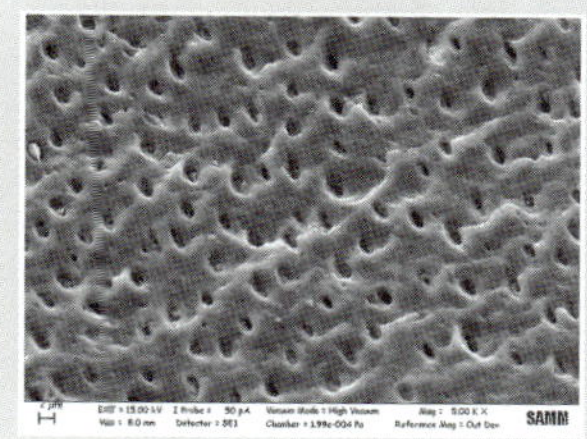
0.01 M HCl	10% H_2O_2	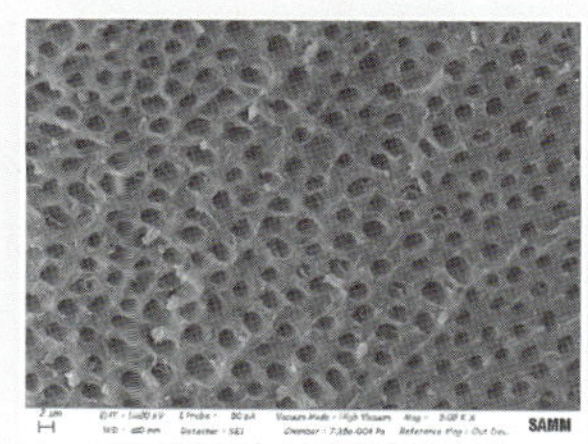
0.01 M HCl	36% H_2O_2	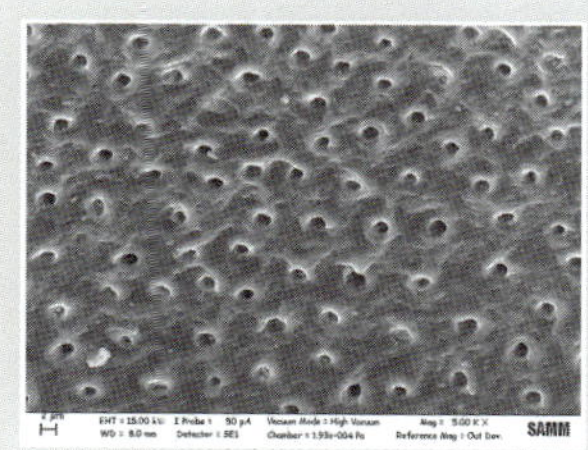
0.1 M HCl	3% H_2O_2	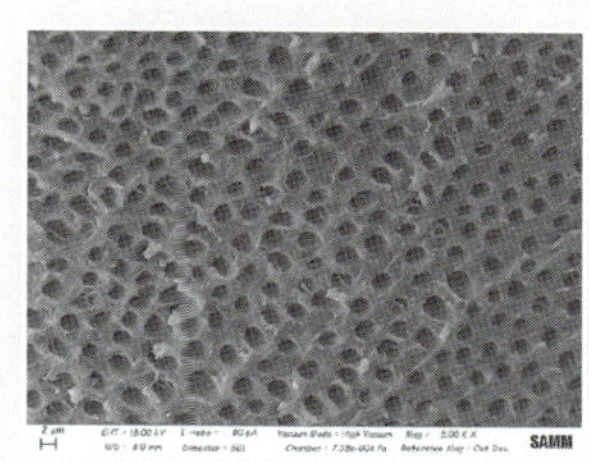
0.1 M HCl	10% H_2O_2	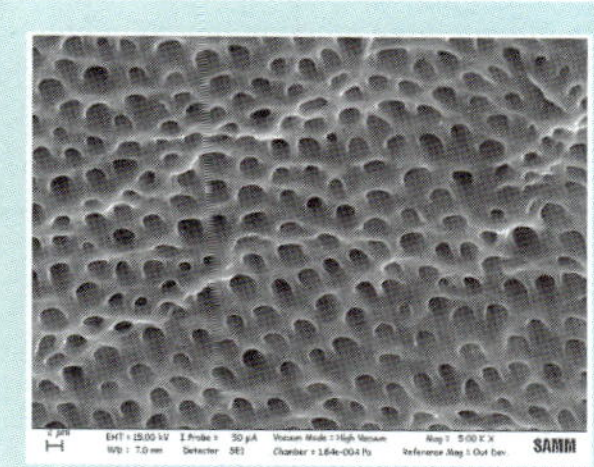

In *aqua green* color: solution that at the end of the tests was considered to be more effective in maintaining proteins and detoxifying.

(Continued on the next page)

5.7 *(Continued from the previous page)*

0.1 M HCl	36% H_2O_2	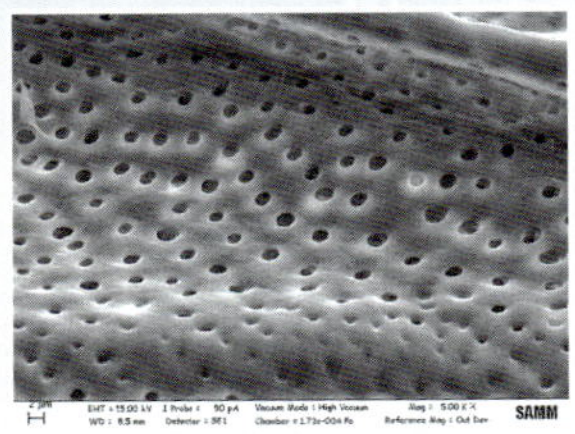
0.6% HCl	3% H_2O_2	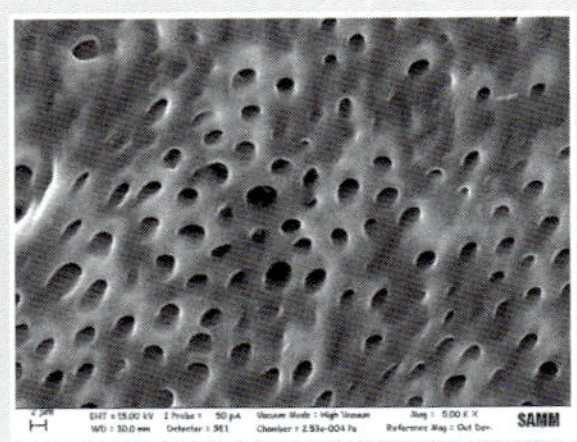
0.6% HCl	10% H_2O_2	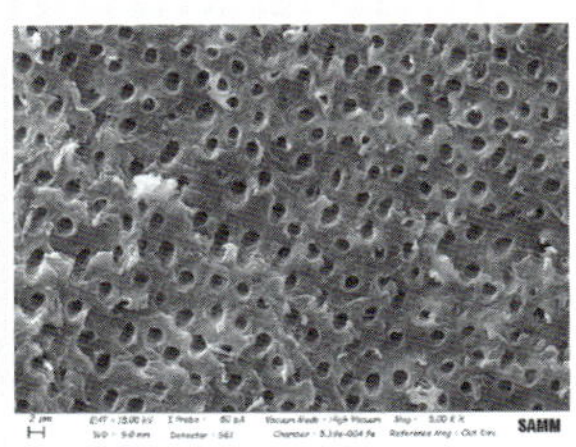
0.6% HCl	36% H_2O_2	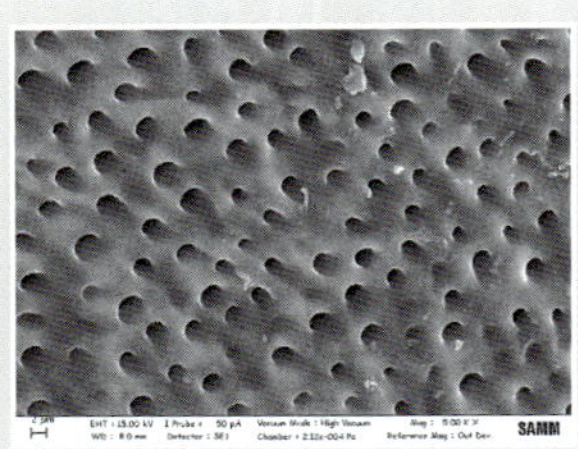
EDTA 17%		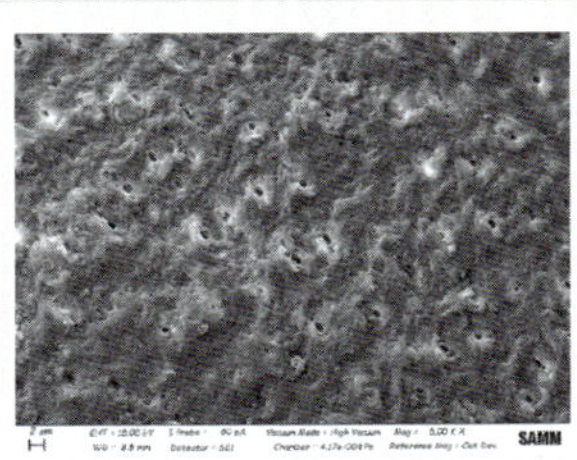
EDTA 10%		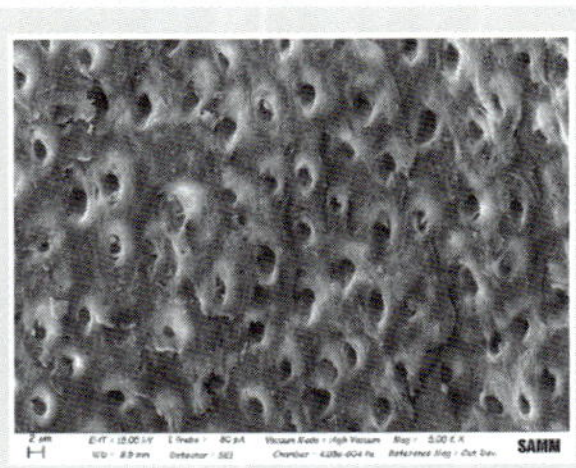
Ethyl alcohol 70%		
Ethyl alcohol 62%		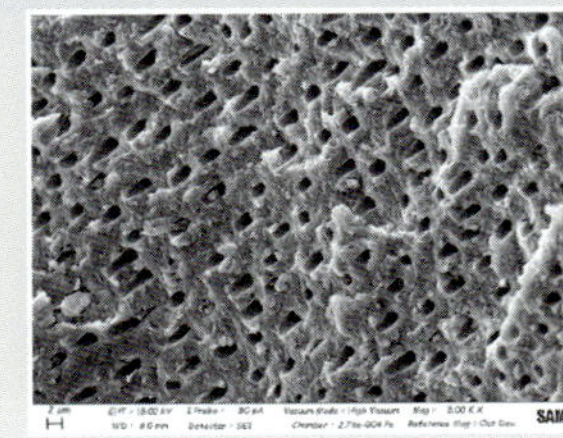
EDTA 17%	H_2O_2 10%	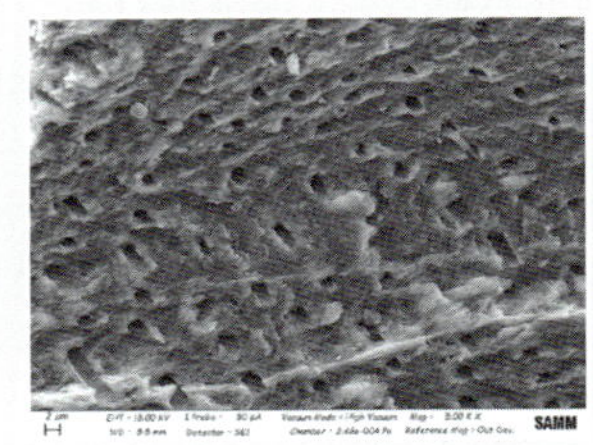
EDTA 10%	H_2O_2 10%	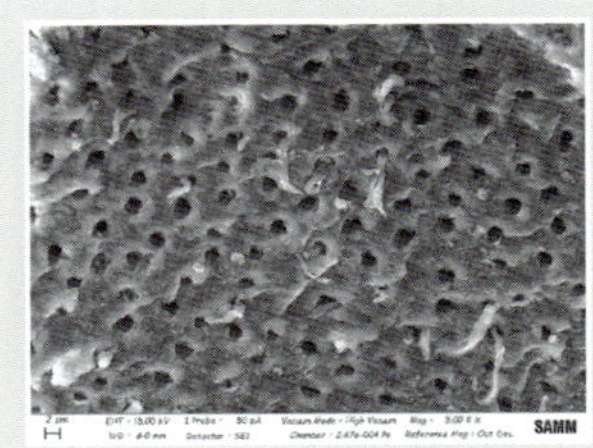
Ethyl alcohol 70%	H_2O_2 10%	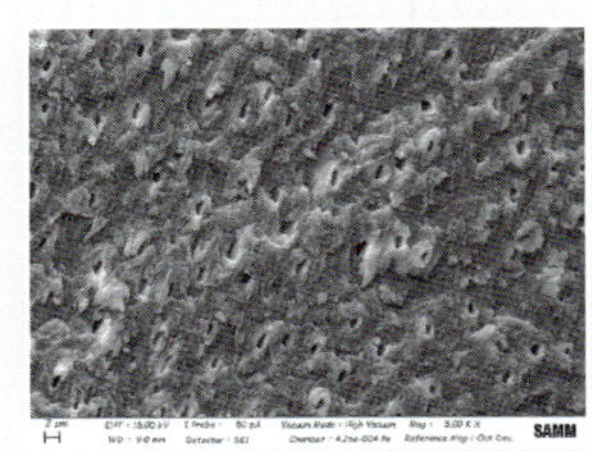
Ethyl alcohol 62%	H_2O_2 10%	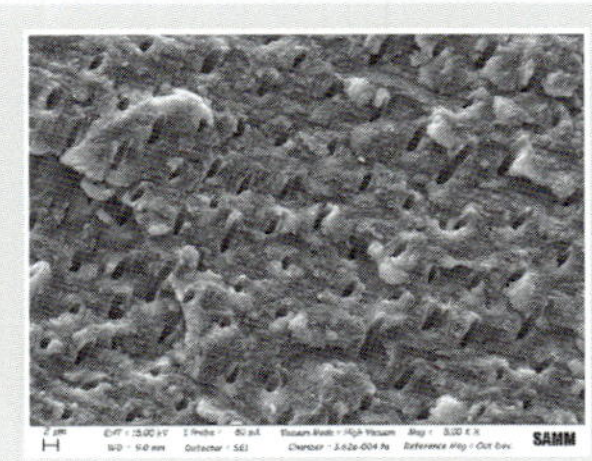
Ethyl alcohol 70%	EDTA 17%	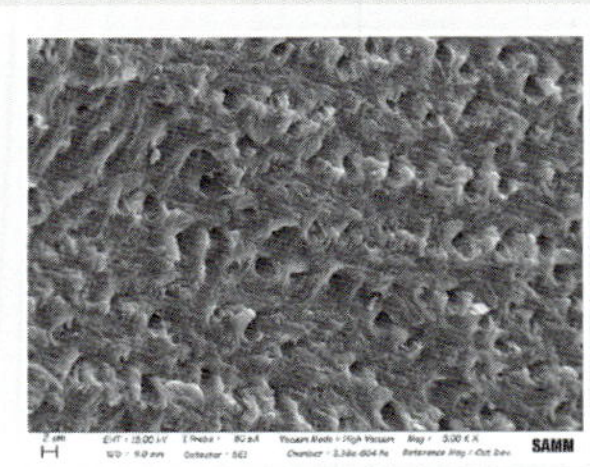
Ethyl alcohol 62%	EDTA 10%	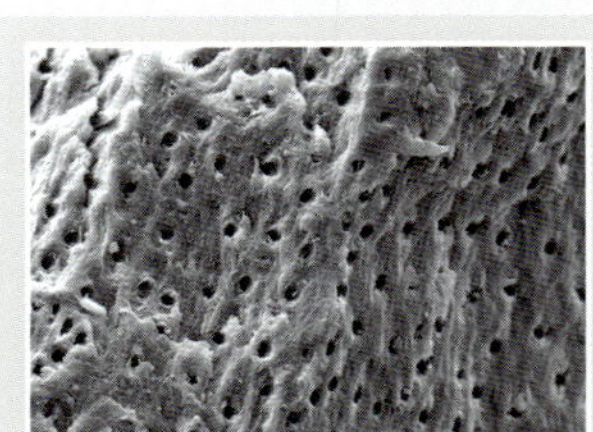

Biological tests

To understand the influence of surface cleaning, biological tests of adhesion and survival of osteoblasts dispersed on the surface of treated, untreated dentin, enamel granules and of the comparative material were carried out (Xenograft, Bio-Oss Geistlich Biomaterials, Baden-Baden, Germany).

Two cell lines (MG63 and SAOS-2) have been selected for this experimental activity.[30]

MG63 are osteoblasts grown at 37° C with an atmosphere of 5% CO_2 concentration, placed in DMEM (minimum essential culture medium) containing 1 mM sodium pyruvate and 10 mM HEPES buffer solution.

SAOS-2 are osteoblasts grown at 37° C with an atmosphere of 5% CO_2 concentration, placed in McCoy culture medium containing 1 mM of sodium pyruvate, 100 U/mL of penicillin, 0.1 mg/mL of streptomycin, 2 mM of glutamine and supplemented with 10% (v/v) of FBS (Fetal Bovine Serum).

After treating the tooth granules, 70 mg of DD (treated dentin) and 70 mg of DnD (untreated dentin) were placed in microtiter plates (5 for DD and 6 for DnD) coated with 120 µL/well of 1% (w/v) phosphate buffered saline solution (UltraPure™ Agarose, ThermoFisher, Monza, Italy). The Agarose solution was used to force the adhesion of the cells to the dentin avoiding adhesion to the well. Thereafter, 400 µL/well were added for each culture; then the plates were incubated at 37° C in a humid atmosphere with 5% CO_2 for 2 hours to allow the stabilization of the dentin.

The cells were then placed on the surface of the dentin granules (5.8-5.10) and incubated at 37° C in a humid atmosphere with 5% CO_2 for 7 days (5.11 and 5.12).

Some cells were placed on plates without granules and used as a control group. Cell survival was measured at different intervals (3 and 7 days) using AlamarBlu assay (Resazurina, Life technologies, Monza, Italy). The absorption was then measured using a microplate reader (Tecan, Segrate, Italy).

The recovered supernatant was used to measure the presence and production of osteocalcin.

Cells had a greater adhesion to the demineralized dentin (*see* 5.10 and 5.11).

It is interesting to note that on the enamel without treatment it seems that the cells have no adhesion (*see* 5.12), while, after the demineralization treatment is carried out, they have adhesion (5.13) and a number of cells per surface similar to the xenograft material

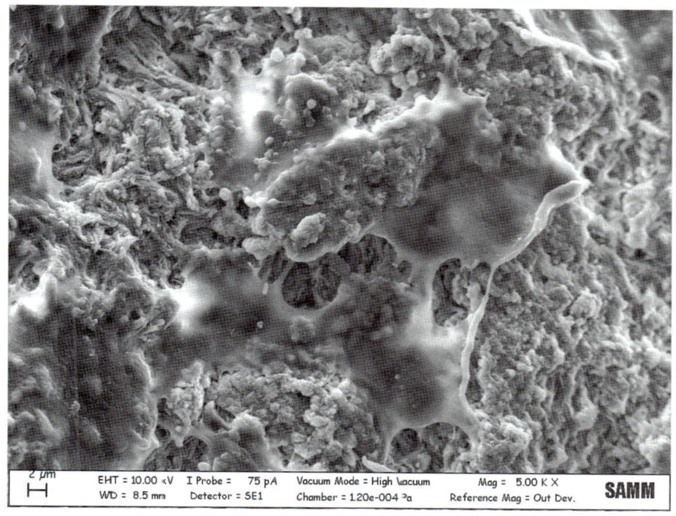

5.8 Osteoblast on the treated tooth surface.

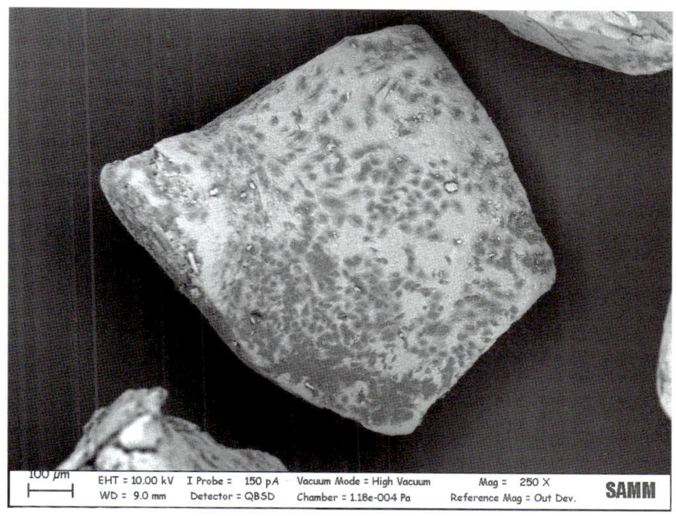

5.9 Demineralized dentine with numerous cells on the surface.

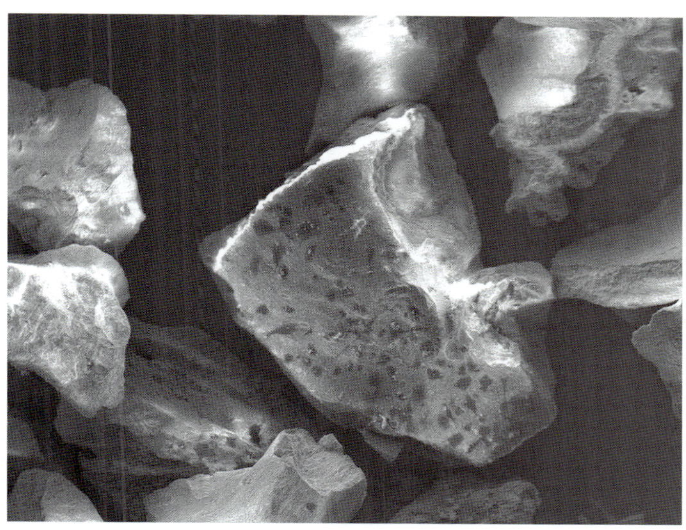

5.10 Non-demineralized dentine. Note the limited number of cells on the surface.

(5.14). By reconsidering the enamel data after treatment, it can be seen that the values of Ca and P (5.8) are very similar to the xenograft material and the behaviour of the cells on the surface seems to reflect these data.

Therefore, it is possible to assume that on surfaces similar to the untreated tooth, one that shows residues of various origins, the cells adhere with difficulty.

Three causes of this "adhesion difficulty" can be hypothesized with:

- residues can disturb the compartment of the cells;
- the greater wettability of the demineralized surface promotes adhesion;
- the high mineralization makes cell adhesion difficult.

The treatments that create a "cleaned" surface with less P and Ca amounts as with the use of HCl, more attractive for cell adhesion confirms Kim's theory.[50]

5.8 Values of the enamel after treatment

Sample	P %	Ca %	Ca/P
Enamel	11.04 ± 0.82	20.25 ± 3.16	1.83
Demineralized enamel	9.99 ± 1.56	15.02 ± 2.52	1.50
Xenograft (Bio-Oss)	8.62 ± 0.20	12.45 ± 0.41	1.44

Quantification of osteocalcin

It should be noted that the presence of dentin leads to a substantial increase in osteocalcin production in both cell lines (5.15 and 5.16). The production increase indicates the overall cell activity.

At what concentrations are proteins eliminated?

Considering that high percentages of calcium or phosphorus indicate a reduction in the organic component, it was decided to analyze the liquids which significantly reduced (>50%) the inorganic part and whose demineralisation was similar in percentage in both minerals.

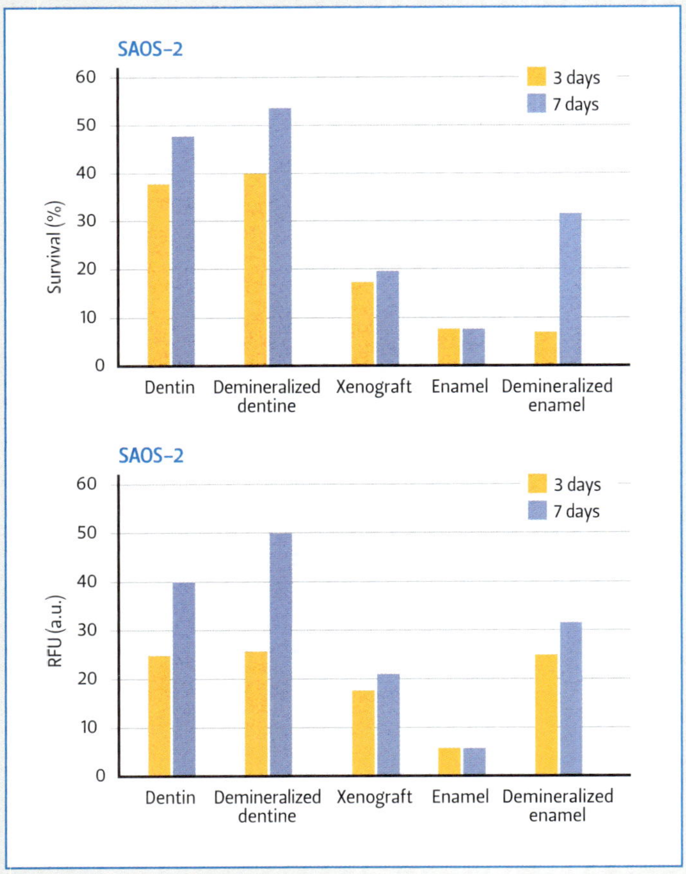

5.11 Titration of cell growth on the different materials at 3 days and at 7 days of the two cell lines. It can be noted that the growth on the DD surface turns out to be the best of the test samples and to be about two times greater than the xenograft material. The cells were cultured on a Polystyrene terrain as a reference (i.e., 100% survival positive control). The data are expressed in RFU as an arbitrary indicator of the number of cells relative to the control. Xenograft (Bio-Oss) was used as a positive control. $P < 0.05$.

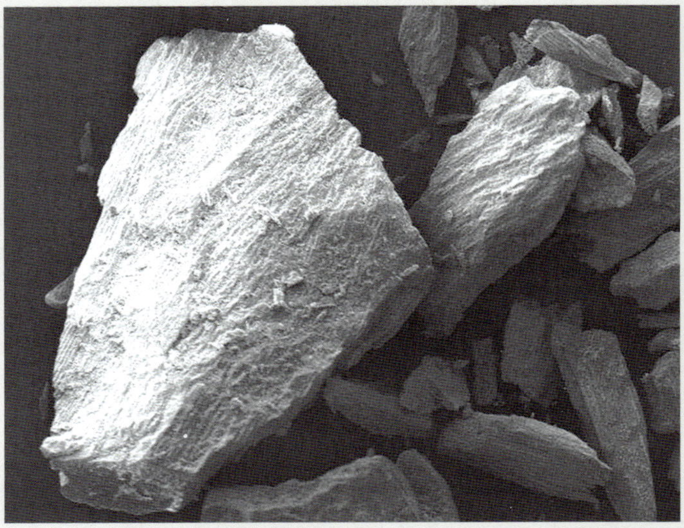

5.12 Enamel before treatment. There appear to be no cells on the surface.

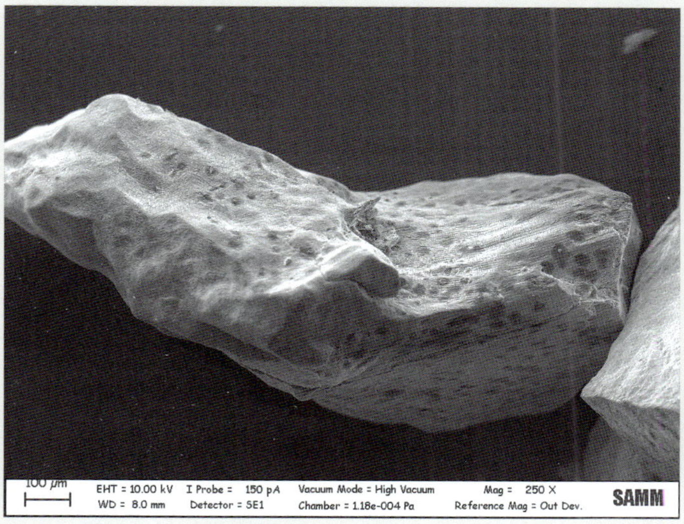

5.13 Demineralized enamel. It can be seen that the number of cells and the surface conformation appear to be similar to the Bio-Oss.

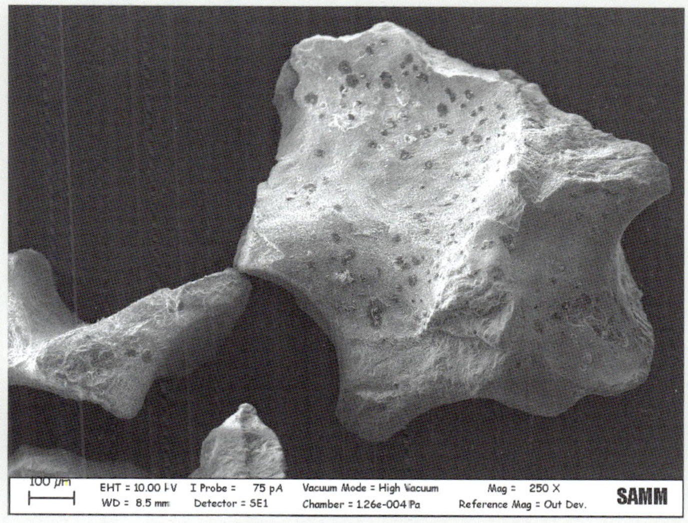

5.14 Granule of xenograft material (Bio-Oss) on whose surface a limited number of cells can be seen.

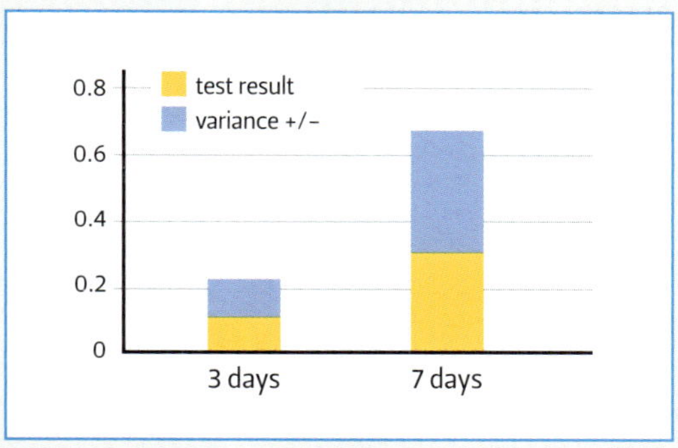

5.15 Quantification of osteocalcin produced after 3 and 7 days by SAOS2.

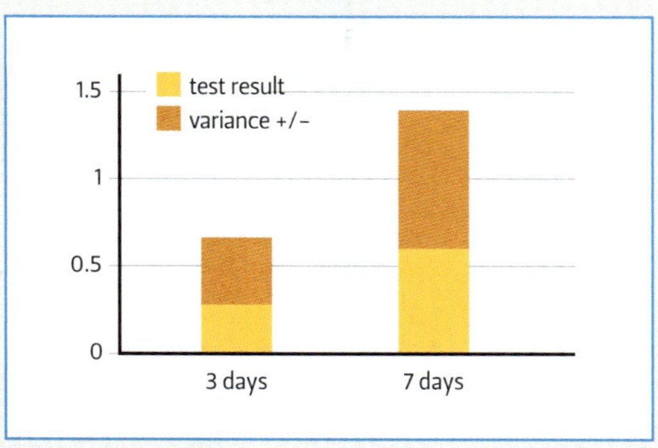

5.16 Quantification of the osteocalcin produced after 3 and 7 days by MG63.

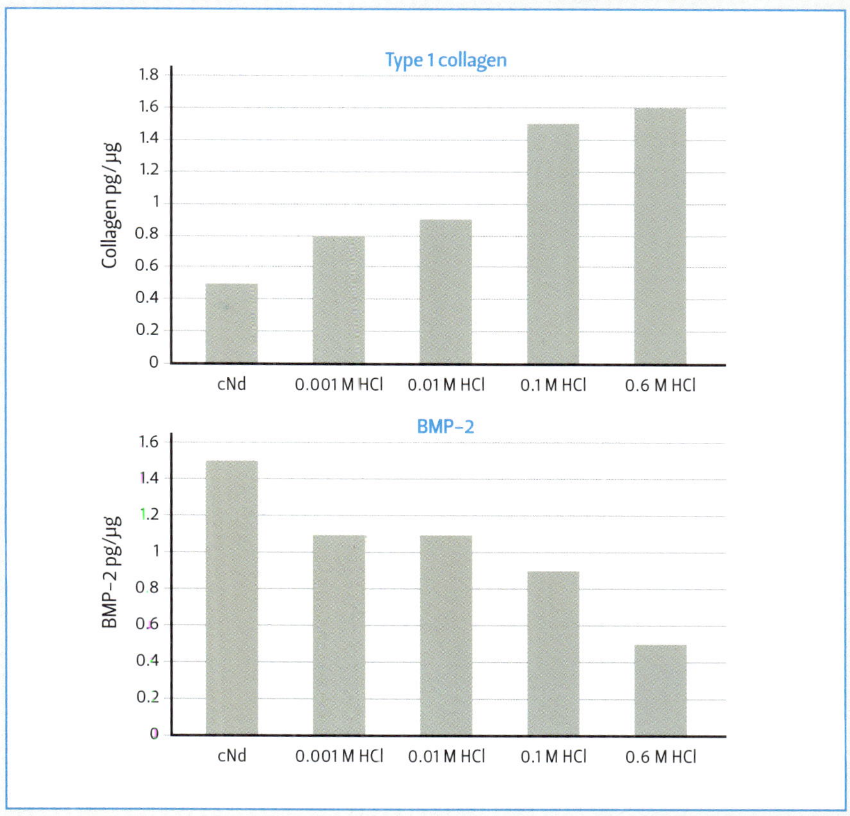

5.17 The proteins contained are normalized with respect to the weight of each sample (expressed as µg per sample of particles).

HCl concentrations were analyzed according to the previous experiments (*see* ■ 5.6).

The ELISA (Enzyme-Linked Immuno-Absorbent Assay) detects the presence of a substance and quantifies it. This test was used to quantify the presence of Collagen type 1 and BMP-2 from the treated samples (📷 5.17). The purpose of this test was to be able to find the best compromise to keep the greatest number of proteins in the treated granules.

After the demineralization/detoxification process, an extraction liquid [500 µL; 50 mM HEPES pH 7.4, 1 mM PMSF, 2 µg/mL leupeptin, 2 µg/mL aprotinin, 1 µg/mL pepstatin, 1% (v/v) Triton X-100] was added to the samples. After an incubation at 4° C for one night, the samples were subjected to ultrasonic treatment in order to extract the proteins. They were then quantified using a BCA Kit (Pierce Rockford, IL, USA) following the manufacturer's instructions. The results were then normalized and expressed with standard deviation (SD).[51]

Highly demineralized (0.1 M and 0.6 M HCl) DD (demineralized dentin) samples have a higher collagen content than cNd dentin (non-demineralized sample) and not fully demineralized dentin (📷 5.17).

A slight decrease in BMP-2 content was found in highly demineralized DD samples (0.1 M and 0.6 M HCl), but this value was significantly lower in 0.6 M HCl treated DD samples only. Unfortunately, there are no data in the literature regarding the demineralization and quantification of BMP-2.

From these data it can be understood that, if the molarity of the acids is excessive (0.6 M), there will be a loss of non-collagenic proteins. The best compromise is the concentration of 0.1 M which guarantees a good concentration of both BMP-2 and type 1 collagen (■ 5.9).

■ 5.9 Sum of the values (Collagen + BMP-2) to understand which option had the greatest amount of protein

Type of treatment	cNd	0.001 M HCl	0.01 M HCl	0.1 M HCl	0.6 M HCl
Sum collagen and BMP-2 present	2.0	1.9	2.0	2.4	2.1

In *aqua green* color: solution that at the end of the tests was considered to be more effective in maintaining proteins and detoxifying.

■ 5.10 Summary of the values expressed by the untreated tissues and by the treated tissues (in bold) by the selected preparations

Sample	P %	Ca %	Ca/P
Native dentine	8.59 ±1.33	16.56 ±3.73	1.92
Demineralized dentine	**5.04 ± 0.60**	**8.59 ± 1.37**	**1.70**
Native enamel	11.04 ± 0.82	20.25 ± 3.16	1.83
Demineralized enamel	**9.99 ± 1.56**	**15.02 ± 2.52**	**1.50**
Xenographic	8.62 ± 0.20	12.45 ± 0.41	1.44

Dentin treatment procedure chosen after the tests carried out

The treatment chosen after the analyzes carried out so far was:

- grinding by a low speed system;
- demineralization and detoxification with concentrations of HCl 0.1 M and H_2O_2 10%.

These are the lowest concentrations that allow either to maintain the maximum of proteins or modifying the tooth surface in a way to promote cell adhesion, as seen above (■ 5.10). Furthermore, these concentrations allow to eliminate the active liquids through simple serial washes and also to eliminate all the bacterial load present in the sample.

P is reduced by 40% and Ca by 39% compared to native dentin. It should be noted that the content of Ca and P in the enamel after treatment is similar to the xenograft one. These tests seem to confirm the Koga data.[2]

An interesting aspect of these data is the Ca and P ratio. In fact, the native bone has a mineral ratio Ca/P = 1.67.[44] A ratio very similar to the natural human bone one indicates that its use will not alter the natural chemical structure of the tissue.

Pre-treatment dentin has a Ca/P ratio = 1.92. After the treatment, it appears to have a Ca/P ratio = 1.70, so the demineralization chosen leads to a result very similar to human bone. On the other hand, the xenograft material tested as a control has a Ca/P ratio = 1.44 that seems a more different value.

It should be noted that only some tests are able to maintain Ca/P ratio values similar to bone, while most display very distant values.

The ELISA test was also carried out to assess whether, after demineralization by HCl and detoxification by H_2O_2, there were variations in the values of collagen and BMP-2 present (📷 5.18). It is interesting to note how the addition of H_2O_2 caused differences in the presence

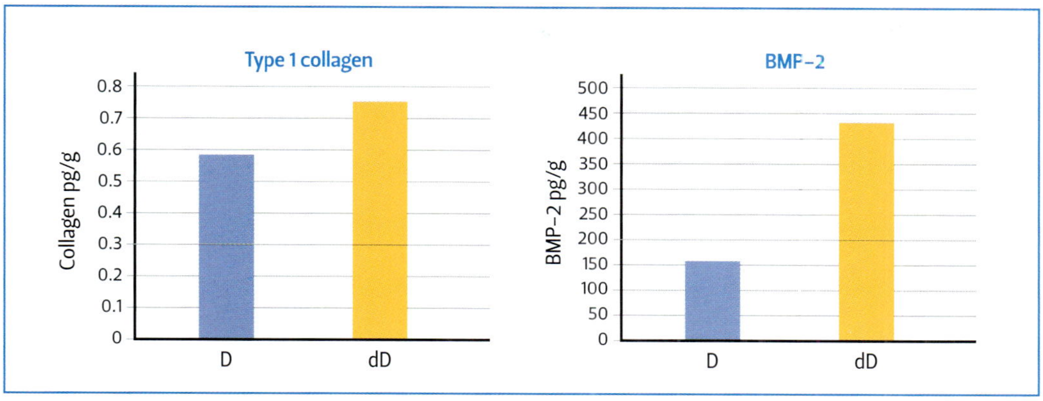

5.18 Values of collagen and BMP2 after treatment. The proteins contained are normalized with respect to the weight of each sample (expressed as grams per sample of particles).

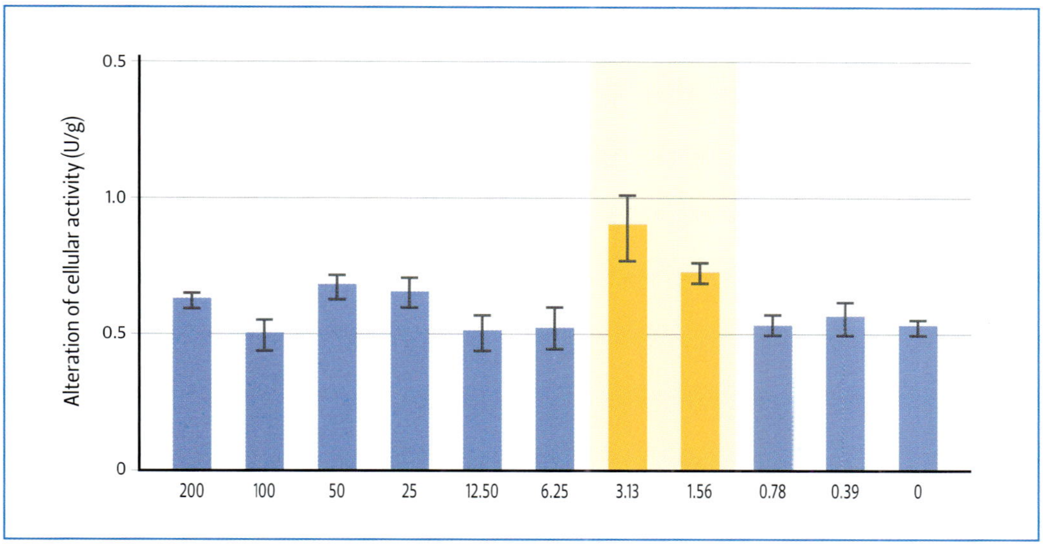

5.19 Alteration of cellular activity following the stimulation of BMP-2 corresponding to those measured in the tests.

of BMP-2 and collagen compared to the evaluations of HCl alone.

In order to understand whether the quantity of BMP-2, which corresponds to 420 pg/g, is sufficient to be able to determine a stimulation, an analysis of the osteodifferentiating effects deriving from exposure to this quantity of BMP-2 was carried out (5.19). The test showed substantial differentiation and stimulation of the cell number.

Bacterial load test

To evaluate the residual bacterial load on the treated and untreated granules, about ≈30 mg for each sample were placed in sterile polypropylene tubes (5.20) and incubated at 37° C for 5 days in a culture broth.

After 5 days of incubation a small bacterial load was found on the untreated granules (original dentin samples), while the granules treated with different concentrations of liquids showed no bacterial load (5.21). These results demonstrate how the combined treatment of HCl and H_2O_2, at any concentration, results in a sort of "sterilization" effect on the dentin.

An evaluation in a Petri dish was also carried out in the same way (5.22) to highlight the presence of bacterial cultures which confirmed the previous results.

Bacterial load over time

For a better understanding it was considered appropriate to report here the study carried out following the development of the Tooth Transformer device at the Laboratory of Chemical, Clinical and Micro-biological Analysis of the IRCCS Galeazzi Orthopaedic Hospital in Milan (Italy) with the collaboration of Dr. De Vecchi.

The goal was to understand if, after the treatment carried out using the Tooth Transformer tool (5.23), the

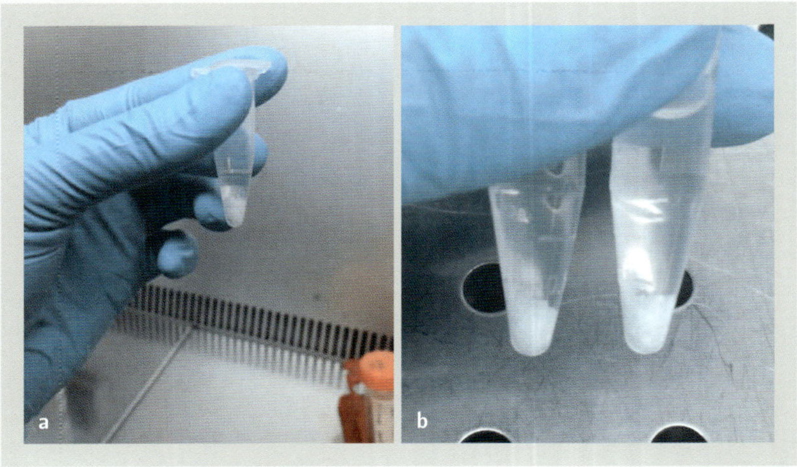

5.20 **(a)** Positioning in a sterile container to carry out demineralization and detoxification. **(b)** Phases of the demineralization and detoxification process.

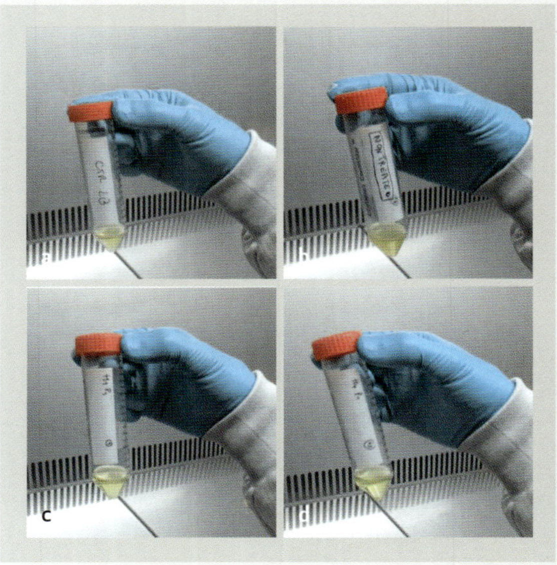

5.21 **(a)** Control culture. **(b)** Untreated culture. **(c)** Culture 0.001 M HCl + 3% H_2O_2. **(d)** Culture 0.6 M + 36% H_2O_2.

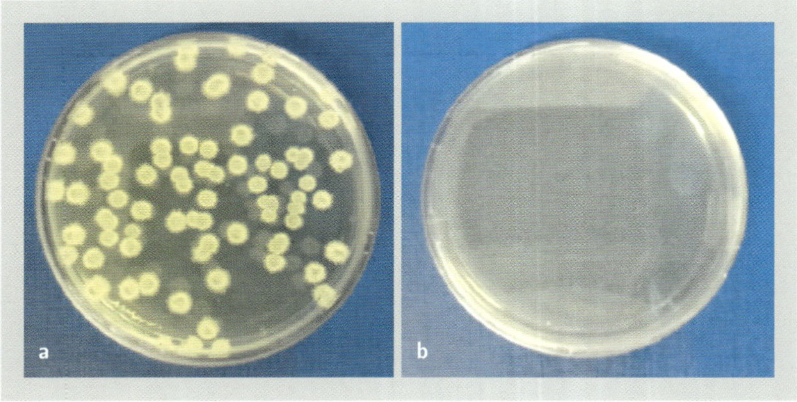

5.22 Cultures in Petri capsules of untreated tooth **(a)** and treated tooth **(b)**.

detoxification expressed in the tests at the Natta Institute of the Polytechnic University of Milan was maintained.

Homogeneous fractions of a preparation obtained after processing with Tooth Transformer were immediately inoculated in thioglycollated broth and 30 minutes after preparation (5.24 and 5.25). During the sampling period, the preparation was kept inside the instrument. Each sample was incubated for 30 days at 37° C. A sample prepared and stored at -20° C (5.26) was placed in the same broth following the same treatment. The treatment broths were checked daily and at different incubation times (7, 14, 21 and 30 days) and parts of 100 µL were seeded on blood agar and Schaedler agar plates. None of the samples prepared on the day of the experiment showed any microbial growth during the observation period. On the contrary, the sample prepared previously and stored at -20° C before sowing in broth was positive after about 10 days. Broth subculture showed the growth of a microbial population consisting of Gram-positive catalase positive cocci identified as coagulase negative staphylococci.

Evaluation of the volume needed to completely remove active liquids (HCl and H_2O_2)

The test was developed in two different phases. The first phase of treatment, using only HCl at a concentration of 0.1 M followed by the washes and, subsequently, the same procedure using H_2O_2 and then the washes (5.11).

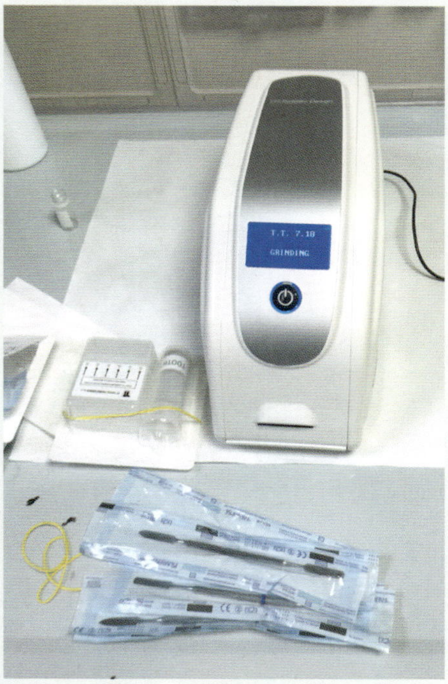

5.23 Tooth Transformer used for testing.

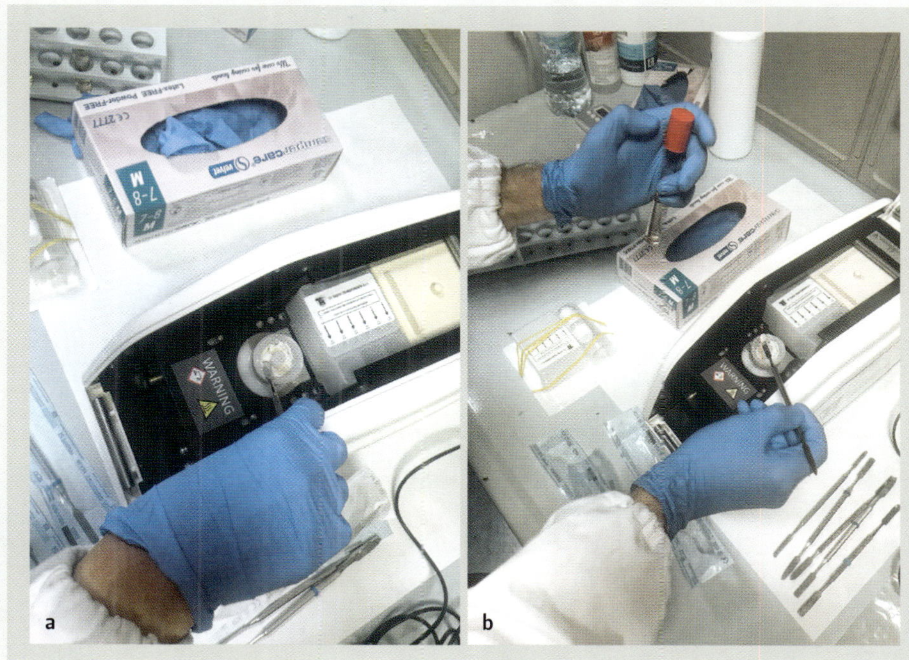

5.24 (a,b) Sampling at set times after preparation.

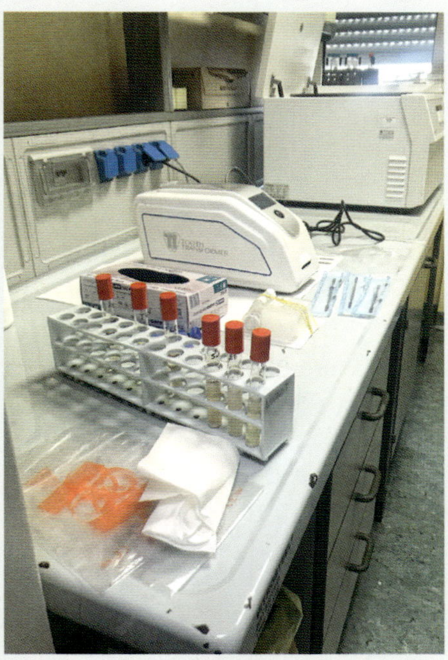

5.25 Tubes containing the samples analyzed after set time intervals.

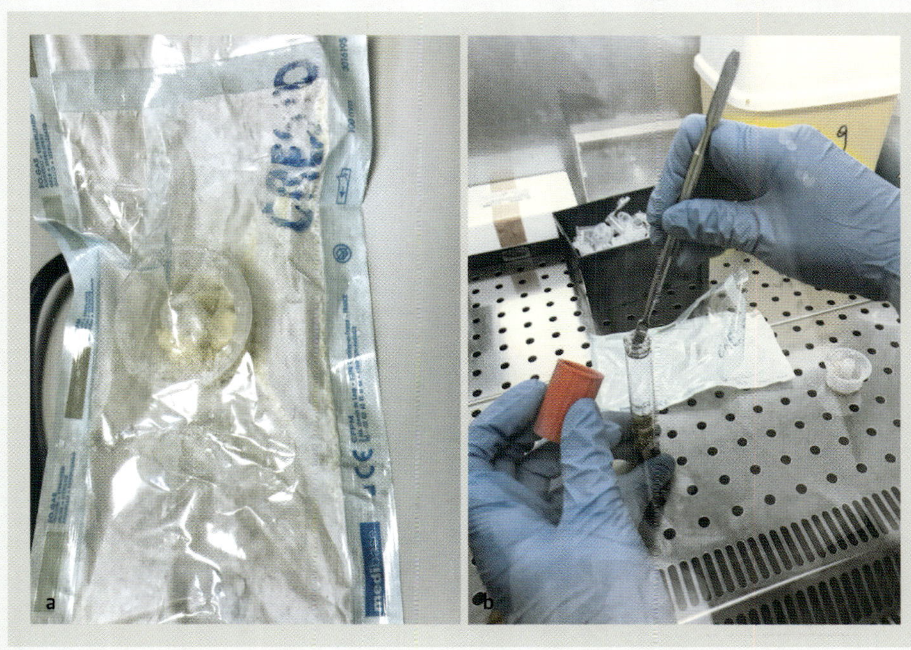

5.26 Frozen sample **(a)**; frozen sample placed in the test tube **(b)**. (Courtesy of Dr. D. Bianco.)

At the end of phase 2 (second wash) the concentration of HCl in saline was already 90 times lower than the 0.1 M HCl used for the treatment (leading to the final concentration of 0.0011 M), and the concentration of HCl decreased up to 200 times at the end of the fourth wash (0.5 mM HCl).

As for the H_2O_2 concentration, at the end of the fourth wash the H_2O_2 concentration in saline was 170 times lower than the starting H_2O_2 solution (w/w) used [the final concentration was 0.06% (w/w)]. The concentration of H_2O_2 at the end of the last wash was 0.002% (w/w), nominally 10% (w/w) (5.12).

To recap, two washes (1 mL each) in step 2 followed by two washes (1 mL each) in step 4 allow to reduce the HCl and H_2O_2 content up to 200 times and 170 times, respectively, in a sample of 50 mg of DD.

Amount of active liquids after the Tooth Transformer treatment

As for the bacterial load, also in this case, after the production of the Tooth Transformer device, the procedure was carried out at the DCMIC chemical analysis laboratory of the Politecnico University of Milan, with the collaboration of Dr. Gelosa, to evaluate the residual quantity of active liquids at the end of the treatment.

The tests were carried out in order to determine the residual content of HCl and H_2O_2 remaining on the tooth sample after the treatment cycle. In order to avoid any variation in the concentration testing, it was decided to carry out the whole process directly in the lab and to analyze the samples immediately after the end of the cycles.

The sample was then taken directly from the machine at the end of the treatment, weighed and analyzed (5.27-5.29) as indicated below. Values are expressed in milligrams of analyte per kilogram of sample (ppm).

Acidity Titration: Titration was performed using standard 0.01 M NaOH and phenolphthalein as indicator.

The purpose is to determine the concentration of HCl present in solution. The results are expressed in three different units of measurement: HCl mg/kg; sample after treatment <50 ppm (parts per million); H_2O_2 titration.

H_2O_2 titration was performed using standardized KMnO$_4$. The purpose is to determine the concentration of H_2O_2 present in solution. The results are expressed in three different units of measurement: H_2O_2 mg/kg; sample after treatment <50 ppm.

This tests pointed out that there are no residual quantities of active liquids at all at the end of the treatment.

5.11 Residues of HCl after washing with physiological solution

Sample		HCl (mM)
Test	1° wash	2.20
	2° wash	1.10
Test	3° wash	0.62
	4° wash	0.50
	5° wash	0.37
	6° wash	0.25

5.12 Residues of H_2O_2 after washing with physiological solution

Sample		H_2O_2 (%w/w)
Test	3° wash	0.53
	4° wash	0.06
	6° wash	0.01
	8° wash	0.002

Deciduous tooth treatment

Particles of deciduous teeth (enamel and dentin), obtained using the Tooth Transformer granulation system, were subjected to the same tests mentioned above for permanent teeth.

50 mg of dentin and 50 mg of enamel derived from deciduous teeth were transferred to a sterile polypropylene test tube and demineralized and detoxified according to the indications of the first part of the project. After the treatment, some granules were placed in a test tube to evaluate their effects, others to be analyzed by SEM-EDS, other ones to carry out ELISA tests and cell cultures.

SEM-EDS tests were performed with the aim of evaluating the differences in the surface of dentin and enamel derived from deciduous teeth.

The scanning electron microscope (SEM + EDS energy dispersive X-ray - ESEM Zeiss EVO50; Carl Zeiss, Milan, Italy) was used as an instrument, with an acceleration voltage of 15 kV, to investigate the surface composition and the image of the surface. The EDS exam consists of an instrumental analytical method that uses the emission of X-rays generated by an accelerated electron beam incident on the sample, which allows to determine the quantification and the list of the individual elements that compose the analyzed material.

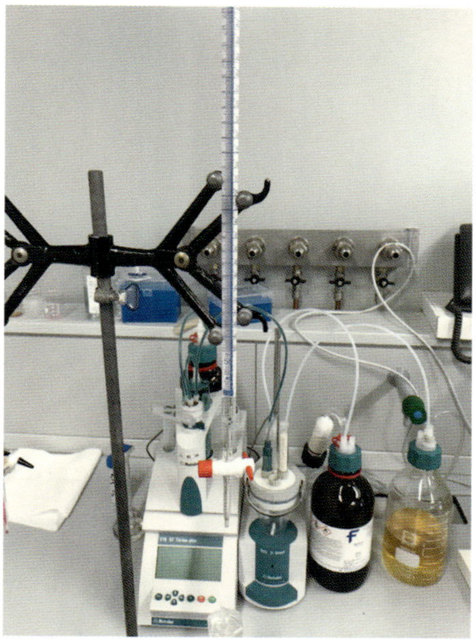

5.27 Class A glassware (0-50 mL burette, flask) + Titrator (Metrohm Titrino Plus) with automatic titration.

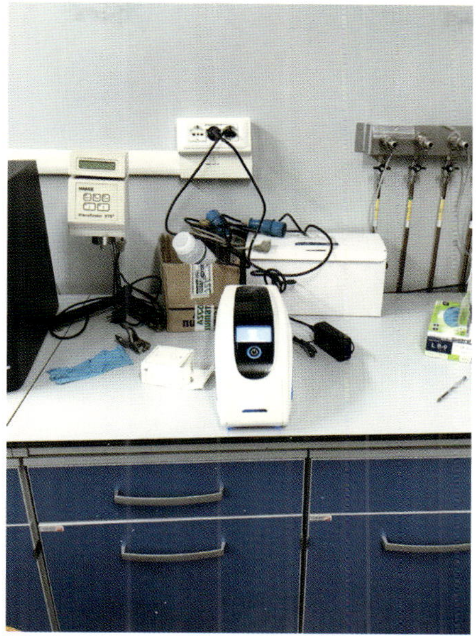

5.28 Tooth Transformer used for testing.

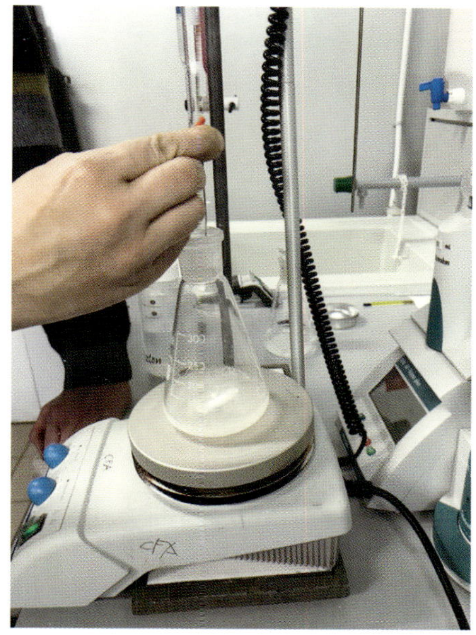

5.29 Magnetic mixer (Fisherbrand).

The samples were first fixed in 1.5% (v/v) glutaraldehyde solution for 20 minutes, then dehydrated in subsequent ethanol baths and, finally, sputtered with gold particles.

The surface of the non-demineralized tooth is characterized by mineral crystals which cover it (5.30).

The treated surface is clean and the dentinal tubules clearly visible as evidenced by the tests on permanent teeth (5.30 and 5.31).

The results of the EDS test are different from the data obtained from the permanent teeth (5.13).[52]

In fact, a significant decrease of Ca and P was found in the treated dentin samples compared to the untreated dentin controls (-75%). The enamel shows a limited reduction, around 9%. The same tests previously performed on the permanent teeth were then reproduced by measuring the quantities of proteins collagen and BMP-2 present, by means of an ELISA test (5.32).

Not too surprisingly, given that part of the primary tooth is structured during the embryonic stages, greater amounts of proteins are found in deciduous dentin than in permanent teeth (5.14).

The same procedures were then performed with cell cultures with permanent teeth (5.33).

5.13 EDS values of the deciduous tooth

Sample	P(%)	Ca(%)	Ca/P
Untreated deciduous enamel	12.99 ± 1.22	21.35 ± 2.45	1.64
Deciduous treated enamel	9.99 ± 1.56	15.02 ± 2.52	1.50
Untreated deciduous dentin	8.54 ± 1.62	12.94 ± 3.06	1.51
Deciduous dentine treated	2.12 ± 0.56	3.35 ± 1.20	1.58

5.14 Comparison of BMP-2 content between primary and permanent tooth

BMP-2 permanent tooth	BMP-2 deciduous tooth
0.4 ng/g	1.2 ng/g

The cells on the surfaces derived from the tooth, both native and demineralized, have shown a higher survival rate compared to the xenograft material (Bio-Oss) (5.34).

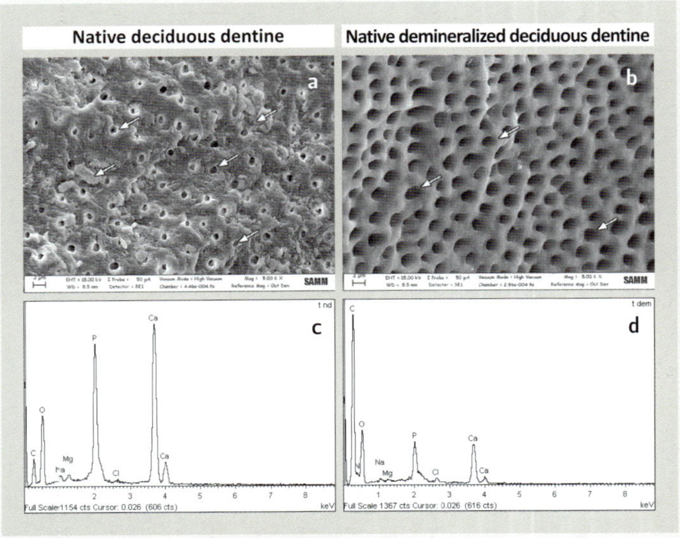

5.30 Native dentin **(a,c)** and treated dentin **(b,d)**. The arrows indicate the dentinal tubules. The size of the tubules varies after treatment.

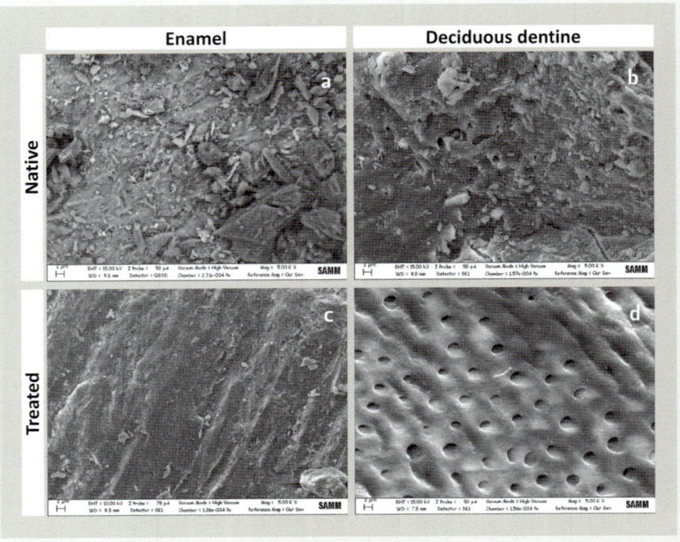

5.31 SEM images of enamel and dentin obtained from a deciduous tooth, before and after treatment.

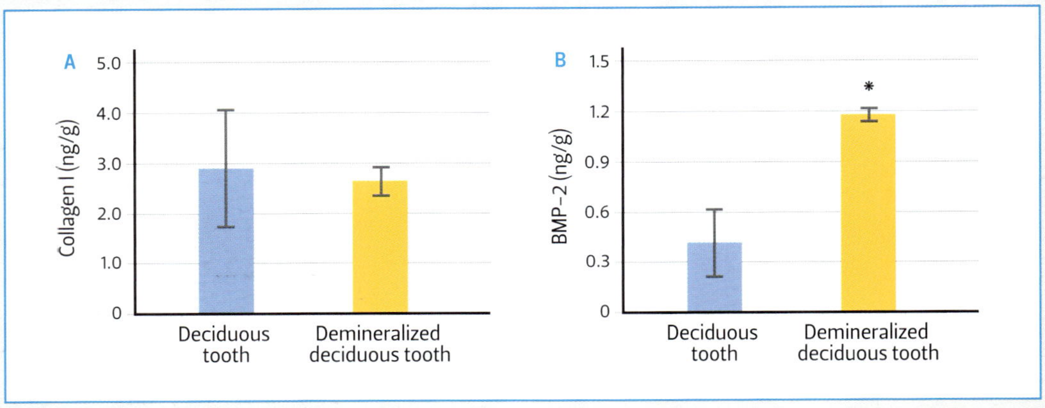

5.32 Quantification by ELISA test of Collagen 1 and BMP-2 present in the granules of deciduous dentin before and after treatment.

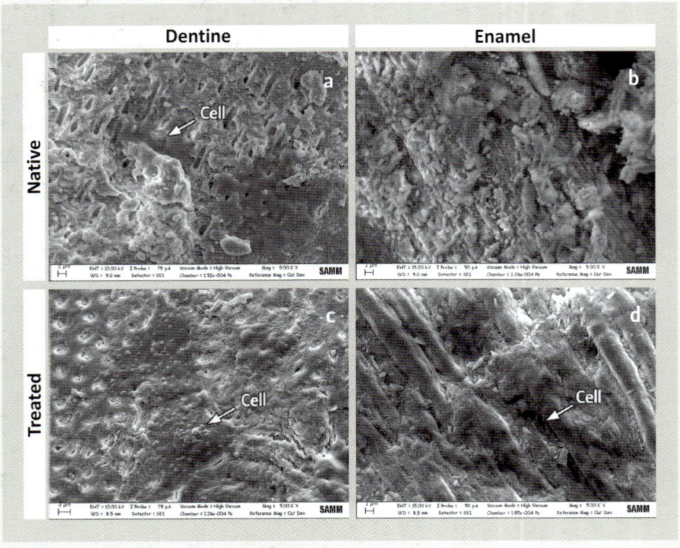

5.33 The cells were dispersed on native and demineralized deciduous dentin, native deciduous enamel and demineralized deciduous enamel. There are only a few cells on the surface of the native deciduous enamel.

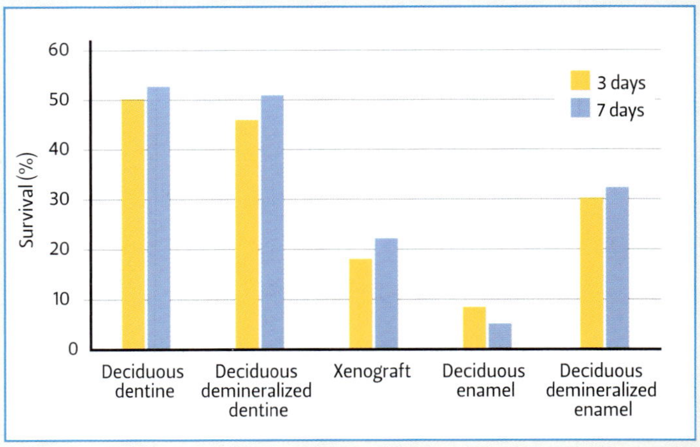

5.34 3 and 7 days survival of cells placed on various materials.

It can therefore be thought that the deciduous tooth may be a good grafting material.[53]

Tooth weight

One of the most obvious problems in the use of the tooth as a graft material is the operator's inability to exactly quantify the size of the final product to fulfil the surgical needs.

In order to identify a method of analysis, the analysis of the weight of the tooth was proposed.[54] In fact, if the needs are to have more quantity you can always add material of other origin. But if the defect is smaller than the amount of material produced, it would be wasted. Therefore, knowing the size of the defect and the volume/weight of the tooth, it would be possible to use only the necessary part of the tooth.

A total of 205 extracted teeth were analyzed using a mini digital scale, to evaluate the weight, and using a millimeter syringe to evaluate the volume. The length of the teeth was measured using a digital caliper (5.35). The average weight varied between 0.68 g and 1.88 g (5.36) and the volume varied between 0.38 cc and 0.96 cc depending on the type of tooth, but the variability was minimal. The minimum weight was 0.4 g and the maximum weight 3.0 g, while the minimum volume was 0.2 cc and the maximum 2 cc (5.37-5.39).

Based on these data it is possible, by weighing or measuring the tooth, to forecast how much graft material will be produced using a system that does not disperse the volume of the tooth.

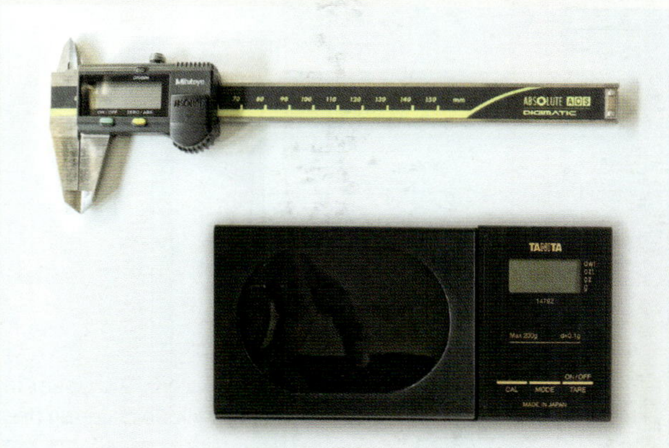

5.35 Gauge and mini digital scale used for the test.

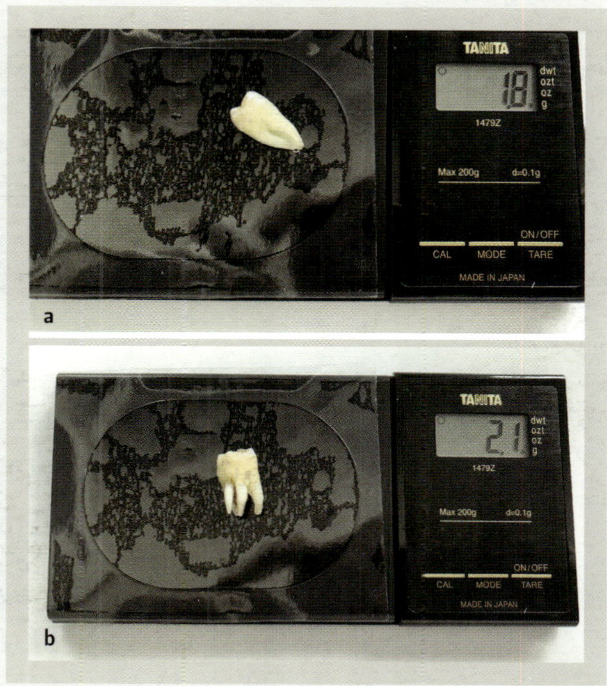

5.36 **(a,b)** Examples of weight of teeth.

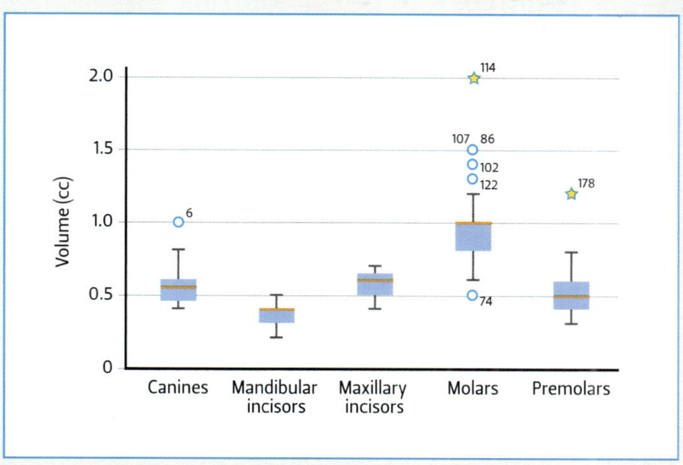

5.37 Average volume of the analyzed teeth.

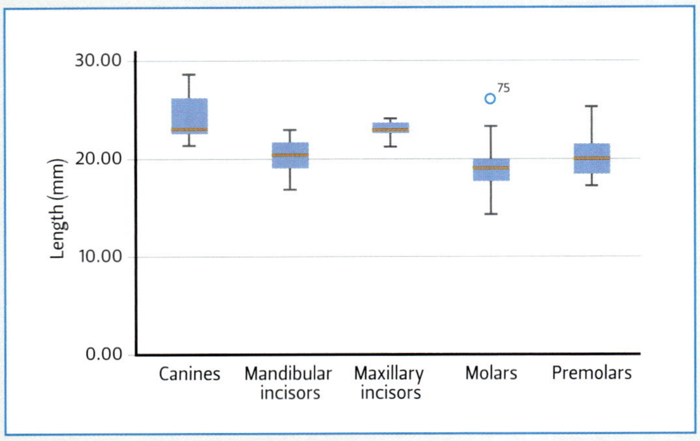

5.38 Average length of the analyzed teeth.

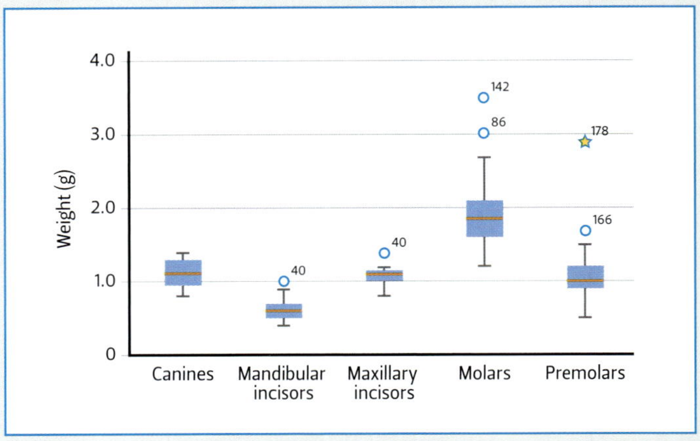

5.39 Average weight of the analyzed teeth.

REFERENCES

1. Dozza B, Lesci IG, Duchi S, et al. When size matters: differences in demineralized bone matrix particles affect collagen structure, mesenchymal stem cell behavior, and osteogenic potential. J Biomed Mater Res Part A 2017;105A:1019-33.
2. Koga T, Minamizato T, Kawai Y, et al. Bone regeneration using dentin matrix depends on the degree of demineralization and particle size. PLoS One 2016;11(1):e0147235.
3. Campana V, Milano G, Pagano E, et al. Bone substitutes in orthopaedic surgery: from basic science to clinical practice. J Mater Sci Mater Med 2014;25:2445-61.
4. Laurencin C, Khan Y, El-Amin SF. Bone graft substitutes. Expert Rev Med Devices 2006;3:49-57.
5. Testori T, Wallace SS, Trisi P, et al. Effect of xenograft (ABBM) particle size on vital bone formation following maxillary sinus augmentation: a multicenter, randomized, controlled, clinical histomorphometric trial. Int J Periodontics Restorative Dent 2013;33(4):467-75.
6. Carano RA, Filvaroff EH. Angiogenesis and bone repair. Drug Discov Today 2003; 8:980-9.
7. Shapoff CA, Bowers GM, Levy B, et al. The effect of particle size on the osteogenic activity of composite grafts of allogeneic freeze-dried bone and autogenous marrow. J Periodontol 1980;51:625-30.
8. Pallesen L, Schou S, Aaboe M, et al. Influence of particle size of autogenous bone grafts on the early stages of bone regeneration: a histologic and stereologic study in rabbit calvarium. Int J Oral Maxillofac Implants 2002;17:498-506.
9. Bhat V, Bhat S. Disinfection methods of extracted human teeth. J Oral Health Comm Dent 2007;1(2):27-9.
10. Park M, Mah YJ, Kim DH, et al. Demineralized deciduous tooth as a source of bone graft material: its biological and physicochemical characteristics. Oral Surg Oral Med Oral Pathol Oral Radiol 2015;120:307-14.
11. Yeomans JD, Urist MR. Bone decalcified dentine implanted into oral, osseous and muscle tissues. Archs Oral Biol 1967;12:999-1008.
12. Huggins C, Wiseman S, Reddi AH. Transformation of fibroblasts by allogeneic and xenogeneic transplants of demineralized tooth and bone. J Exp Med 1970;132:1250-8.
13. Nade N. Bone graft surgery reappraised: the contribution of the cell to ultimate success. Brit J Surg 1970;57:752-6.
14. Bang G. Induction of heterotopic bone formation by demineralized dentin: an experimental model in Guinea pigs. Scand J Dent Res 1973;81:240-50.
15. Kim KW. Bone induction by demineralized dentin matrix in nude mouse muscles. Maxillofac Plast Reconstr Surg 2014;36(2):50-6.
16. Yagihashi K, Miyazawa K, Togari K, et al. Demineralized dentin matrix acts as a scaffold for repair of articular cartilage defects. Calcif Tissue Int 2009;84:210-20.
17. Carvalho VA, Tosello Dde O, Salgado MA, et al. Histomorphometric analysis of homogenous demineralized dentin matrix as osteopromotive material in rabbit mandibles. Int J Oral Maxillofac Implants 2004;19:679-86.
18. Gomes MF, Banzi EC, Destro MF, et al. Homogenous demineralized dentin matrix for application in cranioplasty of rabbits with alloxan-induced diabetes: Histomorphometric analysis. Int J Oral Maxillofac Implants 2007;22:939-47.
19. Gomes MF, Destro MF, Banzi EC, et al. Optical density of bone repair after implantation of homogenous demineralized dentin matrix in diabetic rabbits. Braz Oral Res 2008;22:275-80.
20. de Oliveira GS, Miziara MN, Silva ER, et al. Enhanced bone formation during healing process of tooth sockets filled with demineralized human dentine matrix. Aust Dent J 2013;58:326-32.
21. Jang HS, Kim SG, Lim SC, et al. Osteogenic ability according to the decalcified modality of auto-tooth bone grafts

in peri-implant defects in dogs. Implant Dent 2014;23:482-8.

22. Movin S, Borring-Møller G. Regeneration of infrabony periodontal defects in humans after implantation of allogenic demineralized dentin. J Clin Periodontol 1982;9:141-7.

23. Gomes MF, Abreu PP, Morosolli AR, et al. Densitometric analysis of the autogenous demineralized dentin matrix on the dental socket wound healing process in humans. Braz Oral Res 2006; 20:324-30.

24. Tomson PL, Grover LM, Lumley PJ, et al. Dissolution of bio-active dentine matrix components by mineral trioxide aggregate. J Dent 2007; 35:636-42.

25. Graham L, Cooper PR, Cassidy N, et al. The effect of calcium hydroxide on solubilisation of bio-active dentine matrix components. Biomaterials 2006;27:2865-73.

26. Kim HS, Lee DS, Lee JH, et al. The effect of odontoblast conditioned media and dentin noncollagenous proteins on the differentiation and mineralization of cementoblasts in vitro. Arch Oral Biol 2009;54:71-9.

27. Parmar G, Chhatariya A. Demineralising effect of EDTA at different concentration and pH - A spectrophotometer study. Endodontology 2004;16:54-7.

28. Reis-Filho CR, Silva ER, Martins AB, et al. Demineralised human dentine matrix stimulates the expression of VEGF and accelerates the bone repair in tooth sockets of rats. Arch Oral Biol 2012;57:469-76.

29. Vennat E, Bogicevic C, Fleureau J-M, et al. Demineralized dentin 3D porosity and pore size distribution using mercury porosimetry. Dent Mater 2009;25:729-35.

30. Czekanska EM, Stoddart MJ, Richards RG, et al. In search of an osteoblast cell model for in vitro research. Eur Cell Mater 2012;24:1-17.

31. Cardaropoli D, Nevins M, Schupbach P. New bone formation using an extracted tooth as a biomaterial: a case report with histologic evidence. The Int Jour of Perio & Restor Dentistry 2019;39(2):156-63.

32. Bindermann I, Hallel G. A novel procedure to process extracted teeth for immediate grafting of autogenous dentin. J Interdisciplinar Med Dent 2014;2(6):1000154

33. Joshi CP, Dani NH, Khedkar SU. Alveolar ridge preservation using autogenous tooth graft versus betatricalcium phosphate alloplast: a randomized, controlled, prospective, clinical pilot study. J Indian Soc Periodontol 2016;20:429-34.

34. Tomson PL, Grover LM, Lumley PJ, et al. Dissolution of bio-active dentine matrix components by mineral trioxide aggregate. J Dent 2007;35:636-42.

35. Al-Namnam NM, Shanmuhasuntharam P, Ha KO, et al. Processed allogenic dentine as a scaffold for bone healing: an in vivo study. Aus J Basic Appl Sci 2010;4:5932-40.

36. Kim SK, Kim SW, Kim KW. Effect on bone formation of the autogenous tooth graft in the treatment of peri-implant vertical bone defects in the minipigs. Maxillofac Plast Reconstr Surg 2015;37:2.

37. Tulio AV, Kang CD, Fabian OA, et al. Socket preservation using demineralized tooth graft: a case series report with histological analysis. Int J Growth Factors Stem Cells Dent 2020;3:27-34.

38. Nampo T, Watahiki J, Enomoto A. A new method for alveolar bone repair using extracted teeth for the graft material. J Periodontol 2010;81:1264-72.

39. Moharamzadeh K, Freeman C, Blackwood K. Processed bovine dentine as a bone substitute. Br J Oral Maxillofac Surg 2008;46:110-3.

40. Elkayar A, Elshazly Y, Assaad M. Properties of hydroxyapatite from bovine teeth. Bone Tissue Regen Insights 2009;2:31-6.

41. Huang YC, Lew WZ, Feng SW, et al. Histomorphometric and transcriptome evaluation of early healing bone treated with a novel human particulate dentin powder. Biomed Mater 2016;12:015004.

42. Yagihashi K, Miyazawa K, Togari K, et al. Demineralized dentin matrix acts as a scaffold for repair of articular cartilage defects. Calcif Tissue Int 2009; 84:210-20.

43. Calvo-Guirado JL , Cegarra del Pino P, Sapoznikov L, et al. A new procedure for processing extracted teeth for immediate grafting in post-extraction sockets. An experimental study in American Fox Hound dogs. Ann Anat 2018;217: 14-23.

44. LeGeros RZ. Calcium phosphates in oral biology and medicine. Monogr Oral Sci 1991;15:1-201.

45. Blum B, Moseley J, Liller l, et al. Measurement of bone morphogenetic proteins and other growth factors in demineralized bone matrix. Orthopedics, 2004;27(1 Suppl):161-5.

46. Firschein HE, Urist MR. Enzyme induction, accumulation of collagen, and calcification in implants of bone matrix. Clin Orthop Relat Res 1972;84:263-75.

47. Zhao G, Schwartz Z, Wieland M, et al. High surface energy enhances cell response to titanium substrate microstructure. J Biomed Mater Res 2005;74A:49-58.

48. Lim JY, Taylor AF, Li Z, Vogler EA, et al. Integrin expression and osteopontin regulation in human fetal osteoblastic cells mediated by substratum surface characteristics. Tissue Eng 2005;11:19-29.

49. Eriksson C, Nygren H, Ohlson K. Implantation of hydrophilic and hydrophobic titanium discs in rat tibia: cellular reactions on the surfaces during the first 3 weeks in bone. Biomaterials 2004;25:4759-66.

50. Kim YK , Lee JK, Kim KW, et al. Healing mechanism and clinical application of autogenous tooth bone graft materialIn: Pignatello R. Advances in Biomaterials Science and Biomedical Applications. Rijeka, InTech, 2013; pp. 405-435.

51. Bono N, Tarsini P, Candiani G. Demineralized dentin and enamel matrix as suitable substrates for bone regeneration. J Appl Biomater Funct Mater 2017;15(3):e236-e43.

52. Bono N, Tarsini P, Candiani G. BMP-2 and type I collagen preservation in human deciduous teeth after demineralization. J Appl Biomater Funct Mater 2019;17(2):2280800018784230.

53. Minetti E, Taschieri S, Corbella S. Autologous deciduous tooth-derived material for alveolar ridge preservation: a clinical and histological case report. Case Rep Dent 2020:2936878.

54. Minetti E, Corbella S, Taschieri S. The weight of permanent teeth: an exploratory study on a total of 205 teeth. Quintessenza Internazionale & Jomi 2019;34:85-89

Tools and procedures for processing bone substitute from dental origin

E. Minetti

Proposed procedures

Numerous procedures have been proposed to try to use the tooth as a graft material. Some of these are quite unattainable either due to costs or to the equipment used. It is also clear that chairside use requires a preparation time that is congruent with the needs.

In 2010 Murata[1] presented a high-speed device (12,000 rpm) for grinding teeth, consisting of zirconium oxide blades capable of producing dental particles with dimensions between 0.5 and 5 mm. The tooth was placed in the freezer at -80° C until used, then chopped, placing ice blocks of saline together, and placed in 2% nitric acid solution (pH 1) for 20 minutes and finally lyophilized and filtered. The granules were then inserted into subcutaneous pockets of mice to evaluate bone production after 4 weeks. The results were positive.

Al-Namnam and colleagues,[2] in 2010, in an vivo study on rabbits, suggested the following process, using only root dentin: They placed dentin in a cryotube at -169° C in liquid nitrogen for 2 weeks, they then thawed it at room temperature for 15 minutes and crushed it with a mortar and pestle and, finally, immersed it in a solution of gentamicin and 70% ethyl alcohol for 30-60 minutes.

Obviously, this process cannot be transformed into a *chairside* clinical process and, in any case, the crushing with mortar endangers the proteins and their osteoinductive capacity.

In 2011 Li and colleagues (West China Stomatology Hospital of Sichuan University)[3] used 40 premolars extracted from 10 patients. The protocol used by them was: the immersion of the extracted tooth in distilled water for 5 hours (water replacement every hour); cleaning for 20 minutes every hour using an ultrasonic instrument; immersion in EDTA 17% for 5 minutes; 10 minutes of washing in distilled water; immersion in 5% EDTA for 10 minutes; 10 minutes of washing in distilled water placed in an ultrasonic bath. The treated dentin was immersed in penicillin and streptomycin for 72 hours and rinsed for 10 minutes in distilled water by immersing it in an ultrasonic bath.

As is evident, the tooth processing time was approximately 4685 minutes: a rather long and expensive time for the operators. It is therefore a procedure that cannot be used in normal clinical practice.

In a 2012 publication by Hussain and colleagues[4] (School of Clinical Dentistry, University of Sheffield, Claremont Crescent, Sheffield, UK) used bovine teeth and, after removing the enamel using diamond burs, inserted them into defects on rabbit calvaria. The teeth were crushed into small pieces (5-10 mm) using a pestle and mortar. The fragments were boiled in distilled water for 2 hours, then immersed in isopropyl alcohol for 2 hours and, after rinsing them with sterile distilled water, they were dried at 100° C. Finally, the residues were crushed using a high-speed blender and then placed in sterilization by gamma irradiation.

To all intents and purposes, it is a rather long and complex procedure for the use of bovine teeth, but necessary to eliminate the antigenicity of an allogeneic tissue. Crushing with a pestle can determine the denaturation of proteins due to mechanical trauma, just as the high speed of a blender can cause the same problem. Obviously boiling at 100° C will induce the complete protein component loss.

In 2013, Jianan Li and colleagues[5] (Department of Biotechnology, Life Science College, Jianghan University, Wuhan, China) proposed the following protocol using a human demineralized dentin matrix manufactured by a company that is mentioned in the article (Shen Zhen Guang Ming ChuangBo Biological Products Development Co., Ltd.), but without specifying the method of processing the whole tooth. Granules with a size of 10-140 µm were produced and then mixed with porcine collagen, frozen and dried and then placed for 2 hours at 100° C to form a collagen composite. Finally, they were irradiated with Cobalt 60 at 5 kGy.

It is clear that this procedure appears to be feasible only at an industrial level, not in a clinical setting. Furthermore, the perplexity remains about mixing the tooth, mainly consisting of human type 1 collagen, with porcine collagen. Ethical questions may arise about the possibility of using heterologous teeth to promote a human teeth market!

Another question that will arise in many other procedures concerns the maintenance of proteins after a treatment at 100° C. In fact, proteins denature at about 47° C, thus losing all the osteoinductive potential of the tooth. According to the authors, the use of the tooth must be aimed to produce a material that has better characteristics than the materials on the market.

Bhattacharijya and colleagues,[6] in 2016, considered the dental-derived material as a high quality graft and proposed a treatment similar to that described by Murata in 2010,[1] consisting in placing the extracted tooth in liquid nitrogen at -196° C, then rinsing it in 1 M NaCl physiological solution, demineralizing it using an average power acid, such as acetic acid or hydrochloric acid (pH 2), then immersing it in cold distilled water and freezing it (without specifying the process used) to the final use. This solution is obviously impractical in a clinic that does not have liquid nitrogen.

Kabir and colleagues,[7] in a 2017 publication, analyzed the results of bone defects repaired with whole human teeth perforated and treated in sheep using the following protocol: the teeth, after being cleaned and perforated with calibrated holes of 500 µm, were immersed in an ultrasonic bath with 0.34 M nitric acid at 100 W and 60 Hz for 30 minutes and then rinsed for a long time with distilled water. The results, from the histological point of view, were encouraging and the technique seemed simple, but the amount of dentin was not completely resorbed.

In 2017, Kim (Department of Oral and Maxillofacial Surgery, Section of Dentistry, Seoul National University Bundang Hospital, Seongnam, Korea) and Murata (Division of Oral and Maxillofacial Surgery, School of Dentistry, Health Sciences University of Hokkaido, Sapporo, Japan)[8] have published a procedure consisting in the use of allogeneic teeth. The tooth was extracted and refrigerated with ethyl alcohol, mechanically cleaned of the pulp and ligament residues, with retrograde rotation, reduced to 300-800 µm particles, demineralized using 0.6 M HCl and dehydrated with ethyl alcohol. The powder was rinsed in distilled water and freeze-dried for 3-5 hours. The interesting aspect of this process was the attempt to use an allogeneic tooth (from a donor), but, as in the case described by Jianan Li and colleagues[5] in 2013, important ethical questions arose regarding tooth donation.

To all intents and purposes, the process, apart from the 3-5 hours of waiting for freeze-drying, is identical to the process proposed by Kim.

Also in 2017, Minimizato and colleagues[9] (Department of Regenerative Oral Surgery, Unit of Translational Medicine, Nagasaki University Graduate School of Biomedical Sciences, Nagasaki, Japan) evaluated, on 16 patients, the possibility of producing an autologous demineralized onside dentin particulate.

Vital and non-vital teeth were used, cleaned, immersed twice in a saline buffered solution and then crushed together with ice cubes in a specific high-speed rotating device with ceramic blades (Takigen, Japan; international patent application No. PCT/JP2007/053321, international published No. WO2007/099861 A1). Particulate matter with size between 400 and 800 µm was washed with 1.0 M sodium chloride and partially demineralized with 2% nitric acid (pH 1) for 10 minutes. Finally, they were immersed twice in hydrochloric acid (pH 7.4) for 10 minutes. The process, lasting about 40 minutes, might be appropriate to clinical needs.

In 2009, in Korea, a tooth bank was created, where the extracted tooth could be sent. The tooth was then processed at the bank, placed in a container with ethylene oxide,[10] which guaranteed sterility over time, and redelivered so that it could then be used as needed. The use of a particularly flammable gas, such as ethylene oxide, and potentially dangerous, requires very strict rules in terms of safety during production. This approach guaranteed a qualitative treatment for each patient; however, it had to comply with rather strict rules regarding the recognition of the tooth in the procedure to maintain the nominality.

Alone, in the period January 2009-October 2012, about 38,702 teeth were processed.[11]

Obviously, this whole operation impacts on costs. Two contrasting aspects are represented by the fact that, on the one hand, the material is available only after a certain time from the extraction and therefore all the immediate regeneration procedures are excluded; on the other hand, while later the particulated tooth will be like every other grafting material.

Devices on the market

There are currently four devices on the market for using the tooth as grafting material. These are, in chronological order, Bon Maker, Vacuasonic, Kometabio and Tooth Transformer.

All these devices have three stages, which are described below.

Step 1: tooth cleaning

After the extraction, the tooth must be cleaned of any residues of calculus, caries, soft tissues and restorations (6.1). The fillings of any material must be eliminated, even cleaning in excess the dental tissue on which the reconstruction lays in order to avoid finding resins or other materials in the regeneration material. The prosthetic parts and cements must be cleaned in the same way. Some devices allow the use of teeth with root canal therapies, in which case cleaning performed mechanically is preferred. For some devices (Bon Maker, Vacuasonic and Kometabio), in which the sieve is used to separate the granules according to the size, it is advisable to remove with tweezers the parts not congruent with the dental tissue after grinding.

Tooth Transformer, which requires the tooth to be sectioned (6.2) for grinding, recommends cleaning the root canal treatment residues during the sectioning phase, thus allowing the cleaning of small sections more easily visible by optical magnification (6.3).

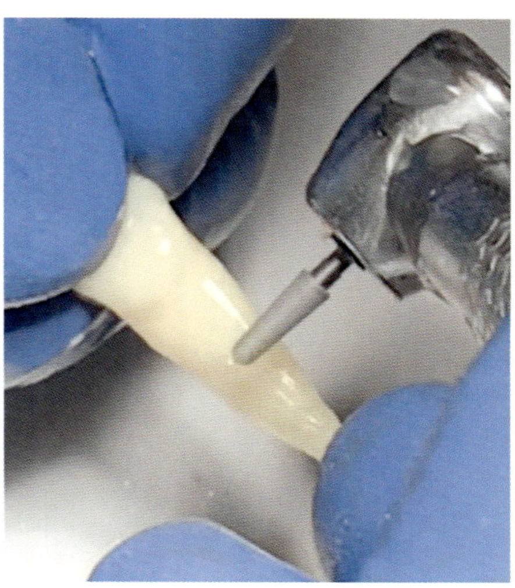

6.1 Tooth cleaning.

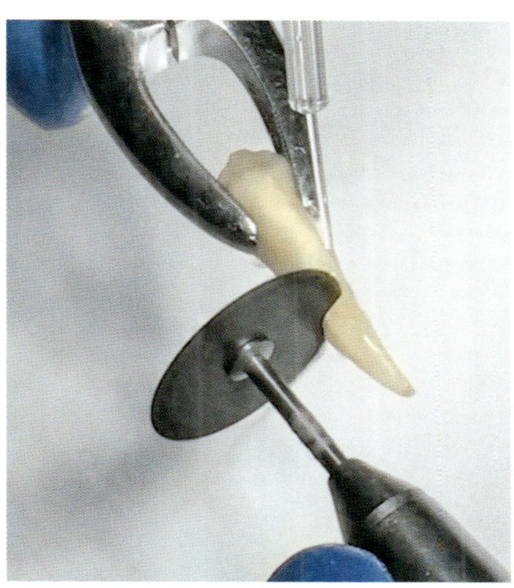

6.2 Sectioning of a tooth with disk.

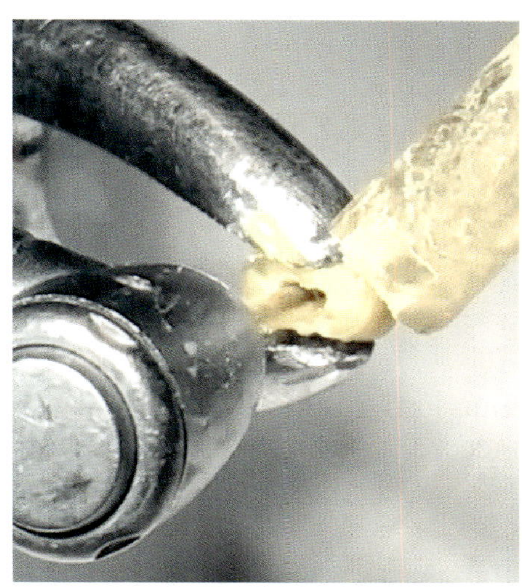

6.3 Cleaning of root canal treatment residues using a rotary drill.

Step 2: tooth grinding

Two devices (Bon Maker and Vacuasonic) involve the use of a hammer and pestle to crush the tooth (6.4).

Particular attention is recommended to this procedure to avoid any trauma to the operator. After crushing, the tooth is placed in a non-sterilizable high-speed mill (6.5a,b). The granules are then separated by a manual sieve (6.5c).

This sieve has two meshes and separates the fragments of different sizes. The larger ones, sized 850 µm, will remain blocked by the first filter, while the thinner ones, sized 450 µm, will pass through the second filter, ending up in the lower plate.

Kometabio also uses a high-speed mill, which however differs from the previous ones as it is disposable (6.6) and contains an automatic sieving and vibrating system. After grinding, a vibration system is activated which filters the tooth through the holes on the bottom of the grinder, blocking granules larger than 1200 µm, while another drawer sieve filters granules larger than 300 µm.

The high-speed crushing ensures rapidity and determines the pulverization of part of the tooth.

Tooth Transformer uses a multi-use sterilizable system (6.7) which works at low speed without loss of pulverized dental substance, but it has the disadvantage of not allowing the insertion of a whole tooth into the grinder and therefore the sample must be sectioned within dimensions before the insertion.

Phase 3: treatment by device

Bon Maker:[12] the tooth, crushed properly, must be inserted manually in a cylindrical container in plas-

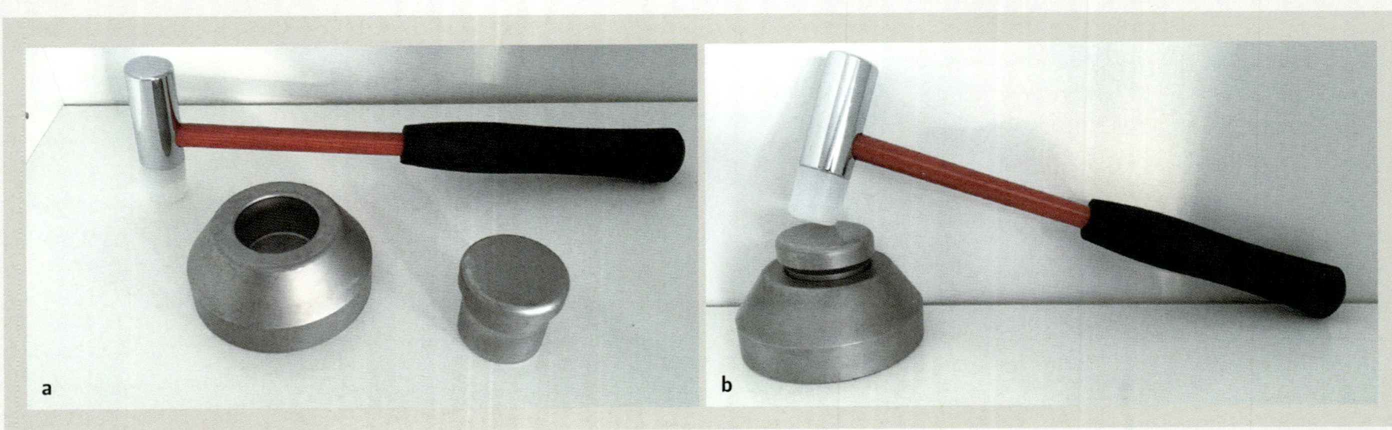

6.4 **(a, b)** Hammer and pestle in Bon Maker device.

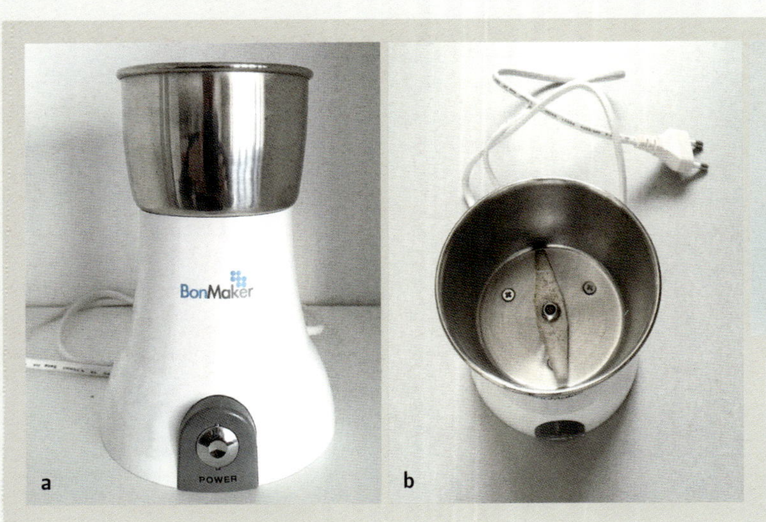

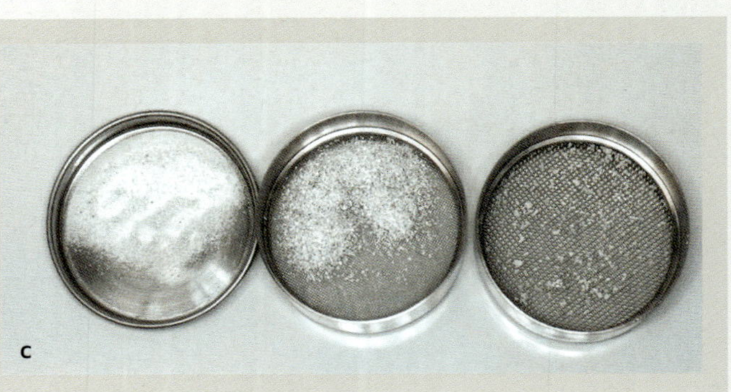

6.5 **(a, b)** High speed grinder in Bon Maker device. **(c)** Manual sieves with different filtrations.

tic sterilized multipurpose material (Bonbin) (6.8). The Bonbin containing the granulate must be inserted in a slot on the upper front part of the machine. The liquids, contained in disposable bottles, must be emptied manually into the respective cavities following a colour code. A bottle to be tightened onto the upper part of the device must also be filled with physiological solution.

The device can treat even whole teeth, to be inserted into the Bonbin, which must previously be perforated with a specifically designed bur. Specific liquids are available, with the same procedure, for treating the block. At the end of the treatment, which lasts about 26 minutes, the material is extracted from the Bonbin. Exhausted and contaminated liquids are collected in a glass bottle situated behind a door in the front of the device, which must be emptied after a few uses. The composition of the liquids has not been clarified in any publication. In 2016, at the Polytechnic University of Milan, the liquids used were therefore subjected to an analysis, and the results were as follows:

- *granular formulation*: HCl 0.45 M-H_2O_2 130 volumes-ethanol 62.6% chloroform 31.3% water 6.1% + washing saline solution;
- *block formulation*: HCl 0.56 M-H_2O_2 120 volumes-ethanol 47.2% chloroform 47.2% water 5.6% + washing saline solution.

Vacuasonic:[13,14] the tooth, made granular, must be inserted manually in a disposable plastic phial. After screwing a cap containing the formulation, according to a sequence numbered from 1 to 3, the disposable phial with the tooth is inserted inside a grid, under a trap door on the upper part of the device (6.9).

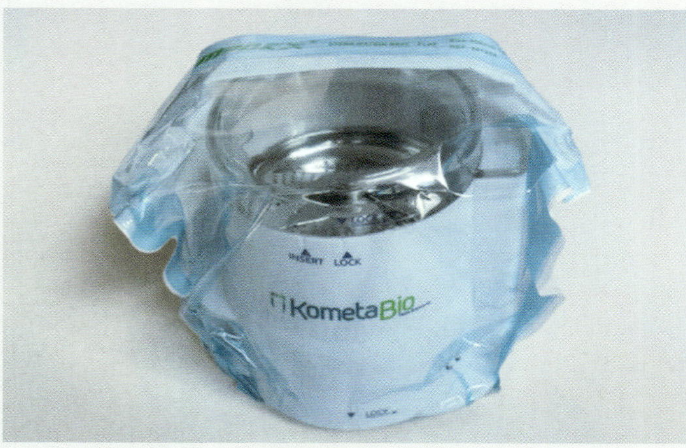

6.6 High speed mill with integrated Smart Dentin Grinder® sieve. (Courtesy of Kometabio Inc., New Jersey, USA.)

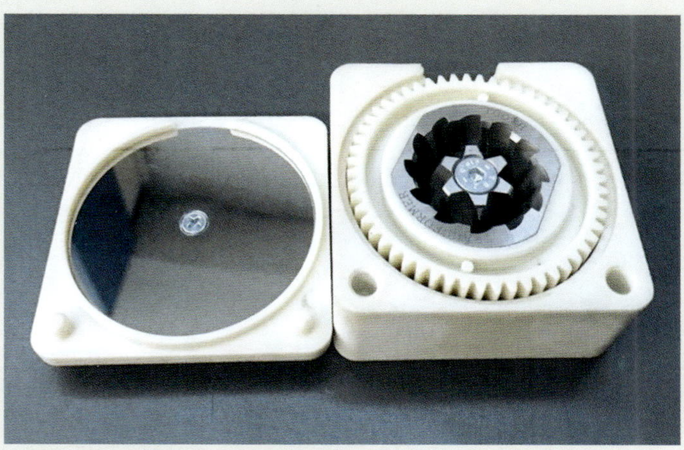

6.7 Low speed grinder.

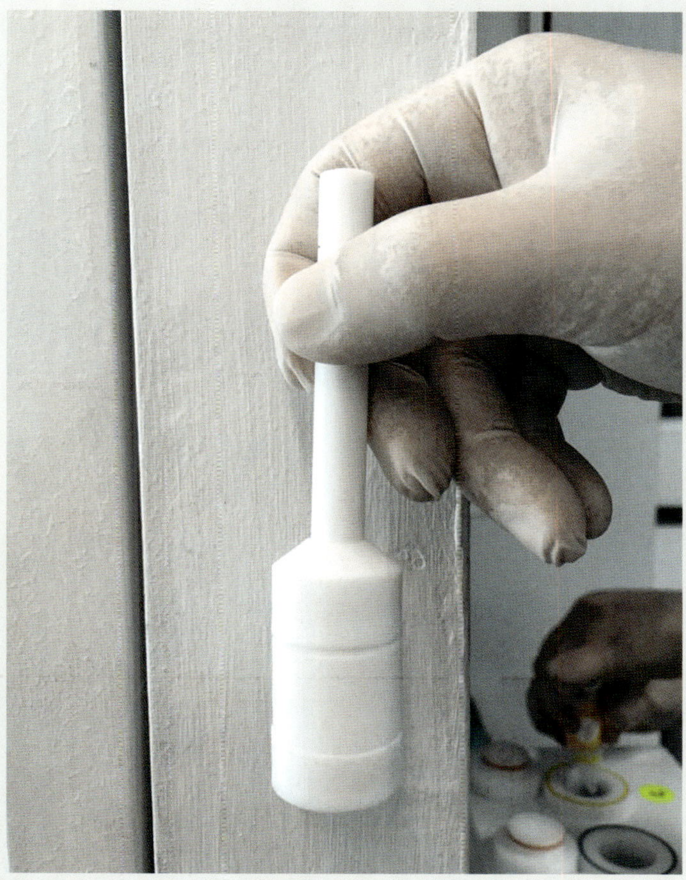

6.8 The Bonbin container and the liquids from colour coded vials poured into the wells.

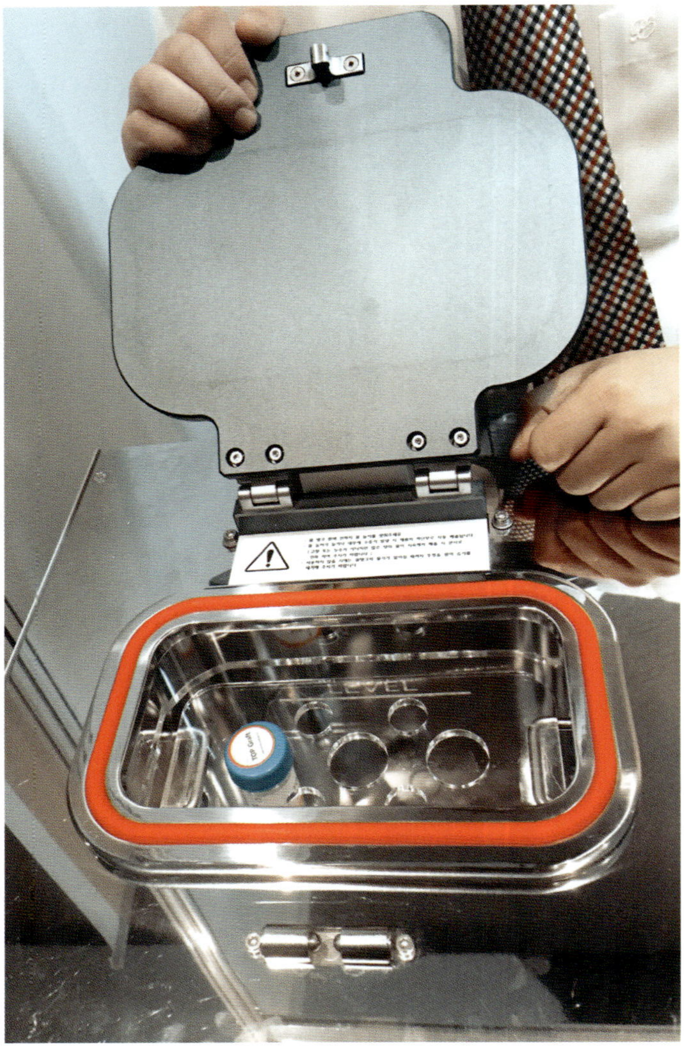

6.9 Top opening in Vacuasonic device.

The device must be previously filled with aqueous solution. The granulate must then be moved to phial no. 2 and no. 3, repeating the procedure.

The device consists of a large ultrasonic tank that amplifies the action of the individual reagents.

The same procedure should be followed with the whole tooth for a block graft. The liquids used are: 0.6 M hydrochloric acid (HCl) + peracetic acid + ethanol + phosphate wash buffer solution (6.10).[13-25]

Kometabio: the granulated tooth from the mill is placed in a glass bowl into which the first liquid contained in plastic bottles is added according to a colour code (6.11).

After the time required for the procedure, the liquid is eliminated using a gauze or a pipette and then the second liquid is introduced. Recently, Kometabio presented a third liquid to be used if you want to have demineralization (EDTA). Liquids need to be added manually and removed manually using gauze or pipettes. It is also possible to dry the mixture with the intention of storing it in a hot plate at 140° C, manually placing the glass bowl over the hot plate.

In the literature there seem to be different methods of use, all made possible by a manual use of the device and varying the times on personal considerations.

In 2014, Bindermann[15] proposed to immerse the particulate matter for 10 minutes in a liquid called alcohol cleanser, consisting of 0.5 M NaOH and 30% ethyl alcohol, and then use after rinsing twice with a PBS buffer solution. Alternatively, the still wet particulate can be placed on a hot plate at 140° C for 5 minutes to have a bacteria-free particulate for a ready or later use.

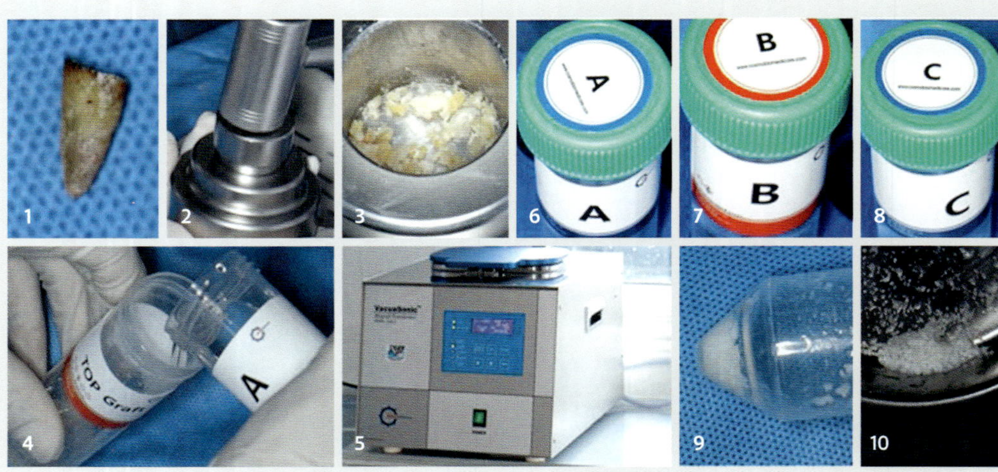

6.10 Steps for preparation using Vacuasonic: immediate preparation of the autologous dental graft material. **1** Minimally invasive tooth extraction. **2–3** Preparation and pretreatment, crushing by hammer. **4–10** The particulates are then demineralized, sterilized and rinsed to produce the tooth-derived autogenous graft material. (From: Wu et al., 2019.)[24]

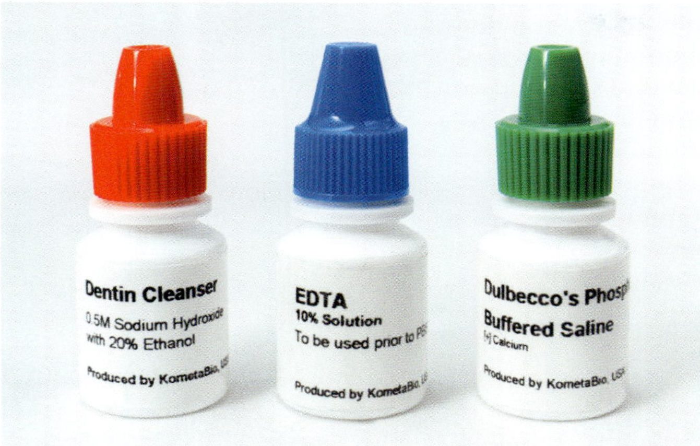

6.11 The bottles of liquids used by Kometabio. (Courtesy of Kometabio Inc., New Jersey, USA.)

In 2016, Hallel[16] stated to immerse the obtained granules in 0.5 M NaOH and 20% ethyl alcohol for 10 minutes and then to eliminate the solution by means of a pipette or gauze and, finally, to rinse all with the PBS buffer solution for 3 minutes.

In 2017, Bindermann[17] indicated that the cleanser consists of 0.5 M NaOH and 20% ethyl alcohol to be used for 10 minutes, followed by PBS for 3 minutes, then eliminated with gauze.

Guirado,[18] in 2018, indicated a 15-minute soaking time, then a 5-minute PBS wash.

Later, in 2019, Guirado,[19] in *Materials* magazine, recommended using the cleanser for 10 minutes, then for 2 minutes in EDTA solution and finally in saline for 3 minutes.

In 2019, Cardaropoli[20] presented the protocol of 0.5% NaOH and 30% ethyl alcohol bath for 10 minutes.

Tooth Transformer: after inserting the sectioned and cleaned tooth inside the grinder (6.12), it is closed and placed in the device (6.13). The disposable part contains a cartridge with liquids and a cylinder with a cup for collecting the granulate (6.14).

Both are inserted into the device in their respective slots, the cartridge is activated by piercing (6.15) and then, once the door is closed and the button is pressed, the process starts. The procedure is completely automatic and repeats the same steps each time. The first phase of grinding at low speed causes the granules to fall into the collection basket The six liquids present in the cartridge tank fall by gravity after the automatic perforation of the lower membrane of the cartridge and start the process. The granules are subjected to UVA rays and ultrasonic vibrations with temperature variations always below 43° C to avoid damage to the proteins. At the end of the process, the used and contaminated liquids remain inside the cylindrical container which can be disposed of.

The liquids used have not been indicated in the literature. In this case the authors received, for the first time, the possibility to publish the liquids used, which are constituted by 0.1 M hydrochloric acid, 10% hydrogen peroxide and demineralized water as a wash.

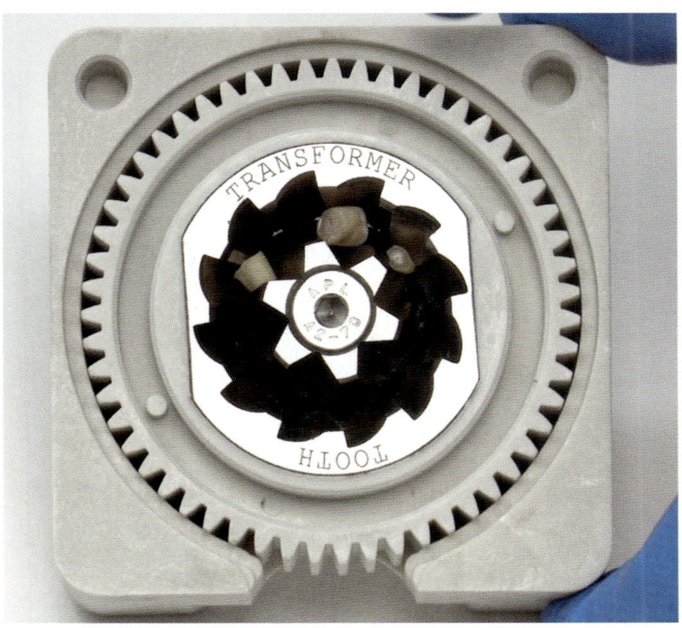

6.12 Sectioned tooth inside low speed grinder.

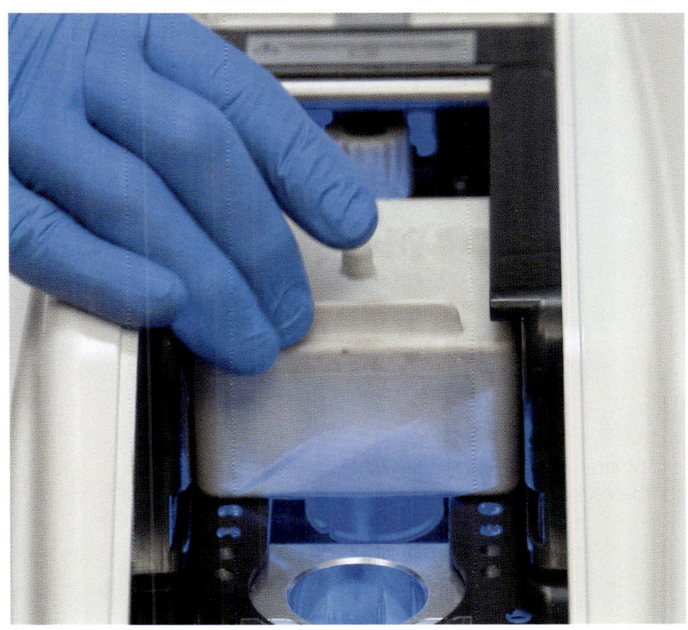

6.13 Insertion of the grinder into Tooth Transformer device.

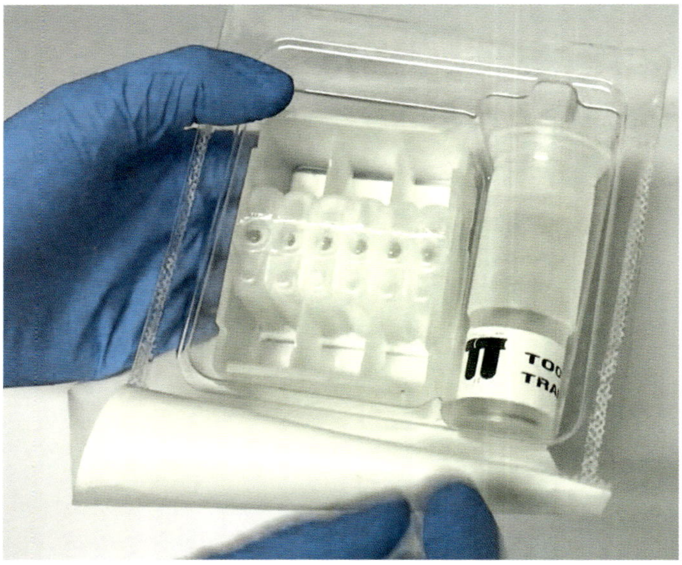

6.14 Disposable Tooth Transformer.

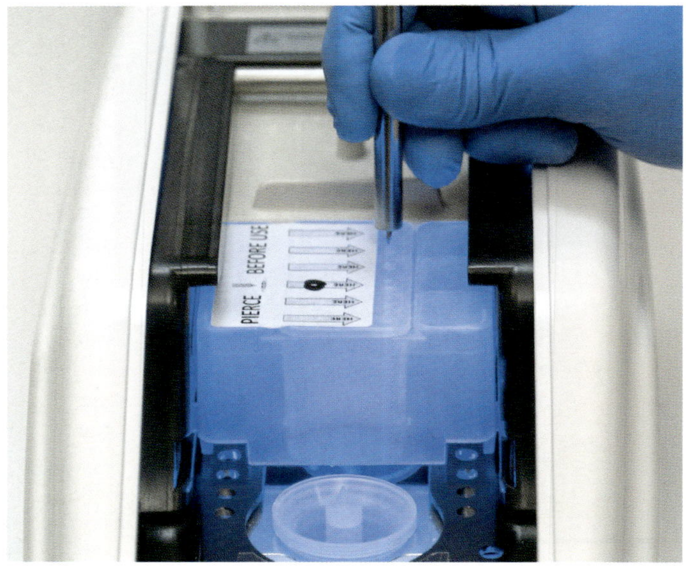

6.15 Disposable part positioned and piercing of the liquid tank of the Tooth Transformer device.

Protein denaturation

One of the focal aspects of tooth use is its protein content, which is quantified in 3.5-4% of the weight of the tooth. Proteins can allow osteoinduction.

It is clear that, to keep the protein content intact, the treatment must be as "gentle" as possible, while guaranteeing, at the same time, the fundamental phases such as detoxification, demineralization and trituration. Therefore, each part of the process must be studied for

Bon Maker

Manufacturing: **Korea;**
Korea Dental Solution Co. Ltd

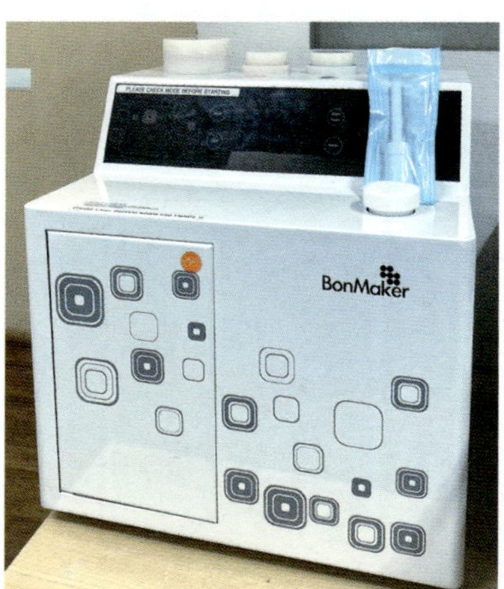

Phase 1	Tooth cleaning using piezoelectric and/or rotating tools
Phase 2	Manual with hammer and with high speed mill
Phase 3	Treatment with three liquids and three washes
Shape of the material	Granular - Block
Dimensions	45 × 45 × 45/60 cm
Weight	Approximately 15 kg
Disposable	Three liquids in bottles to be placed manually Washing liquids to be added in a plastic bottle to be screwed to the upper part of the machine
Usage	Manual/automatic
Composition of liquids	*Granular formulation:* HCl 0.45 M-H_2O_2 130 volumes - ethanol 62.6% chloroform 31.3% water 6.1% *Block formulation:* HCl 0.56 M-H_2O_2 120 volumes - ethanol 47.2% chloroform 47.2% water 5,6%
Duration of treatment	26 min 26 s
Possibility of using endodontically treated teeth	Yes
Recovery of used liquids	Manual. They are discharged into a glass bottle which must be emptied manually

Vacuasonic

Manufacturing: **Korea**
Cosmobiomedicare, Gangnamgu, Seoul, Korea

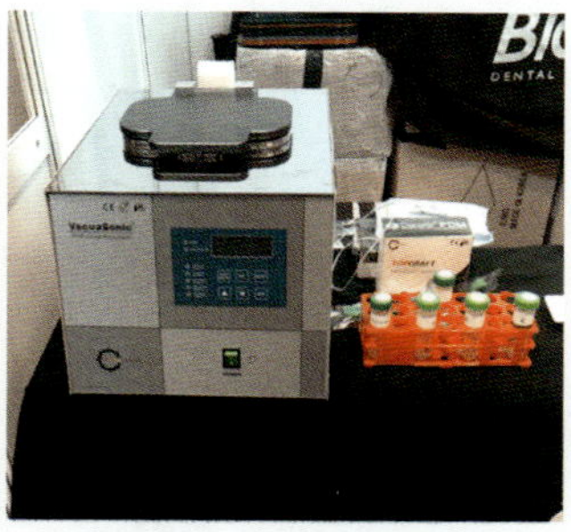

Tooth crushing	Manual with hammer and with high speed mill
Shape of the material	Granular - Block
Dimensions	45 × 45 × 60 cm
Weight	30 kg
Disposable	Three vials in bottles to be placed manually
Usage	Manual/automatic
Composition of liquids	0.6 M HCl + peracetic acid + ethanol - phosphate buffer saline solution
Duration of treatment	30 min per granulate - 2 hours per block
Possibility of using endodontically treated teeth	Yes
Recovery of used liquids	Manual

Kometabio

Manufacturing: **Israel/USA**
Kometabio Inc., NJ, USA

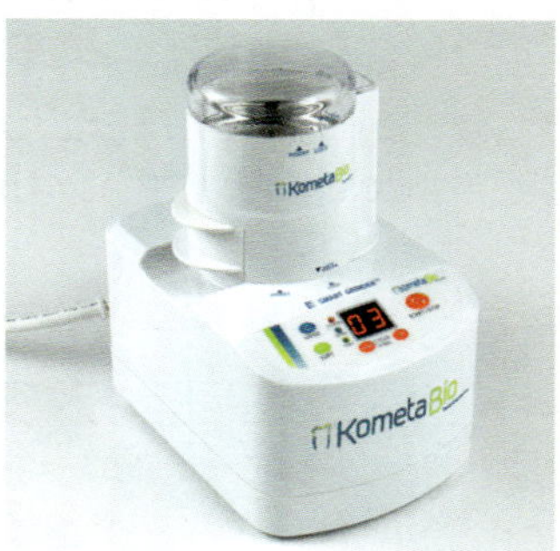

Smart Dentin Grinder®. *(Courtesy of Kometabio Inc., New Jersey, USA.)*

Tooth crushing	With high speed mill
Shape of the material	Granular
Dimensions	20 × 15 × 15 cm
Weight	1 kg
Disposable	Three bottles to be placed manually
Usage	Manual
Composition of liquids	0.5 M NaOH and 30% alcohol
Duration of treatment	20 min
Possibility of using endodontically treated teeth	Yes
Recovery of used liquids	Manual with gauze by soaking it in the used liquid or with a pipette

Tooth Transformer

Manufacturing: **Italy, TT Tooth Transformer srl, Milan**

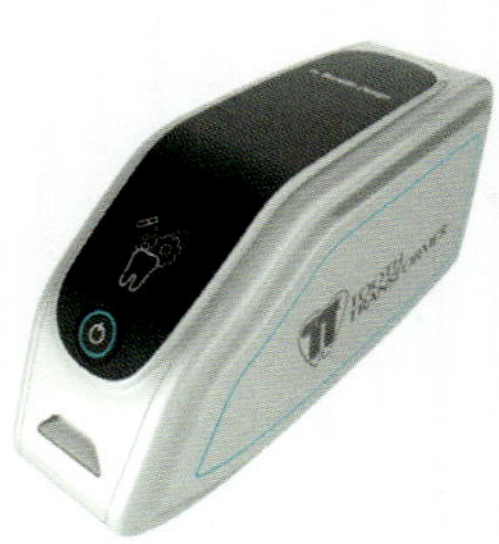

Tooth Transformer®. *(Courtesy of Tooth Transformer, Milan, Italy.)*

Tooth crushing	With low speed grinder
Shape of the material	Granular
Dimensions	39 × 15 × 17 cm
Weight	6 kg
Disposable	Maker and liquids tank
Usage	Automatic
Composition of liquids	0.1 M hydrochloric acid, 10% hydrogen peroxide, demineralized water as wash
Duration of treatment	30 min for granulate
Possibility of using endodontically treated teeth	Yes
Recovery of used liquids	Automatic

the maintenance of 3.5-4% of the tooth weight because, otherwise, a graft material with only osteoconductive characteristics will be obtained. The graft will still be good, because it will consist of an autologous collagenated hydroxyapatite with autologous type 1 collagen, and therefore it will work well.

To understand how it is possible to lose proteins, it is necessary to consider that these are macromolecules with a complex structure at four levels,[23] with a ball structure. If an alteration of the structure occurs through chemical denaturation, thermal denaturation[21,22] above 44/47° C or mechanical denaturation, the functionality of the proteins is lost. A denatured protein (6.16), even if quite similar, as far as the coarse structure is concerned, is no longer able, however, to perform its biological functions. It can be compared to a bent key which no longer fits into the keyhole.

The total loss of the mineral part also implies the loss of proteins, as the acids that dissolve the mineral part also attack the proteins, denaturing them. In tests carried out at the Polytechnic University of Milan it has been seen that changes in molarity or in timings determine large differences in the presence of proteins.

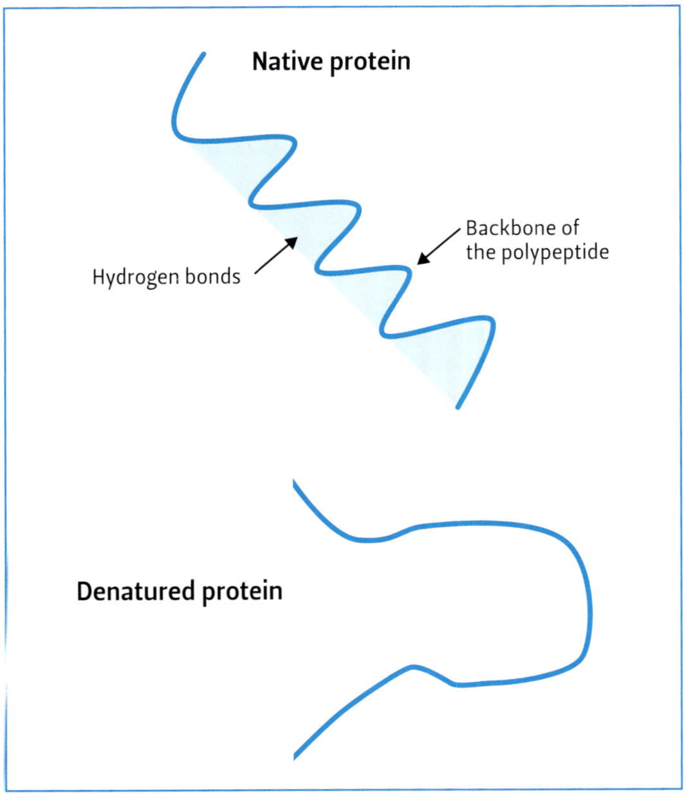

6.16 Differences between natural and denatured proteins.

CE marking

The CE marking names a set of mandatory practices for all products covered by Community directives, which also includes the application of a symbol with the letters "CE" on the product that is subject to marking (hence the name). It is made by the manufacturer of a product regulated in the European Union, who declares, by a declaration of conformity or performance for construction products, that the product complies with the safety requirements laid down by the directives or by the applicable community regulations.

The CE marking, in force since 1993, indicates a compliance with all the obligations imposed on manufacturers (or importers) regarding their products (or those placed on the market under their own responsibility) under the Community directives, allowing free marketing of branded products within the European market.

Differences between CE and medical CE

MEDICAL CE

A medical device is an instrument used in medicine for diagnostic and/or therapeutic purposes. Before being placed on the market, medical devices, like medications, must be able to demonstrate their safety and effectiveness of action considered by clinical studies carried out in suitable structures authorized for the purpose. The CE marking indicates the suitability of the medical device for being placed on the market. It is mandatory according to the EEC directive 93/42 on medical devices.

According to the definition contained in the legislative decree 24 February 1997, n. 46 ("Implementation of Directive 93/42/EEC, concerning medical devices"), a medical device is «*any instrument, apparatus, implant, substance or other product, used alone or in combination, including the software used for functioning properly, and intended by the manufacturer for use in humans for the purpose of diagnosis, prevention, control, therapy or alleviation of disease; to diagnose, control, treat, alleviate or compensate for an injury or handicap; study, replacement or modification of the anatomy or of a physiological process; of intervention on conception, which product does not exert the main action, in or on the human body, for which it is intended, by pharmacological or immunological means or by metabolic process but whose function can be assisted by such means*».

Medical devices are grouped, according to their complexity and the potential risk for the patient, into four classes: I, IIa, IIb, III.

For classes IIa, IIb and III it is necessary to issue a specific certification, which provides the verification of all the necessary procedures by a notified body.

In the event that the CE mark is accompanied by a four-digit number, it means that the medical device is certified by a notified body, identifiable by the corresponding number. The notified body is a body authorized by the competent authorities of the various states of the European Union and designated to carry out the certification procedures.

The list of active medical devices and implantable medical devices notified in the "Medical devices database" system, is available to the public to facilitate the dissemination and use of the registration number in the database established pursuant to the Decree of the Minister of Health, 21 December 2009 (through public consultation).

A manual device can cause errors in its activity and therefore substantially change the result of the treatment due to human errors. A device that involves manual skills cannot be medical.

CE FOR ELECTRICAL DEVICE

A CE marking that covers only the electrical part has no sanitary value and it does not qualify the device as medical.

The CE marking of an electrical device declares the conformity of the electrical equipment with the essential requirements set out in the "Low voltage" directive (Directive 2014/35/EU of the European Parliament and of the Council).

The directive is aimed at ensuring that the electrical equipment involved has adequate protection against electrical hazards of various kinds. Referring to IEC/ISO EN technical standards - which manufacturers of electrical products must comply to - the Directive explicitly specifies the risks to health and safety, defining the parameters for which the devices are safe with respect to their intended use.

This directive forms part of the legislative framework for the free movement and marketing of products in the European Community. Its ultimate aim is to avoid the risks associated with a product or phenomenon, thus defending a common interest of European citizens and companies.

Electrical equipment can be placed on the market if it complies with the requirements of the directive after simple laboratory tests on the machinery.

In the **electrical CE** the CE symbol is without numbers.
In the **medical CE**, the CE symbol is followed by 4 numbers that indicate the body that certified the device by testing it following all the regulations.

Outside the European Community, a medical device, in order to be sold, must be registered within the respective regulatory authority with methods, times and costs that vary greatly from country to country.

The CE certification, internationally recognized as a rigorous process with a long history, starts from the European Directive of 1993 to the new European Regulation defined applicable from 26 May 2021 and it is often considered sufficient for registering a medical device in many countries outside the EU, also considering the tendency to overlap the way of classification of Medical Devices according to risk and similar international technical standards on the basis of the tests to demonstrate the safety essential performance and toxicological assessment of biocompatibility.

Also in the technical field, international standards still regulate the way key investigations such as Risk Analysis, Clinical Evaluation and Device Usability are carried out, while in the context of Quality Management Systems they are similarly recognized standards of address whose contents are common to the architecture and quality management systems and the requirements of such systems.

Following these considerations, even if it is necessary for a foreign country to carry out a real certification process with the request of numerous documents to be drawn up from scratch and technical tests to be redone in full, often on the spot, there is, however, a common matrix that, apart from some exceptions, allows an effective dialogue and action through a transversal lexicon.

Finally, it is essential to consider the requests of a particular country outside the EU regarding the need for local representation through a foreign manufacturer, an authorized representative, a distributor, an importer, an agent or a sponsor that deals with conversations with the local authority throughout the process leading to registration and, subsequently, for the post-sale surveillance of a device.

REFERENCES

1. Murata M, Akazawa T, Takahata M, et al. Bone induction of human tooth and bone crushed by newly developed automatic mill. J Ceram Soc Jpn 2010;118(6):434-7.
2. Al-Namnam NM, Shanmuhasuntharam P, Ha KO, et al. Processed allogenic dentine as a scaffold for bone healing: an in vivo study. Aust J Basic Appl Sci 2010;4(12): 5932-40.
3. Li R, Guo W, Yang B, et al. Human treated dentin matrix as a natural scaffold for complete human dentin tissue regeneration. J Biomaterials 2011;32:4525-38.
4. Hussain I, Moharamzadeh K, Brook IM, et al. Evaluation of osteoconductive and osteogenic potential of a dentin-base bone substitute using a calvarial defect model. Int J Dent 2012;2012:396316.
5. Jianan Li, Juan Yang, Xiaozhong Zhong, et al. Demineralized dentin matrix composite collagen material for bone tissue. J Biomater Sci Polym Ed 2013; 24(13):1519-28.
6. Bhattacharijya C, Gadicherla S, Kamath AT, et al. Tooth derived bone graft material. World J Dent 2016;7(1):32-5.
7. Kabir MA, Murata M, Akazawa T, et al. Evaluation of perforated demineralized dentin scaffold on bone regeneration in critical-size sheep iliac defects. Clin Oral Impl Res 2017;28:e227-e35.
8. Kim YK, Bang KM, Murata M, et al. Retrospective clinical study of allogenic demineralized dentin matrix for alveolar bone repair. J Hard Tissue Biol 2017;26:95-102.
9. Minamizato T, Koga T, Takashi I, et al. Clinical application of autogenous partially demineralized dentin matrix prepared immediately after extraction for alveolar bone regeneration in implant dentistry: a pilot study. Int J Oral Maxillofac Surg 2018;47:125-32.
10. Kim YK, Yun PY, Um IW, et al. Alveolar ridge preservation of an extraction socket using autogenous tooth bone graft material for implant site development: prospective case series. J Adv Prosthodont 2014;6(6):521-7.
11. Kim YK, Um W, Murata M. Tooth bank system for bone regeneration. J Tissue Biol 2014;23(3): 371-76.
12. Kim KW. Bone Induction by demineralized dentin matrix in nude mouse muscles. Maxillofac Plast Reconstr Surg 2014;36(2):50-6.
13. Tulio AV, Kang CD, Fabian OA, et al. Socket preservation using demineralized tooth graft: a case series report with histological analysis. Int J Growth Factors Stem Cells Dent 2020;3:27-34.
14. Dong Wu, Lin Zhou, Jichao Lin, et al. Immediate implant placement in anterior teeth with grafting material of autogenous tooth bone vs xenogenic bone. BMC Oral Health 2019;19:266.
15. Binderman I, Hallel G, Nardy C, et al. A novel procedure to process extracted teeth for immediate grafting of autogenous teeth. J Interdiscipl Med Dent Sci 2014;2:6.
16. Hallel G, Leretter M, Sapoznikov L. Greffe de dentine autologue et preservation de la crete alveolaire. L'Information Dentaire 2016;28(96):20.
17. Binderman I, Hallel G, Leretter M. Alveolar ridge preservation: particulate dentin of extracted teeth are optimal for immediate grafting of extracted site. Dentalife/Viața Stomatologică 2017;4:7-11.
18. Calvo-Guirado JL, Cegarra Del Pino P, Sapoznikov L, et al. A new procedure for processing extracted teeth for immediate grafting in post-extraction sockets. An experimental study in American Fox Hound dogs. Ann Anat 2018;217:14-23.
19. Calvo-Guirado JL, Ballester Montilla A, De Aza PN , et al. Particulated, Extracted Human Teeth Characterization by SEM-EDX Evaluation as a Biomaterial for Socket Preservation: An in vitro Study. Materials 2019; 12(3):380.
20. Cardaropoli D, Nevins M. New bone formation using an extracted tooth as a biomaterial: a case report with histologic evidence. The Int J of Periodontics Restorative Dent 2019;39(2):156-63.
21. Eriksson RA, Albrektsson T. The effect of heat on bone regeneration: an experimental study in the rabbit using the bone growth chamber. J Oral Maxillofac Surg 1984;42(11):705-11.
22. Bischof JC, He X. Thermal stability of proteins. Ann NY Acad Sci 2005; 1066:12-33.
23. Moharamzadeh K, Freeman C, Blackwood K. Processed bovine dentine as a bone substitute. Br J Oral Maxillofac Surg 2008;46(2):110-3.
24. Wu D, Zhou L, Lin J et al. Immediate implant placement in anterior teeth with grafting material of autogenous tooth bone vs xenogenic bone. BMC Oral Health 2019;19:266.
25. Lee E-Y, Kim E-S, Kim K-W. Scanning electron microscopy and energy dispersive X-ray spectroscopy studies on processed tooth graft material by vacuum-ultrasonic acceleration. Maxillofac Plast Reconstr Surg 2014;36(3):103-10.

Histological characteristics of the bone substitute of dental origin: scientific evidence

Biomedical aspects of cyto-histology of bone tissue

A. Casasco, M. Casasco

Histology of the bone tissue

Histology is the study of the tissues that constitute our body. The *tissues* are, by classical definition, four: epithelial tissue, connective tissue, muscle tissue and nervous tissue. Actually, the various tissues do not exist in nature individually, but they exist as combinations of each other in order to generate *organs*.[1-10]

Histological techniques allow to analyze in detail under the microscope how a tissue and an organ are made. The use of the microscope allows you to observe structures at the micrometric (1 thousandth of a millimeter) or the nanometric (one millionth of a millimeter) level. Histological analysis is therefore, still today, unreplaceable in the biomedical field, for the study of both normal and pathological tissues (think, for example, of tumor and histopathological diagnostics). Despite the progresses, bioimaging techniques (with various contrast media), such as computed tomography (traditional or cone-beam), magnetic resonance, positron tomography, ultrasound or other examinations, still do not allow the exact assessment at the cellular and tissue level.

Each organ has specific characteristics (often multiple) and the component responsible for these characteristics constitutes the organ's *parenchyma*, while the other tissues participate in the formation of the organ without having specific functions. Connective tissue, for example, is present in every organ, making up the so-called *stroma*, which contains, among other things, blood vessels, lymphatics and nerves with their endings.

The various tissues are then organized to conceive the *organs*, macroscopically identifiable anatomical structures (i.e. with the "naked eye"), which make up the systems. The study of the organization of tissues in organs represents the microscopic anatomy.

Each tissue is made up of *cells*, which represent the individual, self-sufficient and vital units of the human body. The study of the cell is called *cytology*.

The variety of cells in the body is very wide and there are at least 200 different types of cells in human tissues (without considering the gametic or epigenetic varieties). The entire cell, tissue and organ sample is derived from a single cell, the *zygote*, generated by the fusion of the sperm with the egg cell.

The *cell differentiation process* leads to a cellular biodiversity present in the body. Taking into account that the structural genetic structure of each individual is almost identical in every cell, it is not so much the structural modifications of the DNA that define the fate and activities of each cell type (*cytotype*), but the adjustments that occur at the functional level in DNA and RNA. These aspects have fundamental implications in the possibility of modifying cells according to the activities they may or may not carry out and can be exploited in the artificial modification of the genome to produce cells that can be used in *cell therapy* or *tissue therapy*.

Bone tissue is a type of connective tissue that is distinguished by its marked rigidity and hardness, due to the presence of abundant calcium salts in the fundamental substance. Due to this characteristic, it is delegated to the function of support and protection, although it also has an important task in the field of metabolism, as it represents an indispensable reserve of calcium and phosphorus. Bone tissue constitutes an indispensable component for the survival of any mammal and phylogenetic studies suggest that the bones of the craniofacial region are the ones that first underwent ossification.

Histological methods of studying bone tissue

Histological techniques involve the removal of tissue and its fixation, i.e. the arrest of metabolic and autolysis activities. This usually occurs by immersion in aldehyde aqueous solutions, such as paraformaldehyde (formalyn). After fixation, the organ or tissue sample usually undergoes a hardening process that allows it to be sectioned.

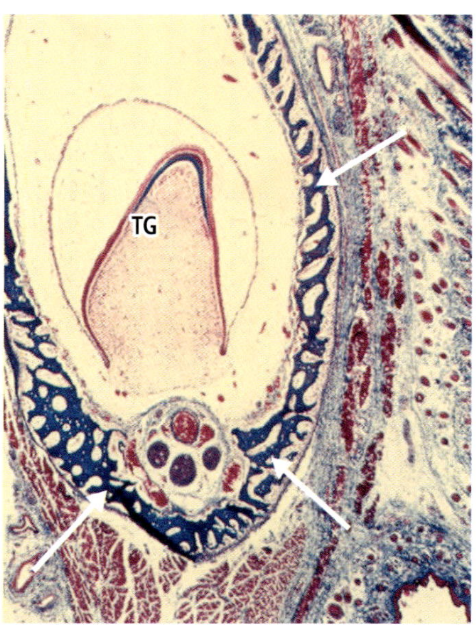

7.1 Microscopic section of a human embryo at the level of the craniofacial region. We observe the outline of a tooth (tooth gem, TG) at the "bell" stage. Around the outline, the formation of the maxillary alveolar bone tissue is evident (*in blue, arrows*). Azan stain. Original enlargement 40×.

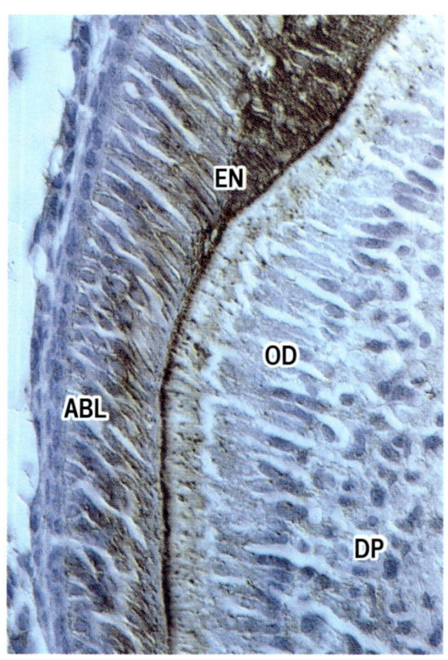

7.2 Immunohistochemical localization of enamel proteins under a light microscope in a newborn rat dental germ. The specific antibodies to enamel proteins allow their recognition both within the ameloblasts (which produce them) and in the matrix of the enamel being formed (*in brown*). Immuno-peroxidase technique and counterstain with hematoxylin (*in blue*). ABL, ameloblasts; DP, dental pulp; EN, enamel; OD, odontoblasts.

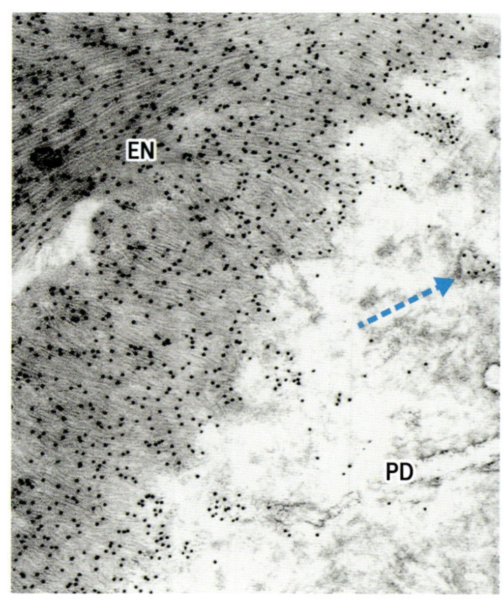

7.3 Immunocytochemical localization of enamel proteins in a newborn rat dental germ under the electron microscope view. Antibodies specific for enamel proteins were conjugated with colloidal gold particles of 15 nm which appear as electrondense pellets. Needlelike mineral crystals are identified in the enamel being formed (EN). The blue arrow indicates the penetration of enamel proteins into the pre-dentine (PD): these proteins play an inductive role on the differentiation of odontoblasts. Original enlargement 60,000×.

This is achieved either through inclusion in substances (such as paraffin or resins) or through freezing.

The sample, fixed and hardened, is then appropriately sectioned. The sections are subsequently stained using various colorants. The simplest and most commonly used staining is made with two colorants, hematoxylin and eosin, which respectively color the acidic and basic substances of cells and tissues. But the histological stains are various and they allow practically to identify every tissue component (7.1). Some stains, called *histochemicals*, allow the selective identification of single cells or molecules in a specific way. This type that are used today are immunohistochemical ones, which, as a strategy, use the antigen-antibody reaction: the antigen is present in the cell or tissue and is localized through antibodies that are placed on the tissue section; these antibodies (which are bound to the antigen) are detected with particular tracking systems, at the level of both optical and electronic microscopy (7.2 and 7.3).

The study of bone tissue - due to its consistency - requires the use of special histological techniques. The cells and the organic part of the fundamental substance can be studied in preparations and stained after decalcification of the bone sample. This procedure consists in depriving the bone of the mineral part by means of dilute solutions of acids or with solutions containing chelating substances (such as ethylenediaminetetraacetic acid, EDTA): the bone loses its hardness and can therefore be reduced into sections. If the bone tissue sample to be observed under the microscope is small enough (as in the case of biopsies), it can be sectioned without decalcifying it, using special cutting systems.

Bone cells and the *bone matrix* (or *fundamental substance*) participate in the constitution of bone tissue.

Specific cells of bone tissue

Like any other connective tissue, bones contain various structures, including vessels and nerves. Furthermore, bones contain another connective tissue, the marrow, which produces blood cells. The specific bone cells are osteocytes, osteoblasts, osteoclasts and osteogenetic stem cells.[1,10]

Osteocytes

The body of osteocytes is contained in the bone lacunae, cavities dug into the calcified basic substance, from which thin channels, the bone canaliculi, branch off, containing the cell extensions.

The extensions are not in direct contact with the calcified fundamental substance that forms the wall of the bone canals, but they are separated from it by a glycoprotein coating. The presence of tight junctions between the extensions of the adjacent bone cells, inside the bone canaliculi, allows the passage of ions and small molecules from one cell to another, allowing for cell to cell communication.

Osteocytes derive from osteoblasts and differ from these due to the lower cytoplasmic basophilia, as they own a smaller quantity of ribosomes and granular endoplasmic reticulum, which are the sites of intracellular protein synthesis. However, under appropriate stimulation, the osteocytes can convert back into osteoblasts as metabolically active cells: therefore, osteocytes and osteoblasts actually represent two functional stages of the same cellular stem.

Osteoblasts

Osteoblasts (7.4), mesenchymally derived, process the organic part of the fundamental substance of the bone and are involved in the deposition process of mineral salts. They are rather large cells (about 25-30 nm) of various shapes, with an eccentric nucleus, provided with a large nucleolus.

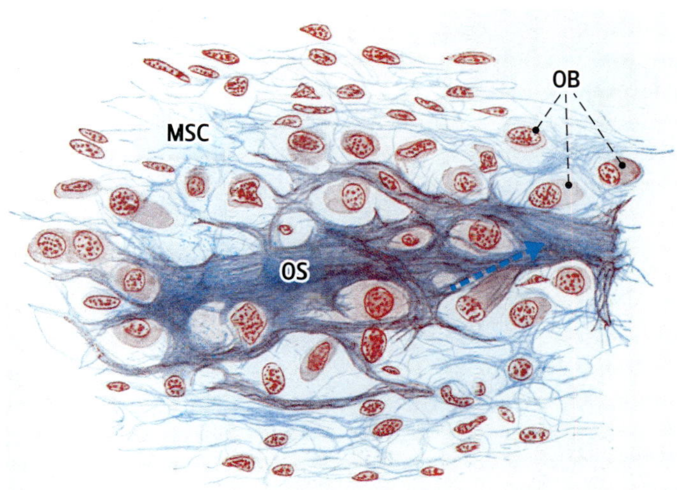

7.4 The drawing, taken from a histological preparation, shows the process of direct ossification at the level of a jawbone, i.e. the transformation from the mesenchyme to the bone without direct involvement of the cartilage. Osteoblasts (OB), mesenchymal stem cells (MSC) and the maturing bone matrix (osteoid substance, OS) are observed. The matrix appears basophilic (*in blue*) because it is still immature and rich in glycoproteins and proteoglycans. Original enlargement 400×.

In the cytoplasm, which is intensely basophilic, there is the presence of an enzyme, alkaline phosphatase, and some granules positive for the PAS reaction for glycoproteins, which can be interpreted as precursors of the vesicles of the matrix whose content will subsequently be secreted in the basic osteoid substance.

The appearance of the osteoblast under the electron microscope is that of a cell with strong protido-synthetic activity: in addition to a very extensive granular endoplasmic reticulum and numerous free ribosomes, in fact, a very developed Golgi apparatus and numerous vesicles are observed, to be interpreted as precursors of the glycoprotein component of the fundamental substance.

Osteoblasts are found wherever bone formation is taking place and tend to aggregate in epithelial-looking laminae, so as to define the formation of the bone lamella.

The secretory activity carried out by the osteoblasts leads these cells to remain imprisoned in the fundamental substance they have elaborated. At this point the osteoblast takes the characteristics of a cell in functional rest modality and it is transformed into an osteocyte.

Osteoblasts/osteocytes possess a cellular extension, called *primary cilium*, which is in fact a mechanism: depending on the mechanical stimulation that the bone receives, the bone cell is activated or deactivated to adapt to the environment, producing or not bone matrix. Hence numerous clinical implications in orthopedics and dentistry regarding the reactivity of bone cells to mechanical stress.[6-8]

Osteoclasts

The bone undergoes continuous modifications throughout its life made possible by the simultaneous carrying out of demolition and reconstructive processes. While the forming elements of the bone tissue are the osteoblasts, the osteoclasts provide for the destruction/remodeling of the bone.

They are cells characterized by considerable dimensions (30-100 micrometers) and by the presence of numerous nuclei inside them (up to 10); therefore, they are easily recognized by osteocytes/osteoblasts. In the abundant cytoplasm, numerous lysosomes are recognized as involved in the destruction of the bone matrix. On the surface facing the bone, the osteoclasts have a structure similar to the striated border, consisting of irregular microvilli, which demonstrate an intense relationship with the surrounding environment.

The action of osteoclasts is influenced by some hormones (in particular parathyroid hormone and calcitonin) and by numerous other homeostatic regulatory factors.

Mesenchymal stem cells and osteogenetic cells

All bone cells derive from the mesenchymal stem cell, from mesodermal or ecto-mesenchymal origin. Once the development of bone tissue in the body has taken place, numerous mesenchymal stem cells remain in the bones. This allows the regeneration of bone tissue in the event of injuries, such as in fractures.

Mesenchymal cells are undifferentiated cells that are difficult to identify at the microscopic level. They have a star-shaped or fusiform shape, little cytoplasm and a relatively large and vesicular nucleus. These cells, in addition to re-supplying the bone with regenerative potential, also act at various levels in the hematopoiesis processes that occur in the spongy bone marrow spaces.

Mesenchymal cells (*see* 7.4) differentiate when they activate a differentiation program, genetic or epigenetic, in an osteogenetic sense: this occurs by the activation of specific genes in the DNA.[2,11,12]

Composition of the fundamental substance of the bone

Like all the connective tissues, bone consists of cells and an abundant intercellular substance. The characteristic of the fundamental substance of bone is that it is "hard", due to the presence of minerals, in percentage being 65% overall, while the organic part is 35%.

In the **organic component** of the fundamental substance, named *ossein*, there is a fibrillar part, composed of collagen fibers and an amorphous part, composed of *osteomucoid*, an interfibrillar substance consisting of glycoproteins and proteoglycans.

The organic matrix of bone contains, first of all, type I collagen (the most represented protein in the human body and which constitutes 90% of proteins in bone) and other molecules including osteonectin, osteocalcin, osteopontin, phosphoproteins, phospholipids and some proteoglycans (in particular, decorin and biglycan). Finally, some growth factors are present in the bone matrix which act at the paracrine level, i.e. locally.

The **inorganic component** is represented by calcium phosphate: for 85%, by calcium carbonate, for 10%, and, to a lesser extent, by magnesium phosphate and calcium fluoride. These salts are found in the form of submicroscopic, needle-like hexagonal crystals, 20-40 nm in length and 3-5 nm in thickness, having the structure of hydroxyapatite, arranged along the course of the collagen fibers.

The bone lamella, an elementary structure of the bone tissue

On macroscopic observation (i.e. without the use of a microscope), two types of bone tissue are distinguished: spongy bone and compact bone tissue. **Spongy bone tissue** is visible in the epiphyses of long bones, in the diploe of flat bones, and in short bones. It consists of *bone trabeculae* interconnected to form a three-dimensional network; the spaces delimited by the trabeculae are called medullary cavities and are occupied by the bone marrow. The orientation of the trabeculae is determined by the mechanical stress to which the bone is subjected, i.e. it corresponds to the trajectories of the lines of force resulting from the mechanical actions acting on the bone skeletal segment. The cavities delimited by the trabeculae of the spongy bone tissue are filled by the bone marrow: red (hemo-poietic tissue) or yellow type (adipose tissue).

The **compact bone tissue** appears, on the other hand, without trabeculae and cavities; it constitutes the body (or diaphysis) of the long bones and the superficial layer of their extremities, as well as the two bone tables that enclose the spongy tissue of the flat bones.

Each bone, except in correspondence with the articular surfaces, is surrounded by a particular connective lamina called the *periosteum*; a similar thinner lamina, called *endosteum*, covers the canal and the medullary cavities. Both the periosteum and the endosteum have osteogenic properties, as they contain osteogenetic cells (mesenchymal and osteoblasts).

At the microscopic level, the bone tissue can be distinguished into "non-lamellar" or "lamellar".

Non-lamellar bone tissue is present only during embryo-fetal development, in some limited areas of the adult skeleton (for example, the insertion areas of tendons) and in areas subject to bone regeneration (as in the case of fractures or surgical wounds). In the latter case, the absence of lamellar organization is an indication of tissue immaturity linked to new bone formation.

Lamellar bone tissue constitutes almost all the mature bone tissue, both spongy and compact. The fundamental histological unit consists of unitary structures called "bone lamellae", that are thin layers of fundamental substance, 5-10 µm thick, on whose surface there are cavities, bone gaps, containing osteocytes. In each lamella, the collagen fibers are arranged parallel, but their direction changes in the adjacent lamellae; in fact, the fibers of a lamella cross those belonging to the adjacent lamella with an angle of about 90°. Osteocytes and the lacunae are placed between one lamella and the other. The bone canaliculi cross the lamellae to anastomize with those originating from the nearby lacunae.

In spongy lamellar bone tissue, the lamellae are united to form trabeculae that delimit the medullary spaces, while, in the compact lamellar bone tissue, the lamellae are aggregated to form particular systems: the external and internal circumferential systems; the Havers systems (or osteons) and the interstitial systems. In particular in long bones (for example, in the upper and lower limbs), the circumferential systems are made up of lamellae arranged in several concentric layers, parallel to the external and internal surfaces of the bone.

The compact bone that constitutes the diaphysis of the long bones is crossed by canals containing the blood vessels and nerves destined for its supply and innervation; some of these canals (Havers canals) have a longitudinal course, while others, which come from the periosteum and endosteum, have a transverse course (Volkmann canals) and lead to the longitudinal ones. Around each Haversian canal, some bone lamellae are arranged concentrically: the canal and the concentric bone lamellae with the related osteocytes form the osteon, which can be considered the structural unit of compact bone.

Histogenesis of bone tissue

Bone tissue in humans derives, in extreme synthesis, from the *mesenchyme*.[1,10,13] Mesenchyma is an immature embryonic tissue that can give rise to numerous cellular jambs. Its derivation is mainly from the *intraembryonic mesoderm* and the ectomesenchyma. It must be taken into account that the human embryo, at the end of the third week, is made up of three laminar structures (primitive sheets: ectoderm, mesoderm and endoderm) which subsequently, in the fourth week of development, organize into a three-dimensional structure. Here begins the first formation of the bone tissue, in particular in correspondence with the mesodermal structures, called *somites*, which will make up the entire axial skeleton. It is the notochord, an organizing structure of the embryo, that guides the first development of the bones. Meanwhile, at the end of the fourth week of development, after the *demarcation of the embryo* has taken place, the *stomodeum* (the primitive buccal cavity) is also formed and, at the beginning of the second month of foetal development the formation of the craniofacial bone structures begins.

There are numerous genetic and molecular mechanisms that regulate the formation and development of the bone tissue, both at the embryonic level and throughout adult life, which will not, however, be discussed here.[12–14] Bone tissue is in fact a metabolically active tissue ready to self-regenerate, as in the case of damage or after appropriate stimulations. This characteristic is the basis of numerous therapeutic approaches in the orthopedic and dental fields. The histogenetic processes of the bone tissue include several phases: 1) the recruitment at the genetic level (*commitment*) of the undifferentiated stem cell into a progenitor bone cell; 2) the activation of the osteogenic cell into an osteoblastic or osteoclastic cell; 3) the modulation of osteoblastic-osteoclastic activities. Each of these phases is determined by the activation and deactivation of tissue-specific genes that find expression at the level of morphology and cellular activity (in particular the production of specific organic molecules of the bone matrix described above).

From the mesenchymal tissue (which should be considered a still immature connective tissue) bone tissue will be generated in two different ways: the mesenchyme differentiates directly into a bone tissue or a cartilage tissue. Named respectively the *direct* (or *free*) *ossification* or the *indirect* (or *chondral*) *ossification*.

Direct ossification takes place in the case of the bones of the cranial vault, the mandible, the tympanic ring, almost all the bones of the face, the clavicle and the sesamoid bones.

If the direct ossification process occurs in the mesenchymal fibrillar connective tissue without any spatial relationship with the cartilaginous skeleton, the ossification is called *membranous*.

On the other hand, in the case in which direct ossification occurs in the mesenchyme surrounding a cartilaginous skeletal segment, we talk of *direct mantle ossification*. However, the cartilage serves only as a support, and not as a model for the bone being formed and therefore the bones develop outside the perichondrium, without tracing the shape and size of the cartilage element. In this way, the mantle bones are formed including the mandible and those that take part in the formation of the skeleton of nasal cavities.

Most of the skeleton, however, is made up of cartilage before becoming bone; the ossification process therefore takes place within the cartilaginous outline and this is the reason why the ossification process is defined as condral. It can take place on the periphery of the cartilage due to the activity of the perichondrium (*perichondral ossification*) or within the cartilage (*endochondral ossification*). In any case, the bone tissue replaces the cartilage that acts as a model and gradually disappears. The bones thus formed are called replacement bones (vertebrae, ribs, sternum, shoulder blades, pelvic girdle, limbs and skull base bones).

A perfect example of chondral ossification is what occurs in the diaphysis of the long bones of the body (7.5) where, in correspondence with the elongation cartilage, the growing cartilage is replaced by bone through extraordinary genetic, molecular and cellular mechanisms which, if altered, can cause serious osteoskeletal pathologies.

The histogenetic events that lead to the formation of mature bone are very different in the case of direct or indirect ossification. From a clinical point of view, it is interesting to observe that some histological aspects of bone generation/regeneration in the case of bone grafting, stimulation (osteoinductive or osteoconductive), guided regeneration, cell or tissue therapy at the level of the jaw bones are similar to what happens in direct ossification where no cartilage is in place to form bone (*see* 7.3).

As already mentioned, the direct or membranous ossification process occurs in the mesenchyme or in the already differentiated connective tissue. It begins in the *ossification centers* and proceeds in a centrifugal direction. The process is characterized by a thickening of the mesenchyme, by an increase in vascularization, consequent to the neoformation of blood vessels and by the differentiation of mesenchymal cells into osteoblasts. These cells begin to produce a soft and viscous intercellular substance, consisting of collagen fibrils and amorphous substance, which takes the name of *osteoid or pre-osseous substance* (*see* 7.1 and 7.3). While the osteoblasts remained imprisoned in the substance they elaborate, they are transformed, achieving long extensions, into osteocytes, calcification of the osteoid tissue takes place and therefore a first bone trabecula is formed. Around the trabecula other osteoblasts are arranged in a row, which gives rise to a new pre-osseous substance in

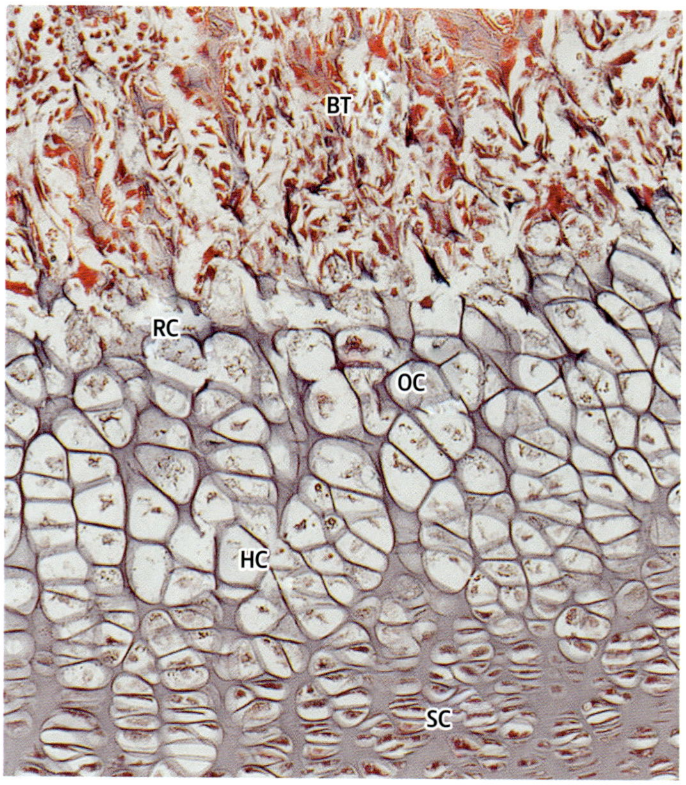

7.5 Chondral histogenesis process in the epiphysis of a long bone of a young rat. The cartilage cells are gradually replaced by bone cells that provide for the formation of the bone head. Cartilage cells ensure both the growth in length of the bone and the tissue matrix for osteogenesis. The various maturation stages that lead to the transformation of cartilage into bone are observed: serial cartilage (SC), hypertrophic cartilage (HC), ossifying cartilage (OC), regressing cartilage (RC) and bone tissue (BT). Staining with hematoxylin and eosin. Original enlargement 200×.

which they end up enclosed, becoming osteocytes. The process, which continues through subsequent deposition of osteoid layers by new series of osteoblasts that differ from the surrounding mesenchyme, leads to a greater extension of the developing trabeculae and to the establishment of an irregular network of trabeculae, between whose meshes (primitive medullary spaces) are the blood vessels that remain imprisoned in the bone and a part of the mesenchyme from which bone marrow, osteoblasts and even osteoclasts will originate. The first developed bone, with intertwined fibers, is then replaced by the lamellar bone. The areas destined to be made up of cancellous bone maintain their trabecular arrangement (formed in any case by lamellae) delimiting the medullary spaces. In the parts where the compact bone will be formed, the lamellae will be arranged concentrically within the medullary spaces, gradually reducing their width: these spaces are the primitive Haversian canals, containing blood vessels and bone marrow.

How bone mineralization occurs

The presence of calcium salts in the form of mineral crystals represents the main characteristic of the so-called "hard tissues" of our organism. These are five: bone, cartilage, dentin, cementum and tooth enamel. With the exception of the dental enamel, which is of ectodermal and epithelial derivation, all the others derive from mesenchyme of mesodermal or ectodermal derivation (ectomesenchyma).

Although the mineralization process of the fundamental substance of bone, cartilage and dentin has been studied for a long time, many aspects still remain unclear, especially regarding the early stages.

This process represents the series of events leading to the formation and deposition of crystalline structures within the intercellular matrix of hard tissues. From a chemical point of view, the process generates hydroxyapathic crystals $[Ca_{10}(PO_4)_6(OH)_2]$ which, under the electron microscope, appear as thin needles about 20-40 nm long and 2-3 nm thick.[15]

Three phases can be recognized in the mineralization of the bone matrix (7.6 and 7.7).

In the first phase, osteoblasts secrete organic matrix (in particular collagen and non-collagenic proteins) and particular vesicles (called *matrix vesicles*) surrounded by a membrane, with a diameter of 50-200 nm.[16,17] These vesicles originate from the Golgi apparatus of the osteoblast and contain numerous substances including enzymes such as alkaline phosphatase, phospholipids capable of binding calcium and growth factors. Furthermore, the vesicle membrane contains some proteins, such as annexins, capable of transporting calcium and phosphorus ions.

In the second phase (vesicular phase), the vesicles – which have accumulated calcium and phosphorus – begin to accumulate the calcium and phosphorus salts to form the first crystalline structures inside them. The action of alkaline phosphatase (which is also a histochemical marker of osteoblasts) seems essential in regulating the availability of phosphorus. The crystalline structures grow due to the entry of phosphorus and calcium ions, resulting in the consequent rupture of the vesicle membrane.

In the third phase (fibrillar phase), hydroxyapatite crystals grow further in the bone extracellular matrix and form the so-called *matrix nodules* (also called *ossifying globules*), which associate with the organic matrix of the osteoid substance, in particular with collagen fibrils (*see* 7.7).

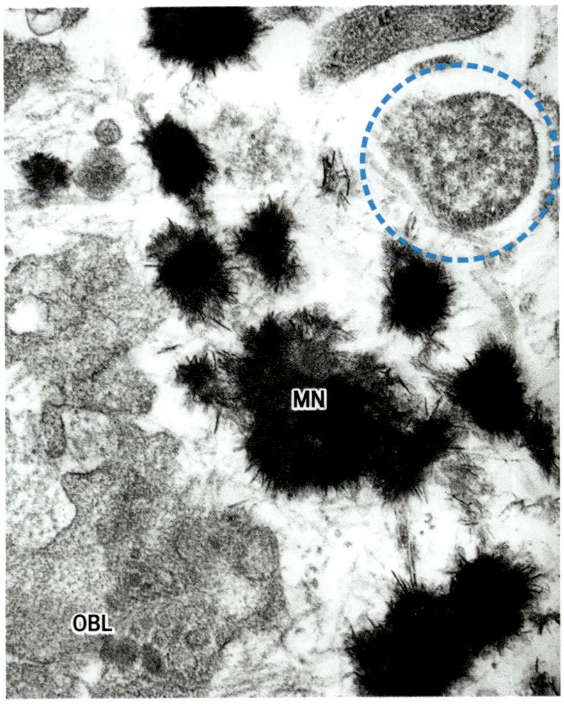

7.6 Process of mineralization observed under the electron microscope. A vesicle of the matrix (circulated in blue) seems to pour its contents outwards. The developing crystalline structures (irregularly shaped and strongly electron-dense) that form the mineralization nucleus (MN) are identified. Around it are identified the collagen fibrils in the process of maturation. Bottom left, the apical surface of an odontoblast (OBL). Dentinogenesis in the dental sketch of a newborn rat. Staining with uranyl acetate and lead citrate. Original enlargement 60,000×.

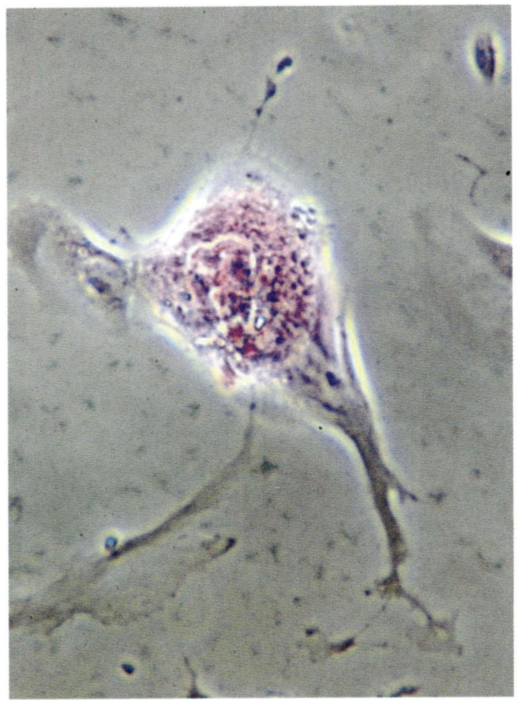

7.7 Development in vitro of bone tissue: a modern biomedical strategy. Mesenchymal stem cells are isolated, cultured and stimulated in an osteo-inductive environment. The Von Kossa reaction (*in red*) shows the osteogenic differentiation of the mesenchymal cell. 100× original enlargement.

It is precisely on the collagen fibers that the hydroxyapatite crystals are deposited and therefore we call them "mineralized collagen".

Some non-collagenic proteins of the bone matrix, such as osteopontin and osteocalcin, play a role in modulating the growth of the nodules of the matrix, while the proteoglycans decorin and biglycan seem to associate peripherally with the growing nodules. Other proteins, such as osteonectin, would take part in the mineralization of collagen. At the level of collagen fibers, the first deposition of the crystals would occur in correspondence with the space between the tropocollagen molecules, which are aligned with each other.

The different embryological derivation of dental enamel (the hardest tissue in our body) determines different mineralization mechanisms; on the other hand, enamel is the only hard tissue free of collagen fibers and its matrix contains different proteins (amelogenins and enameline in particular) involved in the formation initially of crystals and subsequently of enamel prisms[18,19] (*see* 7.3). However, we know that enamel matrix proteins have osteoinductive capabilities and, in the course of development, contribute to dentinogenesis and cementogenesis.[3]

The plasticity of bone tissue and its clinical implications

Bone tissue is extremely dynamic and responsive. As is well known, during our life our bones continue to "remodel", i.e. they undergo modifications that consist of deposition and resorption of bone tissue. Our bone tissue is believed to be completely replaced every 10 years or so. This remodeling is related to various factors, especially metabolic, endocrine (for example, calcium homeostasis) and mechanical. Osteoblasts possess an organ (the primary edge) which represents a sensor for any mechanical stress or strain,[5-7] which causes bone deposition to occur according to the applied load. From this problems related to situations of absence of gravity can origin rather than a therapeutic need to mechanically "load" the bone tissue in the process of formation. The localization and formation of the bone lamellae are in fact induced and regulated by the mechanical stimulation.

But the presence of osteoprogenitor stem cells, especially at the endosteal and periosteal level, allows the bone tissue to regenerate when damaged, such as the healing of fractures or following surgical treatments (orthopedic or dental).

Even in the case of prosthetic interventions (including dental implants) and bone grafts (autologous or heterologous), the bone tissue shows great plasticity.

It is thanks to its great reactivity and resilience that bone tissue constitutes one of the most interesting tissues from a biomedical point of view. Histogenetic knowledge provides the scientific basis for techniques based on natural principles that regulate bone formation. The techniques based on this principle are called "biomimetic" and they include cell therapy and tissue therapy, as well as the use of biological matrices, cell growth and differentiation factors.[9,20-22]

The strategies for bone regeneration are many, but certainly the use of biological material derived from our bone and dental tissues undoubtedly has many advantages and respects the ecological principle: "*re-use, re-fill, re-cycle, re-generated*".

Review of published articles with histological examples

E. Minetti

Our research group has carried out several studies and analyses of the tooth used as a graft material. Seven publications have been published to date in which we have considered the histologies and correlated histomorphometric analyses.

From the data that emerged from the histological examinations, the average of the newly formed vital bone following the regeneration procedures appears to be about 27.46%, a remarkable value.

However, it is necessary to understand and distinguish which values are reported in the histomorphometries.

BV (Bone Volume). This value indicates the amount of mineralized structure present in the analyzed sample. It includes both the regenerated bone tissue and the graft material residues. It is a value that can be very high even in the presence of little vital bone.

RG (Residual Graft). This value indicates the amount of grafting material still present in the analyzed sample. The higher it is, the greater are the residues of grafting material.

VB (Vital Bone). This datum is the most important, because it indicates the amount of bone that is actually newly formed.

It is possible to have a very high VB but which almost entirely contains only grafting material and therefore, for example, does not guarantee integration to an implant. A high VB value, on the other hand, indicates a large amount of regenerated vital bone, bone that will be part of the bone metabolism and therefore will guarantee the following stability and integration.

In the published research, various histological aspects of the use of the tooth as graft material were analyzed, as illustrated in the tables on pages 106-107 (7.1-7.7).

Examples of histological material of dental origin

P. Savadori

In this chapter, the behavior of the tooth treated with the Tooth Transformer (TT) device will be analyzed at a histological level and how this becomes part of the bone regeneration process. Some images, relating to demineralized and non-demineralized samples of newly formed bone tissue, will allow you to view the functional relationships between the dentin, enamel and the bone granules.

The dentin granules, but also the enamel ones, although less represented in terms of quantity, have a marked osteoconductive capacity. They act as the basis for the deposition of a new bone matrix, which is gener-

Multicenter studies and clinical cases

7.1 Comparison between endodontically treated and natural teeth[23]

Title	**Alveolar Socket Preservation with Different Autologous Graft Materials: Preliminary Results of a Multicenter Pilot Study in Human**
Authors	E. Minetti, E. Giacometti, U. Gambardella, M. Contessi, A. Ballini, G. Marenzi, M. Celko, F. Mastrangelo
Publication	Materials 2020;13(5):1153
Kind of activity	Prospective multicenter study
Number of samples analyzed	28 patients – 34 socket preservation – 32 histologies
Type of analysis performed	Histomorphometric analysis
Summary of the results	(see table below) 2 groups: group 1 whole teeth – group 2 devitalized teeth
Material analyzed	Bone biopsy samples taken 4 months after regeneration by dental graft

	BV Bone Volume		RG Residual Graft		VB Vital Bone	
Dataset	1	2	1	2	1	2
Sample size	19	13	19	13	19	13
Average	40.4800	40.2801	19.7017	17.3983	20.7800	22.8900
Standard deviation	8.9032	11.5104	13.7533	7.0935	13.2970	9.7245
T	0.6871		0.5536		0.4887	
Degree of freedom	30		30		30	
p-value (significance level)	0.4973		0.5840		0.6286	

Analyze: $p > 0.05$ No statistical significance value; $p < 0.05$ the hypothesis is wrong

2 groups: group 1 whole teeth – group 2 devitalized teeth

7.2 Endodontically treated teeth used as grafting material[24]

Title	**Autologous Tooth Graft after Endodontical Treated Used for Socket Preservation: A Multicenter Clinical Study**
Authors	E. Minetti, A. Palermo, F. Ferrante, J.H. Schmitz, H.K.L. Ho, S.Ng.D. Hann, E. Giacometti, U. Gambardella, M. Contessi, M. Celko, A. Ballini, C. Mortellaro, P. Trisi, F. Mastrangelo
Publication	Appl Sci 2019;9(24):5396
Kind of activity	Prospective multicenter study
Number of samples analyzed	98 patients – 106 sites treated with socket preservation using endodontically treated teeth – 13 histologies
Type of analysis performed	Histomorphometric analysis
Summary of the results	• VB %: 24.87 ± 9.72 • BV %: 16.6 ± 7.09 • GRAFT %: 41.47 ± 11.51
Material analyzed	Bone biopsy samples taken 4 months after regeneration by dental graft

7.3 Sinus lift using the tooth as graft material[25]

Title	**Autologous Tooth Graft for Maxillary Sinus Augmentation: A Multicenter Clinical Study**
Authors	E. Minetti, A. Palermo, M. Contessi, U. Gambardella, J. Schmitz, E. Giacometti, M. Celko, P. Trisi
Publication	Int J Growth Factors Stem Cells Dent 2019;2(3):45-51
Kind of activity	Prospective multicenter study
Number of samples analyzed	23 patients – 40 sites treated with sinus lift – 5 histologies
Type of analysis performed	Histomorphometric analysis
Summary of the results	• Bone Volume/Total Volume: 36.284 ± 9.77 • Residual Graft/Total Volume: 14.61 ± 14.61 • Vital Bone/Total Bone: 21.5 ± 8.61
Material analyzed	Bone biopsy samples taken 4 months after regeneration by dental graft

7.4 Post-GBR histological analysis (4 months)[26,27]

Title	**Tooth Transformer®: A New Method to Prepare Autologous Tooth Grafts – Histologic and Histomorphometric Analyses of 11 Consecutive Clinical Cases**
Authors	E. Minetti, A. Palermo, P. Trisi, S.L. Taschieri
Publication	Int J Growth Factors Stem Cells Dent 2019;2(3):56-61
Kind of activity	Case series
Number of samples analyzed	11 patients – 11 histologies
Type of analysis performed	Histomorphometric analysis
Summary of the results	• Bone Volume/Total Volume: 43.97 ± 7.38 • Residual Graft/Total Volume: 24.51 ± 15.95
Material analyzed	Bone biopsy samples taken 4 months after regeneration by dental graft

7.5 Post-GBR histological analysis (6 months)[26,27]

Title	**A New Tooth Processing Apparatus Allowing to Obtain Dentin Grafts for Bone Augmentation: The Tooth Transformer**
Authors	E. Minetti, M. Berardini, P. Trisi
Publication	Open Dent J 2019;13(1):6-14
Kind of activity	Case series
Number of samples analyzed	15 patients – 19 implants – 11 socket preservation – 4 sinus lifts – 15 histologies
Type of analysis performed	Histomorphometric analysis
Summary of the results	
Material analyzed	Bone biopsy samples taken 4 months after regeneration by dental graft

7.6 Regeneration using deciduous teeth[28]

Title	**Autologous Deciduous Tooth-Derived Material for Alveolar Ridge Preservation: A Clinical and Histological Case Report**
Authors	E. Minetti, S.L. Taschieri, S. Corbella
Publication	Case Rep Dent 2020; 2020:2936878
Kind of activity	Case report
Number of samples analyzed	1 patient – 2 implants – 1 histology of deciduous teeth extracted 20 years previously used as dental graft
Type of analysis performed	Histomorphometric analysis
Summary of the results	• Bone Volume/Total Volume: 47.22% • Residual Graft/Total Volume: 18.68% • Vital Bone/Total Bone: 28.55%
Material analyzed	Bone biopsy samples taken 4 months after regeneration by dental graft of a deciduous tooth

7.7 Comparison between tooth and tooth mixed with xenographic material[29]

Title	**Autologous Tooth Graft: A Histological Comparison Between Dentin Mixed with Xenograft and Dentin Alone Grafts in Socket Preservation**
Authors	E. Minetti, A. Palermo, P. Savadori, A. Barlattani, R. Franco, M. Michele, F. Gianfreda, P. Bollero
Publication	J Biol Regul Homeost Agents 2019;33(6 Suppl. 2):189-197
Kind of activity	Case series comparison
Number of samples analyzed	6 patients – 6 histologies – 2 groups: • group 1: 3 dentin histologies • group 2: 3 histologies of 50% dentin and 50% Bio-Oss
Type of analysis performed	Histomorphometric analysis
Summary of the results	see table below
Material analyzed	Bone biopsy samples taken 4 months after regeneration by dental graft or dental graft + Bio-Oss The results indicated that using only dentin there was an increase of 85% of vital bone and 83% less residual graft material

	Group 1	Group 2
BV% (Bone Volume)	57.22 ± 8.71	55.5 ± 16.51%
Residual Graft%	18.95 ± 10.99	34.87 ± 9.21%
VB% (Vital Bone)	38.26 ± 6.93	20.63 ± 5.82%

ated by the osteoblasts who are arranged on the perimeter of the granules (7.8 and 7.9).

This deposition does not seem to vary according to whether one is in the presence of dentin or enamel and appears to be an intrinsic property (7.10).

The figure (*see* 7.10) shows newly formed bone that surrounds a granule of enamel and one of dentin.

The newly formed tissue is closely linked to the bone substitute: the distribution appears uniform without the presence of spacing, as can be seen from the detail in the figure (7.11), there is total continuity between the two different types of fabric.

The new bone matrix is able to penetrate deeply into the non-resorbed dentin granules, as shown in the figure (7.12).

A crack completely filled with new bone is clearly visible; a similar situation is shown in the figure (7.13), where a space formed within a dentin granule was filled with new bone tissue.

This osteoconductive capacity seems independent from the age, the type of tooth and the state of the tooth at the time of extraction: no differences attributable to these factors were found in all the analyzed biopsies.

As an example, the figures (7.14 and 7.15) illustrate a regeneration performed using deciduous teeth: the osteoconductive properties are optimal, both in the presence of dentin and in the presence of enamel.

The only difference that can be found in the two types of granules consists in their profile: since the enamel is much harder and more mineralized than dentin, it is not reshaped like the latter, which leads to a different profile due to the maintenance of the breaking lines created by the Tooth Transformer. However, this profile variation does not seem to alter the deposition of the new bone tissue.

Dentin is recognized by the body as its own bone tissue: it is involved in the same bone remodeling processes and it is treated physiologically by osteoclasts and osteoblasts. The granules, when not completely resorbed, show characteristic signs of resorption on their profile as due to the work of the osteoclasts.

In the figure (7.16) it is possible to see a dentin granule which has a very visible resorption zone, while in the previous one (*see* 7.15) it is possible to see an osteoclast, easily recognizable by its multi-nucleated cytoplasm, while degrading a dentin granule.

Dentin can follow different paths, thus not only being completely resorbed or serving as a support function. In the figure (7.17) a dentin granule can be observed which constitutes a sort of "hybrid": the dentinal tubules are visible but have lost their structure; it is possible to distinguish two types of arrangement but they appear intertwined and fused together. Another example of this process can be seen in the figure (7.18).

In the case presented in the figure (7.19), the transition between dentin and bone is "blurred" in comparison to the image shown in the previous figure (*see* 7.18): on the left handside a piece of dentin is recognizable,

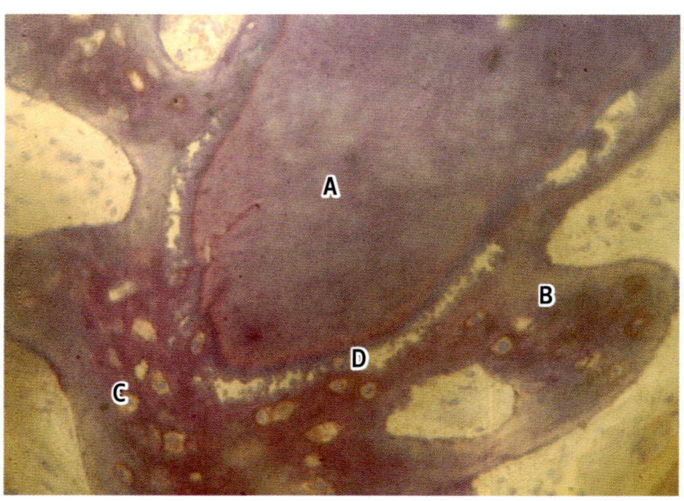

7.8 Dentin granule (A) surrounded by newly formed bone (B). The osteocytes (C) still close together are clearly visible in the bone, indicating a young bone, while calcification nuclei are distinguishable in the bone-dentin interface (D). Ground section, 200× enlargement, color: basic fuchsin. (Histology performed by P. Trisi.)

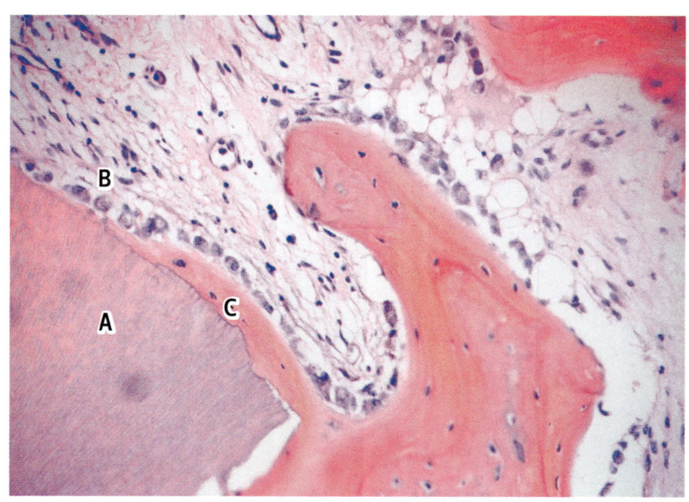

7.9 Dentin granule (A) where osteoblasts arranged in a palisade are depositing the new bone matrix (B). The new tissue is deposited directly on the dentin in successive layers (C). This aspect delineates the osteoconductive capacity of dentin. Transferred section, enlargement 400×, stain: hematoxylin and eosin.

characterized by the presence of dentinal tubules in cross section, which has been converted into bone without a clear separation between the tissues. In this particular case, it is possible to identify an osteocyte located at the interface between the two types of tissue. Another relevant detail, which denotes a very fluid transition between the two arrangements, is the lack of a chromaticity difference. While in general the dentin granules tend to color with a lighter tone than the bone tissue, in this particular case this chromatic discrepancy is not encounterable and this indicates that we are dealing with two tissues of very similar composition.

Although the tooth has proved to be a good bone substitute, capable of guiding the regeneration of a bone defect in a very accurate way, we can find ourselves faced with situations in which regeneration has been insufficient and/or disorganized. The reasons for these failures can be many and are not part of this chapter; however, four different possible regenerations are shown in the figures (7.20-7.23) (where 1 indicates the highest

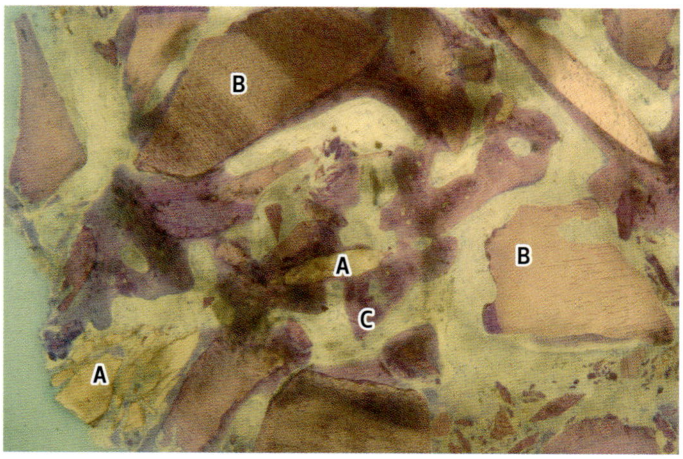

7.10 The enamel (A), light color shaded because unable to retain the colorant due to its very compact structure, shows the same osteoconductive capabilities of dentin (B). Bone tissue (C) has no difference in the way it is deposited regardless of whether it is in front of enamel or dentin. Ground section, 100× enlargement, stain: basic fucsin. (Histology performed by P. Trisi.)

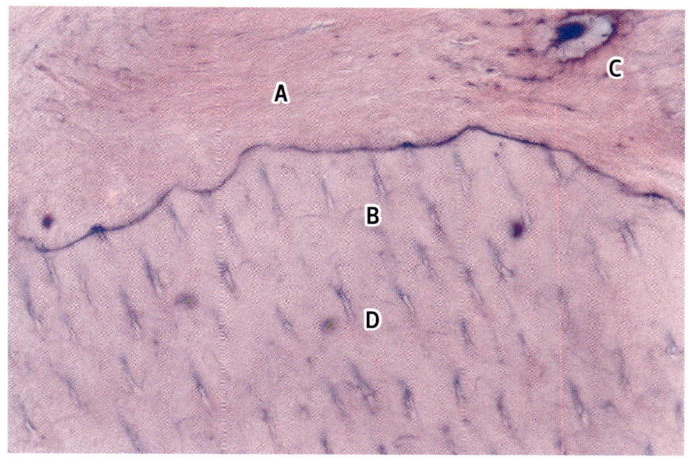

7.11 Junction between newly formed bone anc a dentin granule. In the upper part of the image (A) there is newly formed bone, where it is possible to see an osteocyte with its cytoplasmic extensions, within a bone gap. In the underlying part (B) there is dentin, recognizable by the dentinal tubules (D), firmly attached to the bone: as you can see, the junction between the two tissues does not present any kind of discontinuity. Decalcified section, enlargement 1,000×, stain: hematoxylin and eosin.

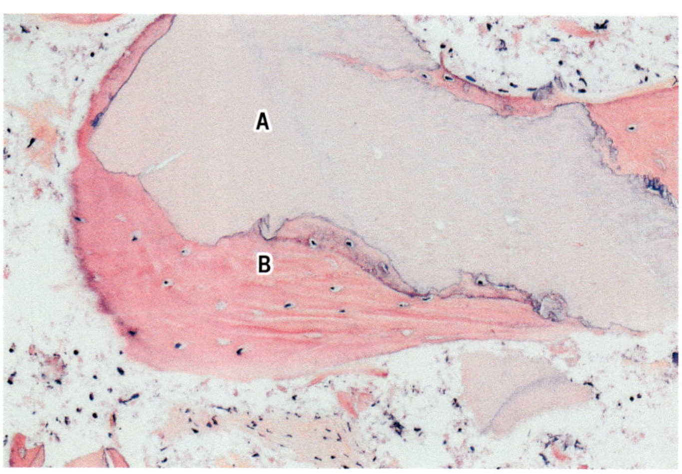

7.12 Example of bone apposition (B) on dentin (A). It is possible to see how osteoblasts are able to deposit new tissue around the entire perimeter of the granule, regardless of the presence of irregularities. Decalcified section, enlargement 200×, stain: hematoxylin and eosin.

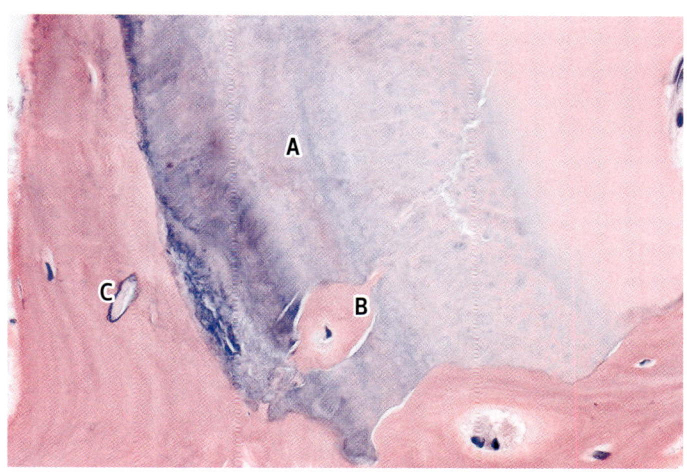

7.13 InfiltrazioneInfiltration of bone tissue (B) within a space present in the dentin granule (A). In this image we can appreciate the ability of dentin to act as an excellent support for osteoblasts, which can penetrate even in very limited spaces. It is also possible to see a small fragment of dentin (C), not resorbed but included in the bone. Undecalcifiec section, enlargement 400×, stain: hematoxylin and eosin.

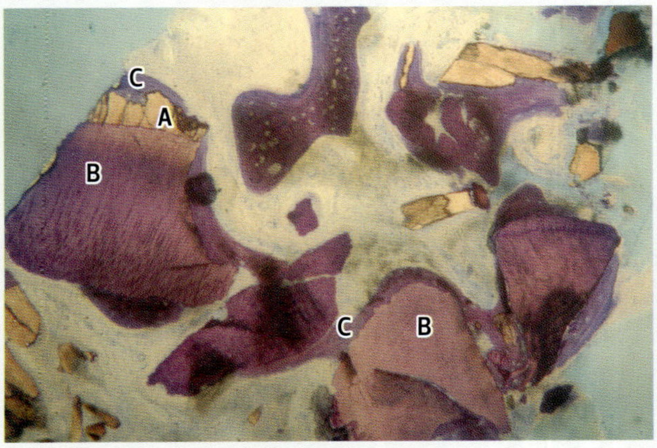

7.14 Deciduous tooth used for bone regeneration: enamel (A) and dentin (B) of deciduous teeth, show characteristics comparable to those of permanent teeth. The bone apposition (C) follows the same dynamics observed in all other cases. Undescaled section, 100× enlargement, stain: basic fuchsin. (Histology performed by P. Trisi.)

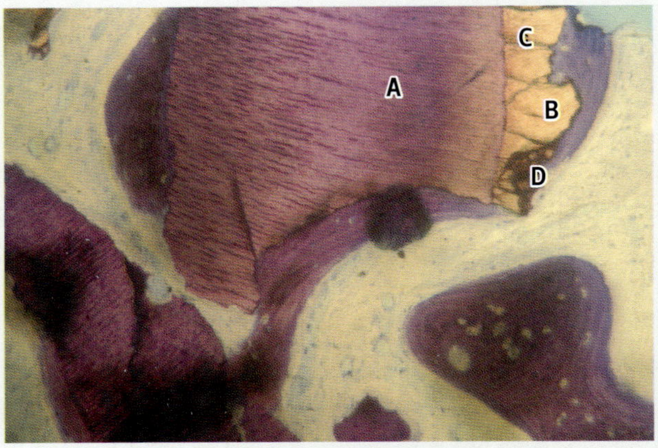

7.15 Detail of Figure 7.14. The structural difference between dentin (A) and enamel (B) can be observed. The dentin forms granules with a regular profile and a homogeneous surface, the enamel has a serrated profile (D) and fracture lines (C). This is due to the greater hardness of this type of structure; however these physical differences do not affect the osteoconductive properties. Not decalcified section, enlargement 200×, stain: basic fuchsin. (Histology performed by P. Trisi.)

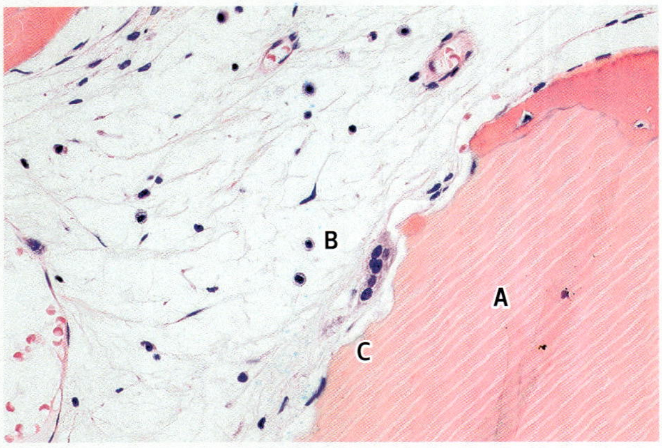

7.16 Dentin granule (A) which is actively reabsorbed by an osteoclast (B), which generates the classic corrugated resorption profile. This image shows how dentin becomes part of the bone tissue homeostasis process. Decalcified section, enlargement 200×, stain: hematoxylin and eosin.

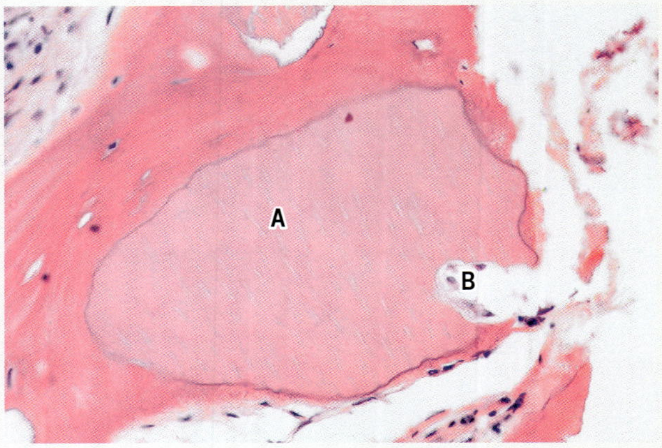

7.17 Dentin granule (A) showing a characteristic sign of resorption by osteoclasts (B). In the reabsorption gap there are some osteoblasts that will fill this newly formed space. Decalcified section, enlargement 200×, stain: hematoxylin and eosin.

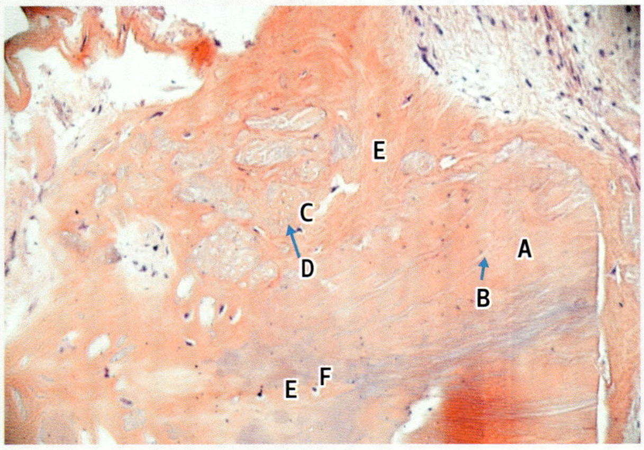

7.18 Hybrid bone-dentin tissue. This image shows a portion where dentin (A) and bone (E) form a kind of hybrid tissue, where the boundary between the two types of tissue is not easily recognizable. The dentin still has the dentinal tubules, visible in longitudinal section (B) or in cross section (D). The area occupied by the bone tissue is highlighted by the presence of osteocytes (C), but the transition between the two different types of tissue is very blurred (F). Decalcified section, enlargement 200×, stain: hematoxylin and eosin.

density level and 4 the lowest density level) according to the quality of the new tissue, where level 4 represents the qualitatively worst one and level 1 the best one.

The quality of newly formed bone is inversely proportional to the amount of residual dentin. This aspect may be quite intuitive and obvious, but unlike the other bone substitutes, which can lead to excellent bone regeneration while retaining their presence, dentin is "converted" into bone, therefore a very good regeneration will have a little residual dentin tissue.

In a level 4 core, the dentin has not been reabsorbed and a real process of osteogenesis has not started: the granules are enveloped by fibroblasts and connective tissue, starting what is called a process of fibro-integration. The resulting tissue is of poor quality and disorganized.

A level 3 core shows a certain amount of bone but, at the same time, a significant amount of non-resorbed dentin. Unlike the previous case, the bone regeneration process was able to begin and continue even if in a non-optimal manner.

At level 2 there is a significant amount of newly formed bone, there are still non-resorbed granules, often due to the presence of dense connective tissue that has infiltrated during the healing of the soft tissues. In this case, the main component is the newly formed bone which shows a good degree of organization and is, therefore, an index of stability.

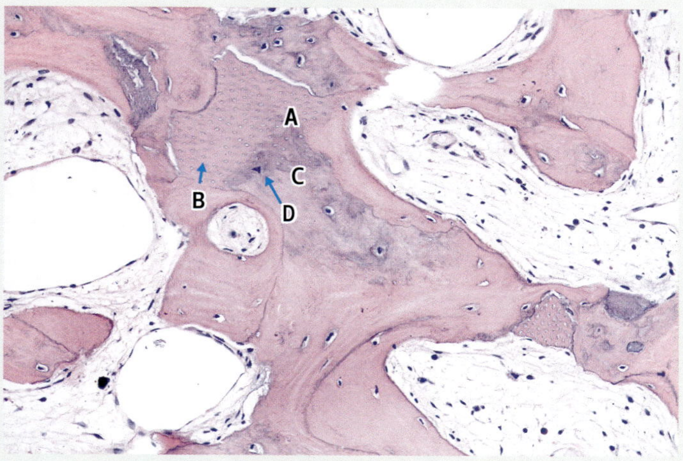

7.19 Dentin-bone transition. In this detail, a piece of dentin (A) can be seen, recognizable by the presence of tubules in transverse section (B), which makes a sort of transition into bone (C). It is a similar situation to that shown in Figure 7.17, but here there is a very "soft" transition, also characterized by the maintenance of the same chromaticity of the tissues, indicating a very similar tissue composition. Also in this case the osteocytes (D) mark the presence of the bone tissue. Undecalcified section, enlargement 200×, stain: hematoxylin and eosin.

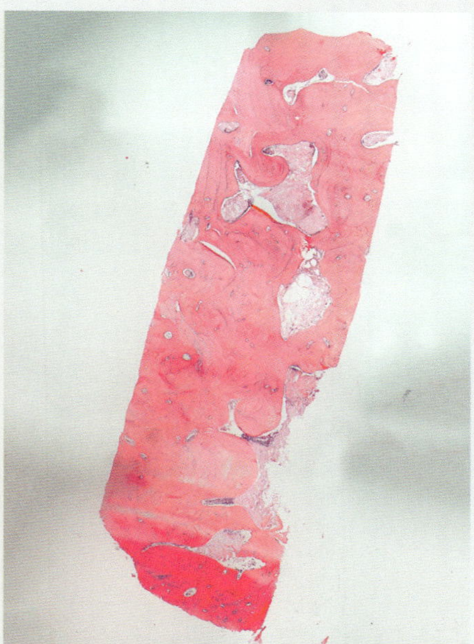

7.20 Level 4 regeneration.

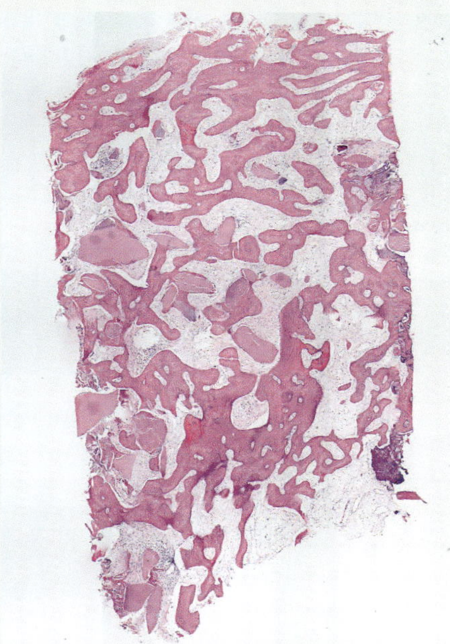

7.21 Level 3 regeneration.

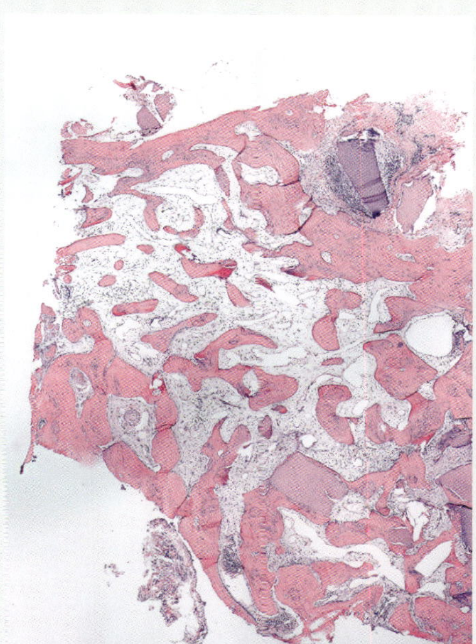

7.22 Level 2 regeneration.

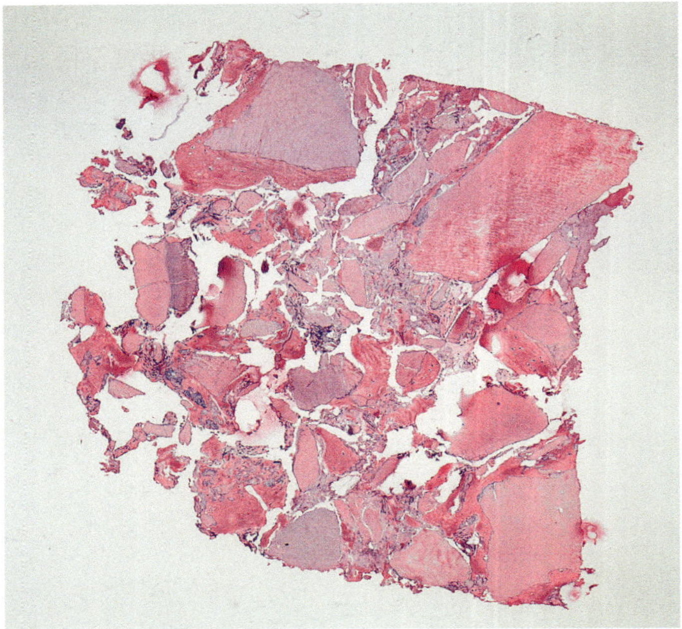

7.23 Level 1 regeneration.

Level 1 shows almost total resorption and conversion of dentin granules. The newly formed tissue is mostly represented by bone tissue which can be very dense, similar to cortical bone. Some dentin granules can be found, but they are usually found well embedded in the bone tissue.

Preliminary data from ongoing studies

E. Minetti

A variable to be taken into consideration with grafting materials which, like the tooth, are reabsorbed over time is precisely the time passing between grafting and biopsy sampling in order to be able to interpret the possible resorption curve.

As known, the biopsy freezes the image of the collected tissue consistent within that single moment. Over time, using resorbable materials, less and less material will remain.

Therefore, carrying on with a sample analysis after 4 months or after 8 months can give different results. This is why the tests shown in the tables on pages 106-107 (*see* 7.1 and 7.7) were all performed at 4 months.

Having available numerous histological samples performed by all the members of the working group, consisting of 11 clinical centers, we analyzed the data with different interpretations. These data represent preliminary analyzes of a larger study that will be completed in the coming years.

Analysis over time (<4 months, 4-6 months, >6 months)

Trying to have an indication of the volumetric changes over time, we divided a sample of 78 histologies into three temporal periods of sampling and their consequent histomorphometric values (up to 4 months, 4-6 months and over 6 months).

With all the possible limitations due to different operators, different procedures, different sites and three-dimensional conformations of the defects and number, we can still make some percentage considerations in the attempt to understand the evolution of the tooth as graft material over time (7.8).

From these data we can conclude that timewise there is an increase in bone tissue inversely proportional to the amount of the residual material. In fact, in the sample under examination, the values of residual material over time have a decrease of 36% and an increase of about 10% in the quantity of vital bone.

7.8 Analysis over time

Biopsy made	No. of biopsy samples	Bone Volume/Total Volume	Residual Graft/Total Volume	Vital Bone/Total Bone
Within 4 months	38	41.8 ± 13.59	12.98 ± 13.14	28.82 ± 19.43
Between 4 and 6 months	24	43.03 ± 7.66	12.69 ± 9.2	30.34 ± 13.19
Over 6 months	16	45.81 ± 13.96	8.29 ± 9.19*	37.52 ± 17.02

* Some samples no longer had granules present on histomorphometric evaluation.

Analysis by operator

The same data were also analysed by different examiners. Each examiner performed histological samples and histomorphometric data were reported (7.9). The analysis was carried out in this way to evaluate the correlation between manual skills and the different results in histomorphometric terms.

Obviously, a greater number allows for a more realistic average since clinical successes and failures are added on average.

7.9 Analysis by operator

Operator	No. of biopsy samples	Vital Bone/Total Bone
A	38	32.70 ± 17.39
B	5	30.97 ± 13.99
C	18	27.37 ± 10.26
D	3	36.86 ± 13.54
E	9	36.91 ± 12.05
F	4	46.27 ± 20.72

Analysis by surgical technique. Membranes and platelet derivatives

The evaluation of the results of the histomorphometries referred to a specific type of surgery that was carried out (7.10). With the limitations linked to the sample size, however, differences have been highlighted regarding some technical details of the individual therapies regarding ridge preservation.

In this preliminary study, similarities were highlighted in the characteristics of the regenerated bone tissue, despite the fact that different types of membranes were used, which instead should have generated very different results.

In the provided information on pages 114-118 (Boxes 7.1 and 7.2), two experts in the field provide us with a quick overview of the characteristics of the membranes used and the platelet derivatives used.

In the provided analysis on pages 118-122 (Box 7.3) an expert shows us a picture of biocentric surgery using only autologous materials.

Distribution of the results of histomorphometric analysis

We evaluated 120 histomorfometries to understand the correlation between the graft material, derived from the tooth, reabsorption and the amount of newformed bone.

Inserted the data in the diagram (7.24) it has been immediately noticed that the greater part of the samples had an amount of residual inferior to 10%.

In addition, these samples were found to be those with the largest amount of newly formed bone.

In the diagram we can understand that there is therefore an inversely proportional correlation between the amount of bone and the residual graft material.

7.10 Analysis by surgical technique

Surgical technique	No. of biopsy samples	Bone Volume/Total Volume	Residual Graft Total Volume	Vital Bone/Total Bone
Collagen membrane[1]	32	46.01 ± 13.91	12.92 ± 13.73	33.09 ± 18.81
Collagen membrane[2]	10	44.62 ± 6.98	8.05 ± 8.38	36.57 ± 11.42
Collagen membrane[3]	6	51.59 ± 11.58	8.14 ± 9.23	43.45 ± 19.54
Collagen membrane[4] + CGF	6	39.54 ± 10.39	8.57 ± 10.70	30.97 ± 13.99
Collagen membrane[5] + PRF	3	40.82 ± 8.78	3.96 ± 3.10	36.86 ± 11.88
PRGF membrane	5	40.46 ± 10.22	15.95 ± 7.89	24.51 ± 7.06
CGF membrane	4	41.71 ± 1.55	12.77 ± 2.51	28.94 ± 0.96
PRGF mixed	18	43.84 ± 10.34	20.19 ± 5.05	23.65 ± 7.45

[1] BEGO OSS: non-cross-linked porcine pericardium membrane; [2] COLLAGEN ZIMMER EXTEND: membrane in bo-vine Achilles tendon collagen;
[3] OSSEOGUARD: bovine Achilles tendon collagen membrane; [4] OSSEOGUARD: bovine Achilles tendon collagen membrane + CGF;
[5] HEART: natural equine pericardium collagen membrane + PRF.

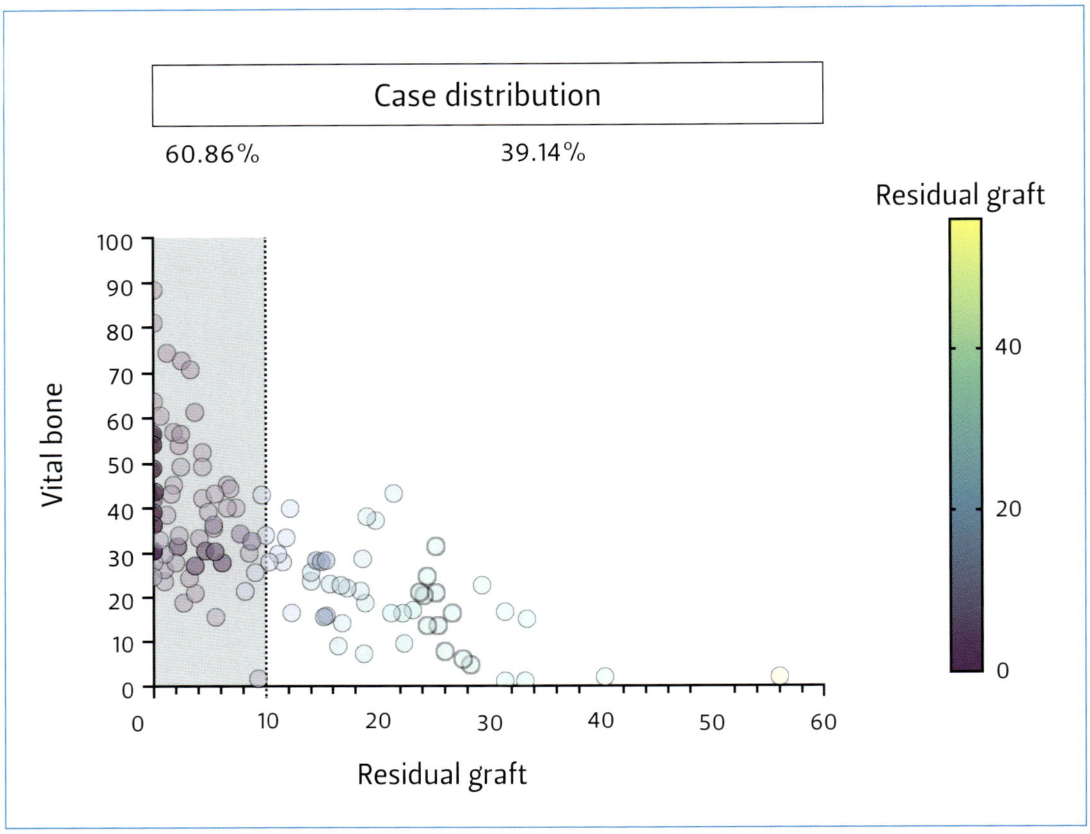

7.24 Results distribution of the histomorphometric analysis.

BOX 7.1

MEMBRANES UTILIZED

E. Giacometti

The use of membranes in bone regeneration (GBR) has been fundamental since the 1990s, as proposed by Jensen et al.[30] The mechanism by which their effectiveness is achieved is twofold: stabilization of the clot and graft, barrier effect preventing or slowing down the migration of epithelial-connective cells within the defect to be regenerated. In all of this, it is essential that the membrane is well stabilized, allowing it to contain the graft and/or the clot in an appropriate manner while maintaining the barrier effect. What is the ideal time of impermeability of the membrane to the migration of epithelial-connective cells has been the object of discussion by several authors, often with different interpretations given.
This is variable and probably depends on several factors:

- dimension of the defect;
- vascular support availability;
- quality, density and persistence over time of molecular signals;
- absence of bacterial contamination.

The membranes are divided into two large **resorbable** and **non-resorbable families**.
As for membranes made of hydrolyzable polyester material, Gotfredsen et al. have shown that during resorption they cause an important inflammatory reaction, similar to a foreign body reaction, complicating the success of regeneration.[31]

The collagen membranes have the advantage of having osteoinductive capacities, in particular type 1 collagen ones, due to their chemotactic effect. The strength of this type of membrane depends on the sampling site and the purification system used, which must preserve as much as possible the presence of proteins such as elastin, laminin and fibronectin.
Equally important, in this regard, is the presence of crossed fibers which improve the strength and extend the absorption times.
Membranes derived from the Achilles tendon are particularly rich in elastin and crossed fibers; many of these are also present in the membranes obtained from the pericardium.
The thickness of the membrane also appears to be important for the resorption times. There are also membranes whose structure, subjected to a particular treatment, presents cross-linked intertwinned fibers, significantly lengthening the resorption times and improving tearing resistance. However, some authors do not agree with this type of treatment. In particular, Annen and colleagues[32] claimed to have obtained, using a native collage membrane, a defect filling of 78%, versus 44% obtained using cross-linked membranes. Becker, on the other hand, in 2009, showed a 60% filling of the defect with a cross-linked membrane, versus 46% of the filling obtained with non-cross-linked membranes.[33]
In 2015, Denusa et al., in an animal study, demonstrated faster healing with cross-linked membranes compared to non-cross-linked ones, while not increasing the inflammation indices.[34]
In the treatment of cases of bone regeneration with demineralized dentin, various types of resorbable membranes have been used by various operators, which have different characteristics.
However, the results obtained were comparable regardless of the type of membrane used. All this seems to depend on the high availability and persistence of the molecular signals contained in the treated dentin.

Bego Collagen Membrane:[35-37] membranes made of non-cross-linked porcine pericardium. The natural cross arrangement of collagen fibers ensures excellent compatibility and a long-lasting barrier function. The fibers create a three-dimensional weave that results in multidimensional stability and good flexibility. Thanks to these characteristics, the membrane, when dry, is stable and rigid, but when wet it becomes flexible and elastic. The Bego Collagen Membrane is cell-occlusive and, like most pericardium membranes, has a smooth side that comes in contact with the soft tissues and a rough side that will come in contact with the clot and the graft, facilitating its stabilization. According to the data provided by the manufacturer, the barrier effect lasts about three months.

Osseo Guard Membranes:[38-40] resorbable membrane derived from highly purified, cross-linked type 1 collagen fibers, derived from bovine Achilles tendon. This membrane has a morphology characterized by dense oriented fibers that guarantee its high mechanical resistance. Some molecular permeability studies have highlighted its permeability to macromolecules, with a porosity able to prevent the migration of connective cells. The manufacturer indicates the resorption time in 26-38 weeks. This particularly long time interval guarantees a prolonged barrier effect, making it suitable for the treatment of particularly unfavourable defects.

Heart Membrane: natural equine pericardium membrane. Deantigenation is obtained by means of a particular enzymatic treatment that maintains the bonds between the collagen fibers and elastin, which the pericardium is composed of, fully unaltered, guaranteeing then a prolonged protection time and particular characteristics of tensile strength that allows no risk of tearing. According to the data provided by the company, the protection time reaches 3/4 months. After this period begins the degradation of the membrane which loses its protective capacity.

Zimmer Biomend Extend Membrane:[41-43] type 1 collagen membrane obtained from bovine Achilles tendon. The characteristics of this membrane change considerably depending on whether it is dry or wet and this allows its handling to be particularly good. The Biomend Extend membrane has an effective pore size of 0.004 µm; this allows the nutrients to pass through it, while preventing the migration of connective cells. The manufacturer indicates the resorption time in about 18 weeks. The strength of this type of membrane allows it to be fixed with sutures or titanium tacks without causing any laceration.

BOX 7.2

GROWTH FACTOR IN PLATELET-RICH PLASMA (PRP), PLASMA RICH IN GROWTH FACTORS (PRGF), ADVANCED PLATELET-RICH FIBRIN (A-PRF), AND CONCENTRATED GROWTH FACTORS (CGF) IN DENTAL SCIENCES

Andrea Palermo

Definition

Platelet-rich plasma (PRP) is a concentrated preparation of platelets now termed "first-generation platelet concentrate". PRP is a rich source of growth factors and promotes significant changes in monocyte-mediated pro-inflammatory cytokine/chemokine release. Leucotriene A4 (LXA4) was increased in PRP, suggesting that PRP may suppress cytokine release, limit inflammation, and, thereby, promote tissue regeneration.[44] Platelet activation allows access to autologous growth factors which by definition are neither toxic nor immunogenic and they are capable of accelerating the normal processes of bone regeneration. In general, a large body of PRP studies demonstrated that PRP stimulates the proliferation and differentiation of fibroblasts, osteoblasts, chondrocytes, and mesenchymal stem cells.[44,45] PRP can thus be considered a useful instrument for increasing the quality of regenerated bone,[47] wound healing,[48] healing of injury-associated soft tissue defects for chronic non-healing tendon injuries including lateral epicondylitis, plantar fasciitis and cartilage degeneration.[49]
In dentistry PRP was originally demonstrated to be effective in the operation of alveolar ridge augmentation and immediately spread to the fields of periodontal and oral maxillofacial surgery.[49] This clinical application was endorsed by the evidence that several major growth factors are contained at high levels in PRP preparations. However, for various reasons, such as low handling efficiency, addition of animal-derived thrombin for clotting, and other fundamental individual differences, it has been indicated that it is difficult to reproducibly control the quality of PRP preparations at similar levels.[50] To overcome these drawbacks, a plasma was developed rich in growth factors (PRGF) by modifying the PRP production procedure[51]. It simplified the preparation protocol and replaced animal-derived thrombin with calcium for clotting.[52]
Platelet-rich fibrin (PRF), a self-clotted preparation of PRP derivative, also overcame these matters. Blood samples collected in the absence of anticoagulants are immediately centrifuged to form fibrin clots. This simple preparation procedure has been widely accepted in various medical fields and spread worldwide. The developer of PRF, further modified it to an advanced form (A-PRF), which is expected to contain a relatively greater number of white blood cells (WBC).[53] Because of a low-speed centrifugation, this fibrin clot is softer than that of the original PRF. On the other hand, concentrated growth factors (CGF), another modified form of PRF, are prepared by repeatedly switching the centrifugation speed and they are characterized as a relatively stiffer fibrin clot.[54] Therefore, it has been anticipated that the difference in mechanical characteristics may produce a difference in the growth factor content.
Novel technologies (as the cell concentrator Silfradent®) make the extraction of the so-called CGF possible. CGF is an autologous leukocyte-rich and platelet-rich fibrin (L-PRF) biomaterial termed "second-generation platelet concentrate". CGF contains autologous osseo-inductive platelet growth factors and an osteoconductive fibrin matrix.[55] There are also present in CGF: TGF-b1, VEGF and CD34 positive cells.[56] The application of CGF resulted in excellent healing of critical-size bone defects *in vivo*,[55] hair loss treatments[57] and promising in periphery and myocardial ischemia treatment.[58]
By definition, PRP must contain a higher concentration of platelets than baseline, however, an increase in platelets is a very approximate description of PRP and it does not accurately describe the variability among different types of PRP. There are several parameters that need to be taken into account when considering PRP including: platelet concentration above the baseline, whether or not leucocytes are included, whether or not the PRP has been anticoagulated and whether it requires exogenous activation.
Platelet count is the first variable to consider. Absolute platelet count varies depending on the platelet concentration in the subject's peripheral blood. PRP devices can be usually divided into lower (2.5-3 times baseline

concentration) and higher (5-9 times baseline concentration) systems. It would seem intuitive that a higher platelet count would yield more growth factors and better clinical results, however this has not been determined yet. Graziani et al. suggested that the optimal concentration of PRP was 2.5 x baseline and above this there might be an inhibitory effect.[59] Optimal concentration was estimated at 2.5-fold to stimulate soft tissues, however, 2.5/3 folds upper baseline was optimal to stimulate regeneration.[59,60]

Classification

PRP containing white blood cells will have different biologic activity than PRP in which they are absent. The lower platelet count systems separate the whole blood into two components: one with the cellular components and the other consisting of serum in which the platelets are suspended. The higher platelet count systems separate the whole blood into three fractions: the red cells, serum and buffy coat. The buffy coat contains both platelets and WBC. WBC can be further classified into different types. These include neutrophils, monocytes/macrophages, and lymphocytes. Their roles in tissue healing are different. Neutrophils are phagocytic cells and contain over 40 hydrolytic enzymes. Their activation leads to phagocytosis of debris and the release of oxygen free radicals and proteases. This release of toxic molecules from the neutrophils can lead to secondary damage to the muscles.[61,62] Whether or not neutrophils have a negative or positive effect on acute or chronically injured soft tissue is unknown. Macrophages are the tissue part of the circulating monocytes. Their role is the removal of debris and they are primarily phagocytic. They also have a role in balancing the proinflammatory and anti-inflammatory aspects of healing.[63,64] Since it is not possible to fractionate different types of white blood cells out of PRP, it may be that the absence of macrophages is more detrimental to healing than any secondary damage inflicted by neutrophils. A classification of the different platelet concentrates into four categories has been proposed depending on their leucocyte and fibrin content: pure platelet-rich plasma (P-PRP), leucocyte- and platelet-rich plasma (L-PRP), pure platelet-rich fibrin (P-PRF), and leucocyte and platelet-rich fibrin (L-PRF). This classification should help to elucidate successes and failures that have occurred so far, as well as providing an objective approach for the further development of these techniques.[65] According to this classification system PRGF, A-PRF and CGF belong to the category of L-PRF.

Considerations about the growth factors preparation

PRGF: blood sample (~9.6 mL) is collected using 18 G needles in contained 0.2 mL sodium citrate. The tubes are centrifuged at 1850 rpm (580 g) for 8 min. A fraction above the buffy coat represent the PRGF.[65]

A-PRF: blood samples (~9.5 mL) are collected without anticoagulants using vacuum plain glass tubes and centrifugated in the device (A-PRF12: Dragon Laboratory Instruments Ltd., Beijing, China). After eliminating the red blood cell (RBC) fractions, the resulting A-PRF clots are used.[66]

CGF: blood samples (~9.5 mL) are collected without anticoagulants using a conventional vacuum plain glass tube (Plain BD Vacutainer Tube; Becton, Dickinson and Company, Franklin Lakes, NJ, USA) and centrifugated in the device: Medifuge centrifugation system (Silfradent S. r. L., Santa Sofia, Italy). After eliminating the red blood cell (RBC) fractions, the resulting CGF clots are used.[66]

Biological effects

The growth factor contents in PRF and CGF preparations and their bioactivities have been demonstrated in in vitro studies by several independent groups[65-77] and it has been clarified that the regenerative effects of PRF/CGF are not solely due to fibrin clots. The major source of growth factors in PRF preparations is the exudate, however, as a minor source, growth factors are thought to be secured by fibrin fibers.[52] The angiogenic activity of PRF/CGF preparations in endothelial cell cultures and in the chick embryo chorion-allantoic membrane (CAM) assay[78] demonstrated that PRF/CGF preparations are somehow more potent in angiogenesis than PRP prepara-

tions. The comparison of the growth factor contents in four types of PRP derivatives (PRP, PRGF, A-PRF, CGF) prepared from the same donors showed that both A-PRF and CGF preparations contained TGF-β1, PDGF-BB, VEGF, IL-1β, and IL-6 at a similar to, or at a higher level than, PRP preparations.[52] The expected proliferative effects of both A-PRF and CGF extracts were demonstrated in the in vitro assay using human periosteal cells which gave rise to osteoblasts involved in periodontal skeletal regeneration. Therefore, as PRP preparations do, these self-clotted PRP derivatives are expected to function not only as a scaffolding material but also as a reservoir to deliver certain growth factors and pro-inflammatory cytokines at the implantation sites.[52]
Another study,[79] found that PRP and A-PRF preparations exert distinguishable actions on periosteal cell proliferation. Because both IL-1β and IL-6 are known to be produced by WBCs,[80] and because WBCs are not included in PRGF preparations, then the bi-phasic effects of PRP preparations may be attributed to WBCs. Further, if WBCs are highly concentrated in A-PRF, it is expected that IL-1β and IL-6 are concentrated at higher levels to exert negative effects at higher doses of A-PRF extracts as this study showed. WBCs, as well as platelets, were highly concentrated in A-PRF.[52-53] Similarly, WBCs were found to be concentrated in CGF preparations.[52] In addition, the inflammatory cytokines were not exceptionally concentrated at higher levels in PRP preparations, and no strong positive correlation between WBC counts and pro-inflammatory cytokine levels was observed in PRP preparations. The negative effects of PRP preparations at higher doses may not be due to these pro-inflammatory cytokines or WBCs.
It has been demonstrated that both A-PRF and CGF contained significant amounts of growth factors, so then both the preparations would not only function as a scaffolding material but also as a reservoir to deliver certain growth factors at the site of application. Accordingly, it is expected that these two preparations are more potently capable of inducing angiogenesis and subsequent wound healing/tissue regeneration than PRP preparations.
PRP was originally demonstrated to be effective in the operation of alveolar ridge augmentation and immediately spread to the fields of periodontal and oral maxillofacial surgery.[50] In addition, PRP is a potentially useful substance in the fight against periodontal pathogens. This might represent a valuable property in adjunct to the enhancement of tissue regeneration.[81] The comparison of the efficacy of PRP and synthetic graft material for bone regeneration after bilateral third molar extraction showed that the PRP was a better graft material than a synthetic graft material in terms of soft tissue and bone healing.[82] PRP has been used in implant dentistry for its remarkable stimulatory effect on oral tissue regeneration, making it a very safe and successful tool.[83] A clinical trial on eleven subjects with Miller's class I and II gingival recessions, concluded that connective tissue graft with PRP was an effective and predictable method.[84]
However, at the present moment, evidence described in the literature on the efficacy of platelet concentrates in oral and maxillofacial procedures are controversial and limited. In order to clarify the real advantages and priorities for the patients, when the blood-derived products are applied, further in vitro and in vivo research about the activity of PRP on the dental cells biology should be conducted.[85]

BOX 7.3

BIOCENTRIC CONCEPT IN GBR

H.K.L. Ho

Traditionally, guided bone regeneration (GBR) is performed using a barrier membrane to grow new bone at sites with insufficient volume. In order to be able to insert an implant, it is mandatory to restore an adequate bone volume and a suitable support to achieve good results in terms of survival and success. With adequate volume in an edentulous area, the surgeon more has more options and greater regenerative possibilities by means of an implant treatment or a pontic site. GBR is also done to correct peri-implant fenestration and dehiscences. To achieve that, it is essential to block the growth of adjacent tissue using various kinds of barrier membranes to form an adequate space for bone regeneration. GBR is a well-documented and widely used procedure in implant treatment of alveolar bone defects. To increase the chance of a successful outcome, it is critical to stabilize the blood clot,[86–87] good primary intention closure, isolation of gingival tissue from defect with a barrier, and space provision.[88–89] However, GBR is still challenging in sites with advanced horizontal and vertical bone defects.[90–93] The original hypothesis of GBR derives from the concept of guided tissue regeneration (GTR).[94] GTR is based on the concept of selective growth of cells derived from periodontal ligament by placing a physical barrier which prevents the apical migration of cells from epithelium and gingival connective tissue.[95–97] Also, the physical barrier is believed to provide protection to the blood clot during the early phases of wound healing and ensure space maintenance for the ingrowth of newly formed periodontal apparatus.[90,92,95,98–102] This principle of wound compartmentalization and that cells from the periodontal ligaments may populate the root surface, and with the landmark study performed by Nyman and coworkers[103] demonstrating that with the use of a membrane to filter out the epithelial and fibroblast cells from populating the area of treatment, has led to periodontal regeneration. This treatment concept was well accepted and embraced by the industry to develop non-resorbable and resorbable membranes to support this surgical protocol. Therefore, the roles of the barrier membrane has been emphasized for successful outcomes. There are three reasons to use membranes for GBR procedures:

- to block the invasion of unwanted epithelium and connective tissue;
- to induce vascular ingrowth from bone and marrow; and
- to form a "chamber" for stable growth of new bone.[99,102]

Presently there are many types of barrier membrane in the market. The clinician has to select the material suitable for the surgical procedure. There are characteristics of the membrane that should be considered. They are, biocompatibility, space making and maintenance, cell occlusion, tissue integration, clinical handling, and limited susceptibility to complications.[104,105]

Biocompatibility is the basic requirement of any implantable device. The biocompatibility test parameters include cytotoxicity, histocompatibility, genotoxicity, mutagenicity, and microbial effects. Cell occlusion property has been extensively studied and researched and as mentioned earlier, established by a landmark study by Nyman et al. However, the concept of cell occlusion has been challenged by numerous studies and questioned the importance of this property. The topography, porosity and chemical properties of the membrane affects the tissue integration at the defect site. It must have the capacity to provide mechanical stability to the defect site. More studies are now helping us to understand the importance of space maintenance rather than the occlusivity of the barrier membrane. The stiffness of the membrane to resist the collapse and loss of space at the surgical site is of utmost importance. This is particularly important for resorbable membranes because of their loss of mechanical strength during degradation. Ease of handling of the membrane is important in clinical practice for obvious reasons. Managing the use of a nonresorbable membrane is tedious and more demanding. Proper trimming, removal of sharp edges is critical to prevent soft tissue damage. Securing of the non-resorbable membrane with screws or tags because of its stiffness are essential. Resorbable membranes are softer and hydrophilic and adapt to the surrounding bone and blood. Non-resorbable membranes have a significant risk of premature exposure and may result in infection and poor outcome in terms of bone regeneration.[106–107]

Comparison between non-resorbable and resorbable membranes in terms of bone fill, when no complication has occurred, non-resorbable membranes performed better than resorbable membranes.[108–109] This is perhaps because ePTFE membrane can provide better maintenance of space, and a longer and controlled barrier effect, absence of inflammation, and its lack of resorption products (polymeric membranes gives acidic by-products during degradation).

Due to the avoidance of a second surgery and good biocompatibility when using collagen membrane, it has become a preferred choice by many clinicians. However, because of its quick resorption, and hence its lack of barrier effect, industry has worked on improving it by prolonging the resorption time by cross-linking process. However, this cross-linking process whilst it increases the biomechanical property of the membrane, it also can increase the possibility of a foreign body reaction, decreasing its biocompatibility. For additional information on the characteristics and use of barrier membranes, readers are encouraged to refer to the earlier chapter on this topic. The present dogma which emphasizes the importance of barrier function has been challenged by some researchers. The use of titanium mesh by numerous clinical studies have shown acceptable clinical outcomes and bone formation. These mesh designs with large perforations has not provided any barrier function to prevent the invasion of epithelial or connective tissues. Furthermore, new evidence by Susin et al.[110] has highlighted numerous studies that the expected sequelae of migration of epithelial cells is not a certainty in periodontal healing and regeneration even if a barrier membrane has not been used. These studies have thrown new light on our understanding of biology and processes of periodontal regeneration.

To take the concepts of GTR and transfer to GBR procedure, in light of the new evidence, shows more needs to be done to relook at our understanding and also change our clinical practice. Thus, GBR needs to be reviewed from a biophysiological point of view with regards to surrounding tissues involved in bone grafting healing. Polimeni et al. in a study on animals has looked at the role of barrier membrane in alveolar bone regeneration. They have showed the importance of wound stability and the space provision by the membranes and critical for the bone formation. They added that the types of barrier membranes used in their study comparing the occlusive ePTFE membrane to a more porous form of the same make, had better bone regeneration compared to the latter. The results showed statistical significance but clinically outcome for both were satisfactory. They concluded that the occlusivity of barrier membrane may have an adjunctive role in bone formation only.[111]

Wikesjö UMet al. have also shown similar results in their study. These studies have shown that the main contribution of barrier membranes, regardless of their occlusivity, is to stabilize the wound and space maintenance.[112] In fact, there is a lack of research on the surrounding tissues which could participate in alveolar bone regeneration. Especially, while researchers have focused on the role of periodontal ligament in the periodontal tissue regeneration, they overlooked that the periosteum has the same nature as the periodontal ligament in alveolar regeneration. In fact, in many experimental studies, researchers have not considered the role of periosteum in GBR. The use of a barrier membrane has actually excluded the periosteum from the bone defect. In addition, the blood supply of the mucoperiosteal flap covering the barrier membrane when performing guided bone procedure is reduced, increasing the incidence of wound dehiscence.[113] In addition, the influence of various graft materials on bone regeneration cannot be excluded. Biocompatibility,[114] bone forming ability,[115-116] resorption by bone cells,[117] and maintenance of space[118-120] can affect bone regeneration results. Both the performance of these graft materials and membranes used affect regenerated bone, and the nature of the graft material affects the membrane's effect on bone regeneration. If the graft material has a good space maintenance ability and biocompatibility, such as the autogenous block bone, the effect of the membrane would not be significant. However, when using fast-absorbing materials, such as cancellous allograft powder bone or demineralized freeze-dried bone (DFDB), titanium reinforced membrane or titanium mesh, which has an excellent space maintenance function, it will show better results. In the case of graft materials that have poor biocompatibility and hardly resorbed by human cells, blocking the external tissue environment using a non-permeable membrane may determine a better result.

In the earlier chapter, the different graft materials available for clinicians today have been discussed and the characteristics of different classes of graft material will help the clinician to employ the adequate steps to achieve the desired outcome. Of particular interest in recent years, the use of the patients' teeth as an alternative graft material has gained increased attention and numerous studies and clinical reports have been published. The positive clinical outcome and experiences by these clinicians and researchers can give both patients and practitioners an additional option, with a more effective, lessened morbidity, lower cost pathway to achieve the treatment outcome. Bone healing is a dynamic, well-orchestrated physiological process that involves complex and spatiotemporally coordinated function.[121]

The complex physiological process of bone healing involves various cells, molecules, and the cascade multistep process of intracellular and extracellular molecular signaling of surrounding tissue is essential role for successful bone healing.[121–124] The functions of the different growth factors and active proteins are discussed in the preceding chapter. Traditional GBR procedure using membranes did not consider the surrounding biological tissue involved in bone regeneration. Moreover, the results of these studies do not explain the exact role of the membranes in promoting healing events within the membrane covered defects.[125]

The periosteum is composed of two distinct layers. The inner cambium layer contains osteoprogenitor cells which participate in bone growth, healing, and regeneration.[121,122,126–128] The remarkable regenerative capability of periosteum was realized centuries ago.[127] However, researchers did not focus on the role and function of periosteum as an important contributing factor in bone regeneration.[126–127] Only recently, biologists are starting to focus and understand the precise roles played by the periosteum in bone healing.[129,130] Unfortunately, not much attention given and only few sporadic reports on the use of the strong osteogenic capacity of the periosteum in alveolar bone regeneration have been provided in dentistry. In addition, the cellular, molecular, and mechanical mechanisms of the periosteum that govern the sequence of biological events during bone regeneration, and the possible bioactive role of the periosteum in modulating these events have scarcely been investigated.

The Biocentric concept focuses on the characteristics of the tissue around the alveolar bone defect that affect bone regeneration and relook at the "compartmentalization concept" of using membrane to perform the traditional GBR. Sambrook and coauthors stated the reaction of the periosteum when it is lifted from the underlying bone by trauma, tumour or pus, will lay down bone. They stated that it is an activation of the normal process of bone formation. The bone formation is the result of activity of osteoblasts in the inner cambium periosteal layer. This bone formation under the lifted periosteum is also evident in osteosarcoma, a tumour of the bone.[131]

Ueno et al. performed an animal study on rabbits by removing periosteum from the tibia and further removed the inner cambium layer of the periosteum, leaving only the fibrous layer, and transplanted to the suprahyoid muscles area. They were able to induce cartilage tissue formation and then the bone trabeculae. They concluded that grafted periosteum form bone by endochondral ossification and the cells from the fibrous layer plays an important role in chondrogenesis that precedes bone formation.[132]

A study was conducted by Zhang et al. using mice as a model to understand the cellular mechanisms for bone grafting healing and repair and to devise a strategy to enhance allograft performance. They found that removal of the periosteum from the live bone graft resulted in a 73% decrease in new bone and cartilage formation on the graft and a 10-fold decrease in neovascularization measured using histomorphometric analysis and micro-CT. The absence of periosteum also resulted in a 75% reduction of osteoclast numbers on the bone graft, which correlated with poor bone remodelling activity of the allograft or autograft. In contrast, removing cells from the bone marrow had minimal effects in the new bone formation on the donor bone graft.[133]

Clearly the role of the periosteum in providing cells and blood supply for bone regeneration with new bone formation and remodelling is critical. It is frequently advocated by clinicians to release the tension when closing the wound for bone grafting procedures. The tension reduction in the flap will prevent wound dehiscences and it will provide a secure environment for bone regeneration. However, in the study conducted by Raab-Cullen and his colleagues on rats, the effects of bending strains on the tibial were observed using a four point bending model. They found that bending loads caused the greater mineral apposition rate (MAR) as compared to the static pressure. Cyclic pressure has no effect on the periosteal MAR or formation surface.[134]

Conclusions

A proposed new approach, the Biocentric Guided Bone Generation is a method which involves making minimally invasive horizontal crestal incision, creating space under the periosteum with adequate flap elevation, and putting the graft material into the space form without the using of any barrier membrane. This creates a strain stress to the periosteum. The intact periosteum with the strain stimulates a positive effect to the local environment starting a chain of events resulting in a strong bone formation. The principle of this perspective is to utilize the natural function of the bone and its related structures together with the natural behaviour of the material under the ideal conditions that trigger and positive effect on bone regeneration.

Comparison of resorption with other materials mixed with the tooth

E. Minetti

Six three-wall ridge preservation cases were analyzed[29] in six biopsy samples: in three samples only the tooth was used as graft material while in the others 50% tooth and xenographic material (Bio-Oss) were mixed (7.25 and 7.11).

Starting from the observations derived from this publication, in order to identify the average resorption of the tooth in the same regeneration by comparing it with an already known material (Bio-Oss), we first evaluated the volume occupied by the material formed by 50% of the tooth by TT Tooth Transformer treatment and 50% from Bio-Oss xenographic material (7.26).
The material thus mixed was inserted into a graduated syringe and, drop by drop, the water solution was poured to occupy the same volume. In the tests carried out, the volume occupied by the graft material corresponds to about 60%, and 40% is an empty space (7.27). Therefore, if a cavity is filled fully with the graft material we can assume that 60% of the space will be occupied by the granules. The histomorphometric examination performed at the established time intervals (4-8 months) will evaluate a 100% volume which, compared to the starting volume, will allow to derive the average resorption rate of this sample, with all the limits deriving from the reduced number (7.12; 7.28 and 7.29).

It must be said that each sample has a value that can also vary greatly as the condensation of the material can bring a greater quantity of tooth or xenograft into that portion of the cavity which will then be analyzed by the histological sample.

In order to have definitive data, the number must be greater than the cases carried out so far. Analyzing the data collected up to now in this preliminary study, the tooth is very resorbed in almost all the samples both at 4 and at 8 months.

However, it is interesting to note that deproteinized bovine bone (Bio-Oss Geistlich Biomaterials, Baden-Baden, Germany) had minimal resorption when comparing the samples at 4 months and the samples at 8 months.

This implies, as specified by Lindhe, that "the placement of a biomaterial in a post-extraction socket delays the healing; the Bio-Oss particles are not resorbed but surrounded by bone"[135] since the material itself, occupying the space, prevents the growth of further bone (7.30). It can be noted that in the sample taken, each space is occupied and only the resorption of the granules can allow a greater presence of bone. Considering that in this image the tooth should have been at 50% of its content, it can be understood how the space occupied by the bone is determined by the resorption of the tooth.

7.11 Comparison between first group and second group

Comparison	Bone Volume/ Total Volume	Residual Graft	New Bone Volume/ Total Volume
First group only tooth	57.21 ± 8.71	18.99 ± 10.99	38.22 ± 8.71
Second group 50% tooth + 50% xenograft	55.50 ± 16.51	34.874 ± 9.21 (12.99 ± 6.26 tooth + 21.88 ± 3.22 xenograft)	20.630 ± 5.82

7.12 4-8 month comparison of samples with 50% dentin + 50% Bio-Oss

Withdrawal months	Numerousness	Bone Volume/ Total Volume	Residual dental Graft/ Total Volume	Residual xenograft Graft/ Total Volume	Vital Bone/ Total Bone
4 months	5 samples	47.26 ± 8.71	6.15 ± 4.33	20.47 ± 6.76	20.64 ± 4.96
8 months	5 samples	51.29 ± 10.77	3.48 ± 1.65	17.03 ± 13.19	30.78 ± 12.57

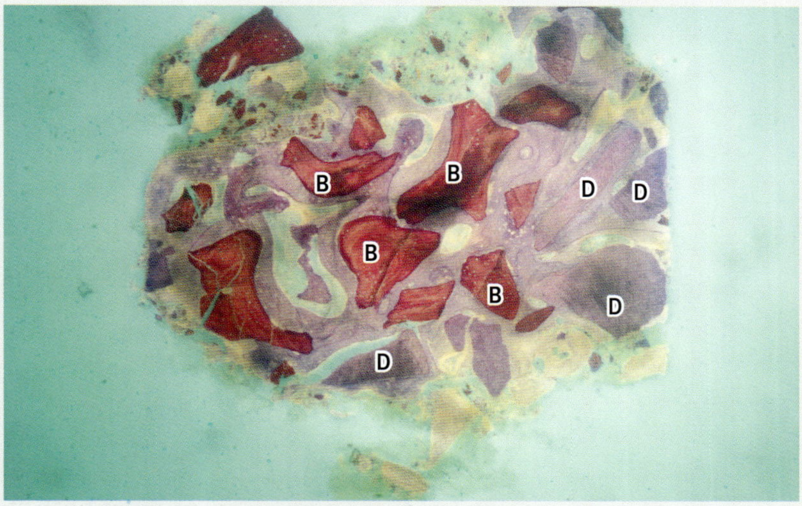

7.25 After 4 months histological preparation 50% tooth (D) + 50% Bio-Oss xenograft material (B).

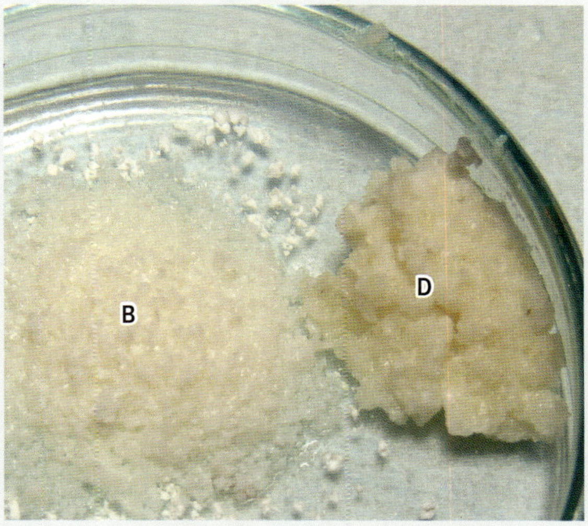

7.26 50% dentin (D) and Bio-Oss xenograft material (B).

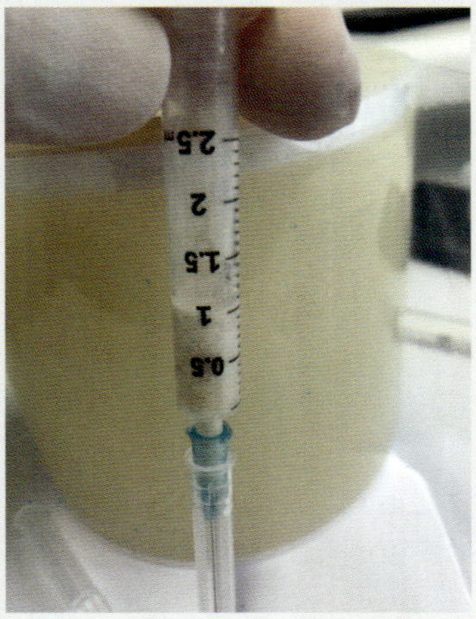

7.27 Syringe used for testing the volume occupied by the grafting material 60% and water 40%.

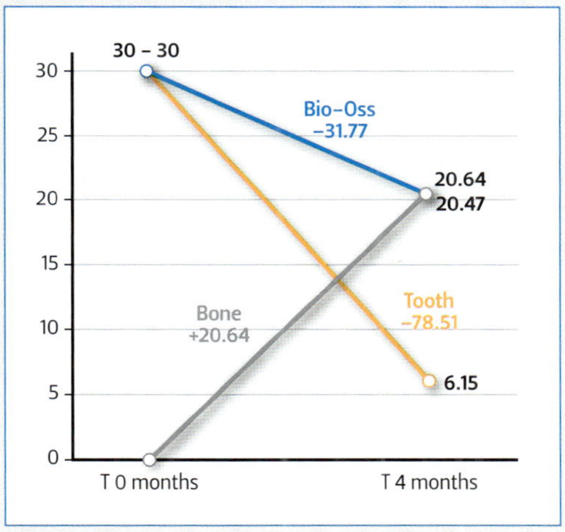

7.28 Tooth and Bio-Oss resorption chart and new bone at 4 months.

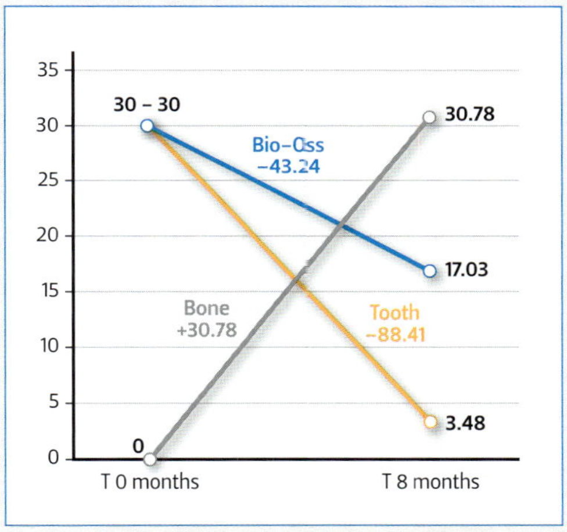

7.29 Tooth and Bio-Oss resorption chart and new bone at 8 months.

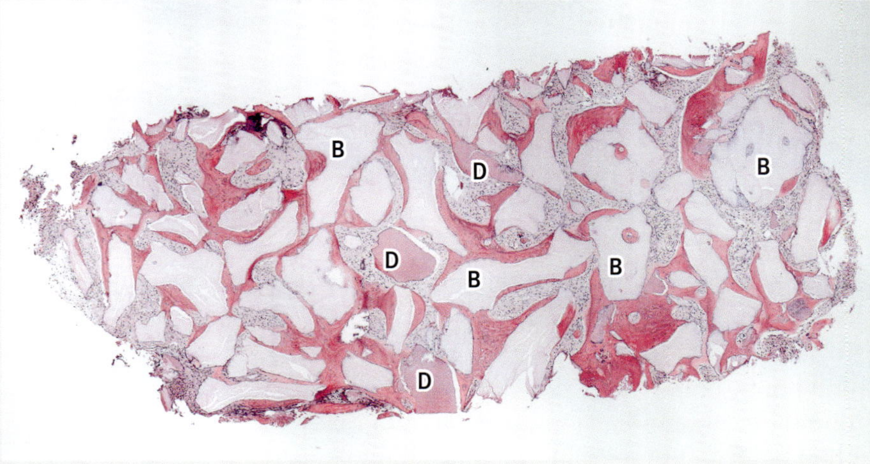

7.30 Histology at 8 months with a mix of 50% dentin (D) and 50% xenograft material (Bio-Oss) (B).

Analyzing the literature review carried out by Corbella and collaborators,[136] in which the author reviewed 802 articles, of which 40 were within the inclusion criteria (each article indicated histomorphometric measurements of numerous graft materials on the market), it was possible to visualize the average residue of grafting material (7.13).

Comparing it with our available data about all the histologies we performed (7.14), it is possible to highlight the remarkable tooth resorption index as already mentioned.

Radiographic images

The tooth is very similar to the bone also radiographically. The evolution over time of the graft means that the image is very similar to the patient's native bone, also because the tooth is completely reabsorbed and replaced by bone. The evolution of bone tissue and graft material can be clearly seen in the radiological images ranging from 2016 to 2019 (7.31).

The enamel in the radiographic images is radiopaque (7.32) and can easily be recognized as whiter spots within the regenerated tissue and over time it does not resorb or change (7.33).

7.13 Residue of the various grafting materials on the market

Biomaterial	Histo samples	Residue
Bovine bone	273	19.35 ± 9.35
Porcine bone	84	27.63 ± 6.93
Allograft	91	13.92 ± 10.25
FDBA	112	22.27 ± 12.7
HA	84	22.7 ± 9.02
Calcium sulfate	56	14.7 ± 2.75
HA + tricalcium phosphate + EMD (Enamel Matrix Derivate)	14	12 ± 6.75

7.14 Average tooth residue

	Histo samples	Residue
Tooth TT	112	11.31 ± 7.57

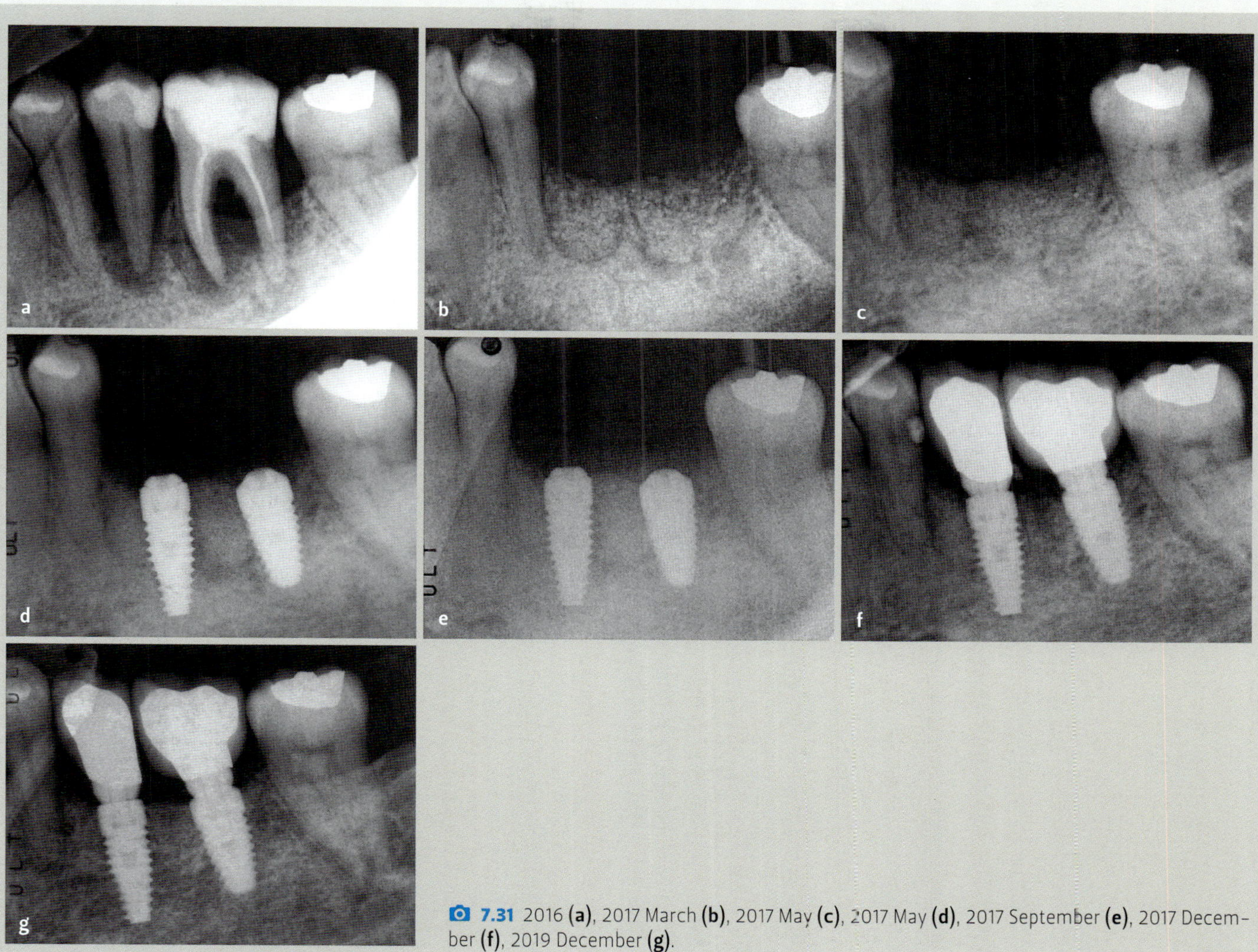

7.31 2016 (**a**), 2017 March (**b**), 2017 May (**c**), 2017 May (**d**), 2017 September (**e**), 2017 December (**f**), 2019 December (**g**).

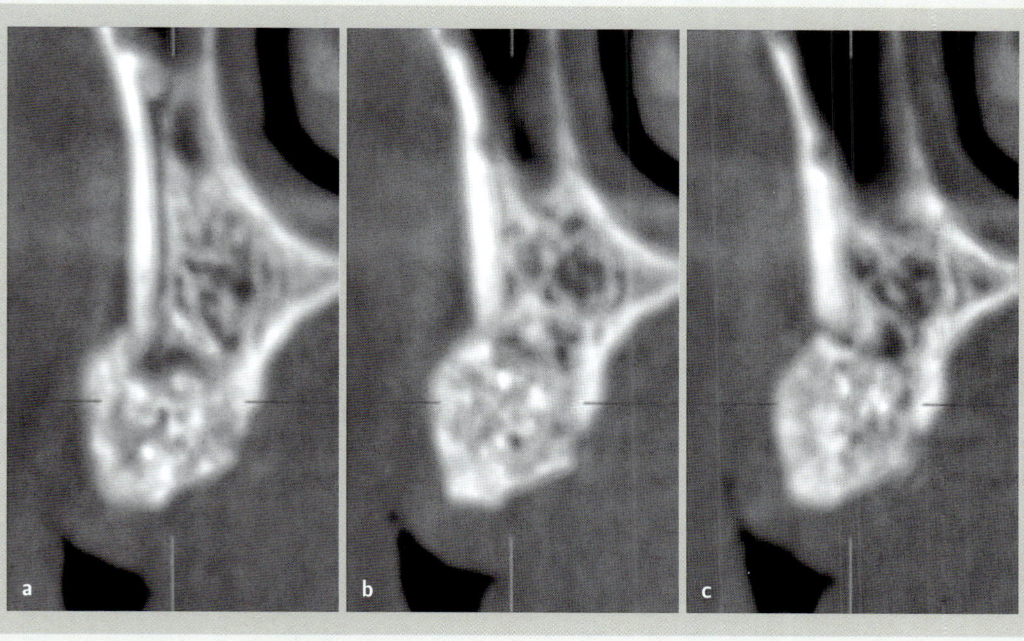

7.32 Postoperative radiography: regeneration with vertical component. Radiopaque granules can be seen.

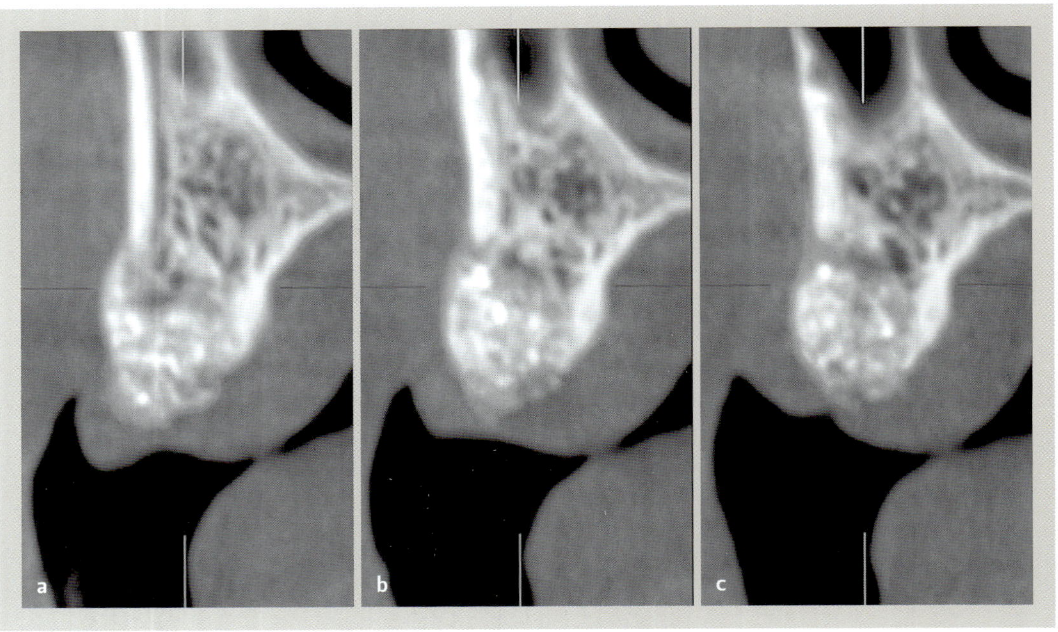

7.33 Radiography after 4 months: healing. The same radiopaque granules can be seen.

REFERENCES

1. Casasco E. Citologia Istologia. Pavia, La Goliardica Pavese, 1989.
2. Florencio-Silva R, da Silva Sasso GR, Sasso-Cerri E, et al. Biology of bone tissue: structure, function and factors that influence bone cells. Biomed Res Intl 2015;2015:421746.
3. Hammarström L, Heijl L, Gestrelius S. Periodontal regeneration in a buccal dehiscence model in monkeys after application of enamel matrix proteins. J Clin Periodontol 1997;24:669-77.
4. Icaro Cornaglia A, Casasco A, Casasco M, et al. Dysplastic histogenesis of cartilage growth plate by alteration of sulphation pathway: a transgenic model. Connect Tissue Res 2009;50:232-42.
5. Icaro Cornaglia A, Casasco M, Riva F, et al. Stimulation of osteoblast growth by an electromagnetic field in a model of bone-like construct. Eur J Histochem 2006;50:199-204.
6. Ingber DE. Tensegrity: the architectural basis of cellular mechanotransduction. Ann Rev Physiol 1997;59:575-99.
7. Leucht P, Kim J-B, Wasen R, et al. Effect of mechanical stimuli on skeletal regeneration around implants. Bone 2007;40:919-30.
8. Listgartnen MA. Soft and hard tissue response to endogenous dental implants. Anat Rec 1996;245:410-25.
9. Minetti E, Palermo A, Trisi P, et al. Tooth transformer: a new method to prepare autologous tooth grafts. Histologic and histomorphometric analyses of 11 consecutive clinical cases. Int J Growth Factors Stem Cells Dent 2019;2:56-61.
10. Adamo S, De Felici M, Dolfi A, et al. Istologia di Monesi (7ª edizione). Padova, Piccin, 2018.
11. Berendsen AD, Olsen BJ. Bone development. Bone 2015;80:14-18.
12. Young MF. Skeletal biology: where matrix meets mineral. Matrix Biol 2016;52:1-6.
13. Sadler TW. Langman's Medical embryology (12ª edizione). Philadelphia, Lippincott Williams & Wilkins, 2012.
14. Bianco P, Robey P. Skeletal stem cells. Development 2015;142:1023-7.
15. Nanci A. Ten Cate's oral histology (9th edition). Development, structure, and function. St. Louis, Elsevier, 2018.
16. Anderson HC. Vesicles associated with calcification in the matrix of epiphyseal cartilage. J Cell Biol 1969;41:59-72.
17. Bonucci E. Fine structure of early cartilage calcification. J Ultrastrut Res 1967;20:33-50.
18. Casasco A, Calligaro A, Casasco M. Proliferative and functional stages of rat ameloblast differentiation as revealed by combined immunocytochemistry against enamel matrix proteins and bromodeoxyuridine. Cell Tissue Res 1992;270:415-23.
19. Nanci A, Bendayan M, Slavkin HC. Enamel protein bio-synthesis and secretion in mouse incisor secretory ameloblasts as revealed by high-resolution immunocytochemistry. J Histochem Cytochem 1985;33:1153-60.
20. Ripamonti U. Biomimetism, biomimetic matrices and induction of bone formation. J Cell Mol Med 2009;13:2953-72.
21. Sculean A, Nikolidakis D, Nikou G, et al. Biomaterials for promoting periodontal regeneration in human intrabony defects: a systematic review. Periodontology 2015;68:182-216.
22. Zheng C, Chen C, Liu S, et al. Stem cell-based bone and dental regeneration: a view of microenvironmental modulation. Int J Oral Sci 2019;23:11-23.

23. Minetti E, Giacometti U, Gambardella M, et al. Alveolar socket preservation with different autologous graft materials: preliminary results of a multicenter pilot study in human. Materials 2020;13(5):1153.

24. Minetti E, Palermo A, Ferrante F, et al. Autologous tooth graft after endodontical treated used for socket preservation: a multicenter clinical study. Appl Sci 2019;9(24):5396.

25. Minetti E, Palermo A, Contessi M, et al. Autologous tooth graft for maxillary sinus augmentation: a multicenter clinical study. Int J Growth Factors Stem Cells Dent 2019;2:45-51.

26. Minetti E, Palermo A, Trisi P, et al. Tooth Transformer®: A new method to prepare autologous tooth grafts - histologic and histomorphometric analyses of 11 consecutive clinical cases. Int J Growth Factors Stem Cells Dent 2019;2:56-61.

27. Minetti E, Berardini M, Trisi P. A new tooth processing apparatus allowing to obtain dentin grafts for bone augmentation: the tooth transformer. Open Dent J 2019,13:6-14.

28. Minetti E, Taschieri SL, Corbella S. Autologous deciduous tooth-derived material for alveolar ridge preservation: a clinical and histological case report. Case Rep Dent 2020; 2020:2936878.

29. Minetti E, Palermo A, Savadori P, et al. Autologous tooth graft: a histological comparison between dentin mixed with xenograft and dentin alone grafts in socket preservation. J Biol Regul Homeost Agents 2019;33(6 Suppl. 2): 189-97.

30. Jensen OT, Greer RO, Johson L et al.Vertical guided bone-graft augmentation in a new canine model. Int J Oral Max Impl 1994;9:644-52.

31. Gotfredsen K, Nimb L, Hjørting-Hansen E. Immediate implant placement using a biodegradable barrier, polyhydroxybutirate-hydroxyvalerate reinforced with poliglactin 910. An experimental study in dogs. Clin Oral Implants Res 1994;5(2):83-91.

32. Annen BM, Ramel CF, Hämmerle CH, et al. Use a new cross-linked collagen membrane fo the treatment of peri-implant dehiscence defect: a randomised controlled double-blinded clinical trial. Eur J Oral Implantol 2011;4(2):87-100.

33. Becker J. At all use a new cross-linked collagen membrana for the treatment of theiscencer-tipe defect at titanium implants: a prospective rondomized-controlled duble-blinded clinical multi-center study. Clin Oral Implants Res 2009;20(7):742-9.

34. Denusa M Verissimo, Renata FC Leitao, Sonia D Figueirò, et al. Guided bone regeneration produced by new mineralized and reticulated collagen membranes in critical-size rat calvarial defects Exp Biol Med 2015;240(2):175-84.

35. Al-Maawis, Gnanaati S. Biologization of collagen-based biomaterials using liquid. platelets-rich fibrin: new insights into clinically applicable tissue engineering. Materials 2019;12(23):3993.

36. Barbeck M, Gnanaati S. Porcine dermis and pericardium-based, non-cross-linked materials induce multinucleated giant cels after their in vivo implantation: a physiological reaction? J Oral Implantol 2015;41(6):e267-81.

37. Liebaug F, Wu N. 20 Jahre membrangeschützte Knochen-regeneration - ein Erfahrungsbericht. ZWP Spezial 2014; 10:12-7.

38. Wallace S, Froum S, Cho S, et al. Sinus augmentation utilizing anorganic bovine bone (biooss) with absorbable and nonabsorbable membrane placed over the lateral window: hystomorphometric and clinical analyses. Int J Periodontics Restorative Dent 2005; 25(6):55-69.

39. Weinländer M, Krennmair G, Schmidinger S, et al. The Mirror Study. A propective randomized controlled study of Endobon and Bio-Oss in maxillary sinus augmentation. Histological evaluation. Clinical Oral Implant Res 2011;22(9):1033.

40. del Castillo RA. Grafting of an extracted maxillary first-molar socket using a new, flexible resorbable collagen membrane for ridge preservation in advance of implant placement. Inside Dentistry 2011;7(9):94-6.

41. Shu-Tung L, Hui-Chen C, Natsuyo SL, et al. A Comparative Study of Zimmer Biomend® and BioMend® Extend™ Membranes made at two different manufacturing facilities. Zimmer Dental INC 2013. ZD1218, Rev. 05/13.

42. Tae-Ju Oh, Meraw SJ, Lee EY, et al. Comparation analysis of collagen membranes for the treatment of implante dehiscence defect, Cl Oral impl Res 2003;14(1):80-90.

43. Coic M, Placet V, Jacquet E, et al. Mechanical properties of collagen Membranes Used In Guided Bone regeneration: a comparative study of three models. Rev Stomatol Chir Maxilofac 2010;111(5-6):286-90.

44. El-Sharkawy H, Kantarci A, Deady J, et al. Platelet-rich plasma: growth factors and pro- and anti-inflammatory properties. J Periodontol 2007;78:661-9.

45. Sampson S, Gerhardt M, Mandelbaum B. Platelet rich plasma injection grafts for musculoskeletal injuries: a review. Curr Rev Musculoskelet Med 2008;1:165-74.

46. Lee KS, Wilson JJ, Rabago DP, et al. Musculoskeletal applications of platelet-rich plasma: fad or future? AJR Am J Roentgenol 2011;196:628-36.

47. Pacifici L, Casella F, Maggiore C. Platelet rich plasma (PRP): potentialities and techniques of extraction. Minerva Stomatol 2002;51:341-50.

48. Gao F, Wang JX, Han Y. Research advance on application of platelet-rich plasma in wound repair - review. Zhongguo Shi Yan Xue Ye Xue Za Zhi 2009;17:840-3.

49. Cieslik-Bielecka A, Bielecki T, Gazdzik TS, et al. Autologous platelets and leukocytes can improve healing of infected high-energy soft tissue injury. Transfus Apher Sci 2009;41(1):9-12.

50. Kawase T. Platelet-rich plasma and its derivatives as promising bioactive materials for regenerative medicine: basic principles and concepts underlying recent advances. Odontology 2015;103:126-35.

51. Anitua E. The use of plasma-rich growth factors (PRGF) in oral surgery. Pract Proced Aesthet Dent 2001;13: 487-93.

52. Masuki H, Okudera T, Watanebe T et al. Growth factor and pro-inflammatory cytokine contents in platelet-rich plasma (PRP), plasma rich in growth factors (PRGF), advanced platelet-rich fibrin (A-PRF), and concentrated growth factors (CGF). Int J Implant Dent 2016;2(1):19.

53. Choukroun J. Advanced PRF & i-PRF: platelet concentrates or blood concentrates? J Periodont Med Clin Practice 2014;1:3.

54. Corigliano M, Sacco L, Baldoni E. CGF-una proposta terapeutica per la medicina rigenerativa. Odontoiatria 2010;1:69-81.

55. Honda H, Tamai N, Naka N et al. Bone tissue engineering with bone mar-

row-derived stromal cells integrated with concentrated growth factor in Rattus norvegicus calvaria defect model. J Artif Organs 2012;16:305-15.

56. Rodella LF, Favero G, Boninsegna R, et al. Growth factors, CD34 positive cells, and fibrin network analysis in concentrated growth factors fraction. Microsc Res Tech 2011;74:772-7.
57. Kang S, Zheng Z,Choi MJ, et al. The effect of CD34+ cell-containing autologous platelet-rich plasma injection on pattern hair loss: a preliminary study. J Eur Acad Dermatol Venereol 2014;28:72-79.
58. Mackie AR, Losordo DW. CD34-positive stem cells: in the treatment of heart and vascular disease in human beings. Tex Heart Inst J 2011;38:474-85.
59. Graziani F, Ivanovski S, Ce, S, et al. The in vitro effect of different PRP concentrations on osteoblasts and fibroblasts. Clin Oral Implants Res 2006;17:212-9.
60. Weibrich G, Hansen T, Kleis W, et al. Effect of platelet concentration in platelet-rich plasma on peri-implant bone regeneration. Bone 2004;34:665-71.
61. Smith C, Kruger MJ, Smith RM, et al. The inflammatory response to skeletal muscle injury: illuminating complexities. Sports Med 2008;38: 947-69.
62. Tuomi H, Best T. The inflammatory response: friend or enemy to muscle tissue? Br J Sports Med 2003;37:284-6.
63. Tidball JG,Wehling-Henricks M. Macrophages promote muscle membrane repair and muscle fibre growth and regeneration during modified muscle loading in mice in vivo. J Physiol 2007;578:327-36.
64. Dohan Ehrenfest DM, Rasmusson L, Albrektsson T. Classification of platelet concentrates: from pure platelet-rich plasma (P-PRP) to leucocyte- and platelet-rich fibrin (L-PRF). Trends Biotechnol 2009;27:158-67.
65. Takeda Y, Katsutoshi K, Matsuzaka K et al. The effect of concentrated growth factor on rat bone marrow cells in vitro and on calvarial bone healing in vivo. Int J Oral Maxillofac Implants 2015;30:1187-96.
66. Kobayashi M, Kawas T, Horimiz M, et al. A proposed protocol of the standardized preparation of PRF membranes for clinical use. Biologicals 2012;40:323-9.
67. Nishimoto S, Fujita K, Sotsuka Y, et al. Growth factor measurement and histological analysis in platelet rich fibrin: a pilot study. J Maxillofac Oral Surg 2015;14:907-13.
68. Lundquist R, Dziegiel MH, Agren MS. Bioactivity and stability of endogenous fibrogenic factors in platelet-rich fibrin. Wound Repair Regen 2008;16:356-363.
69. Su CY, Kuo YP, Tseng YH et al. In vitro release of growth factors from platelet-rich fibrin (PRF): a proposal to optimize the clinical applications of PRF. Oral Surg Oral Med Oral Pathol Oral Radiol Endod 2009;108:56-61.
70. Clipet F, Tricot S, Alno N, et al. In vitro effects of Choukroun's platelet-rich fibrin conditioned medium on 3 different cell lines implicated in dental implantology. Implant Dent 2012;21:51-6.
71. Gassling VL, Acil Y, Springer IN et al. Platelet-rich plasma and platelet-rich fibrin in human cell culture. Oral Surg Oral Med Oral Pathol Oral Radiol Endod 2009;108:48-55.
72. He L, Lin Y, Hu X, et al. A comparative study of platelet-rich fibrin (PRF) and platelet-rich plasma (PRP) on the effect of proliferation and differentiation of rat osteoblasts in vitro. Oral Surg Oral Med Oral Pathol Oral Radiol Endod 2009;108:707-13.
73. Kang YH, Jeon SH, Park JY et al. Platelet-rich fibrin is a bioscaffold and reservoir of growth factors for tissue regeneration. Tissue Eng Part A 2011;17:349-59.
74. Passaretti F, Tia M, D'Esposito V, et al. Growth-promoting action and growth factor release by different platelet derivatives. Platelets 2014;25:252-6.
75. Roy S, Driggs J, Elgharably H, et al. Platelet-rich fibrin matrix improves wound angiogenesis via inducing endothelial cell proliferation. Wound Repair Regen 2011;19:753-66.
76. Lucarelli E, Beretta R,Dozza B, et al. A recently developed bifacial platelet-rich fibrin matrix. Eur Cell Mater 2010;20:13-23.
77. Zumstein MA, Berger S, Schober M, et al. Leukocyte- and platelet-rich fibrin (L-PRF) for long-term delivery of growth factor in rotator cuff repair: review, preliminary results and future directions. Curr Pharm Biotechnol 2012;13:1196-206.
78. Kobayashi M, Kawase T, Okuda K, et al. In vitro immunological and biological evaluations of the angiogenic potential of platelet-rich fibrin preparations: a standardized comparison with PRP preparations. Int J Implant Dent 2015;1:31.
79. Nishiyama K, Okudera T, Watanabe T, et al. Basic characteristics of plasma rich in growth factors (PRGF): blood cell components and biological effects. Clin Exp Dent Res 2016;2:96-103.
80. Sonnenschein SK, Meyle J. Local inflammatory reactions in patients with diabetes and periodontitis. Periodontol 2000 2015;69:221-54.
81. Badade PS, Mahale SA, Panjwani AA, et al. Antimicrobial effect of platelet-rich plasma and platelet-rich fibrin. Indian J Dent Res 2016;27:300-4.
82. Nathani DB, Sequeira J, Rao BH. Comparison of platelet rich plasma and synthetic graft material for bone regeneration after third molar extraction. Ann Maxillofac Surg 2015;5(2):213-218.
83. Anitua E, Troya M, Zalduendo M, et al. Progress in the use of autologous regenerative platelet-based therapies in implant dentistry. Curr Pharm Biotechnol 2016;17:402-13.
84. Srinivas BV, Rupa N, Halini Kumari K.V, et al. Root coverage using subepithelial connective tissue graft with platelet-rich plasma in the treatment of gingival recession: A clinical study. J Pharm Bioallied Sci 2015;7:S530-8.
85. Mihaylova Z, Mitev V, Stanimirov P, et al. Use of platelet concentrates in oral and maxillofacial surgery: an overview. Acta Odontol Scand 2017;75(1):1-11.
86. Wikesjö UM, Nilveus R. Periodontal repair in dogs: effect of wound stabilization on healing. J Periodontol 1990;61(12):719-24.
87. Haney JM, Nilveus RE, McMillan PJ, et al. Periodontal repair in dogs: expanded polytetrafluroethylene barrier membrane support wound stabilization and enhance bone regeneration. J Periodontol 1993;64(9):883-90.
88. Polimeni G, Xiropaidis AV, Wilesjö UM. Biology and principles of periodontal healing/regeneration. Periodontol 2000 2006;41(1):30-47.
89. Retzepi M, Donos N. Guided bone regeneration: biological principle and therapeutic applications. Clin Oral Implants Res 2010;21(6):567-76.

90. Masquelet AC, Begue T. The concept of induced membrane for reconstruction of long bone defects. Orthop Clin North Am 2010;41(1):27-37.

91. Giannoudis, PV, O, Thomas, Goff T, et al. Masquelet technique for the treatment of bone defects: tips-tricks and future directions. Injury 2011;42(6): 591-8.

92. Dimitriou R, Mataliotakis GI, Calori GM, et al. The role of barrier membranes for guided bone regeneration and restoration of large bone defects: current experimental and clinical evidence. BMC Med 2012; 10(1):81.

93. Marolt D, Knezevic M, Vunjak-Novakovic G. Bone tissue engineering with human stem cells. Stem Cell Res Ther 2010;1(2):10.

94. Hitti RA. Kerns DG. Guided tissue regeneration in the oral cavity: a review. Open Pathol J 2011;5:33-45

95. Beanish B, Jawahir A, Reyaz AM, et al. Guided tissue regeneration - Rationale and factors affecting its outcome. IOSR-JDMS 2018;17(6);44-61.

96. Pellegrini G, Pagni G, Rasperini G. Surgical approaches based on biological objectives: GTR versus GBR techniques. Int J Dent 2013; 2013:521547.

97. Bottino MC, Thomas V, Gudrun Schmidt G, et al. Recent advances in the development of GTR/GBR membranes for periodontal regeneration - a materials perspective. Dent Mater 2012;28(7):703-21.

98. Rakhmatia YD, Ayukawa Y, Furuhashi A, et al. Current barrier membranes: titanium mesh and other membranes for guided bone regeneration in dental applications. J Prosthodont Res 2013;57(1):3-14.

99. Dahlin C, Sennerby L, Lekholm U, et al. Generation of new bone around titanium implants using a membrane technique: an experiment study in rabbits. IntJ Oral Maxillofacial Implants 1989;4(1):19-25.

100. Buser, D, Dahlin C. Schenk R. Guided bone regeneration in implant dentistry. Quintessence Publishing 1994:32-4.

101. Meinig RP. Clinical use of resorbable polymeric membranes in the treatment of bone defects. Orthopedic Clinics 2010;41(1):39-47.

102. Retzepi M, Donos N. Guided bone regeneration: biological principle and therapeutic applications. Clinical Oral Implant Research 2010; 21(6):567-76.

103. Nyman S, Lindhe J, Karring T, et al. New attachment following surgical treatment of human periodontal disease. J Clin Periodontol 1982;9:290-6.

104. Hardwick R, Scantlebury TV, Sanchez R, et al. Membrane design criteria for guided bone regeneration of the alveolar ridge. In: Buser D, Dahlin C, Schenk RK. Guided bone regeneration in implant dentistry. Chicago, Quintessence, 1994;101-36.

105. McAllister BS, Haghighat K. Bone augmentation techniques. J Periodontol 2007;78:377-96.

106. Machtei EE. The effect of membrane exposure on the outcome of regenerative procedures in human. A meta-analysis. J Periodontol 2001; 72:512-6.

107. Nowzari H, Slots J. Microbiologic and clinical study of polytetrafluroethylene membranes for guided bone regeneration around implants. Int J Oral Maxillofac Implants 1995;10:67-73.

108. Simion M, Misitano U, Gionso L, et al. Treatment of dehiscences and fenestrations around dental implants using resorbable and nonresorbable membranes associated with bone autografts: a comparative clinical study. Int J Oral Maxillofac Implants 1997;12(2):159-67.

109. McGinnis M, Larsen P, Miloro M, et al. Comparison of resorbableand nonresorbable guided bone regeneration materials: a preliminary study. Int J Oral Maxillofac Implants 1998;13(1): 30-5.

110. Susin C, Wikesjö UME. Regenerative periodontal therapy: 30 years of lessons learned and unlearned. Periodontol 2000 2013;62:232-42.

111. Polimeni G, Koo KT, Qahash M, et al. Prognostic factors for alveolar regeneration: effect of tissue occlusion on alveolar bone regeneration with guided tissue regeneration. J Clin Periodontol 2004;31:730-5.

112. Wikesjö UM, Lim WH, Thomson RC, Hardwick WR. Periodontal repair in dogs: gingival tissue occlusion, a critical requirement for GTR? J Clin Periodontol 2003;30:655-64.

113. Zanetta-Barbosa D, Klinge B, Svensson H. Laser doppler flowmetry of blood perfusion in mucoperiosteal flaps covering membranes in bone augmentation and implant procedures. A pilot study in dogs. Clin Oral Implants Res 1993;4(1):35-8.

114. LeGeros RZ. Properties of osteoconductive biomaterials: calcium phosphates. Clin Orth Relat Res 2002;395:81-98

115. Titsinides S. Agrogiannis G, Karatzas T. Bone grafting materials in dentoalveolar reconstruction: a comprehensive review. Jap Dent Sci Rev 2019;55(1): 26-32.

116. Sheikh Z, Hamdan N, Ikeda Y, et al. Natural graft tissues and synthetic biomaterials for periodontal and alveolar bone reconstructive applications: a review. Biomater Res 2017;21(1):9.

117. Wang W,. Yeung KW. Bone grafts and biomaterials substitutes for bone defect repair: A review. Bioact mater 2017;2(4):224-47.

118. Liu J, Kerns D. Mechanisms of guided bone regeneration: a review. Open Dent J 2014;8:56-65.

119. Elgali I, Omar O, Dahlin C, Thomsen P,et al. Guided bone regeneration: materials and biological mechanisms revisited. Eur J Oral Sci 2017;125(5): 315-37.

120. Venkataraman N, Bansal S, Bansal P, et al. Dynamics of bone graft healing around implants. J Int Clin Dent Res Organ. 2015;7(3):40-47.

121. Wang T, Zhang X, Bikle DD. Osteogenic differentiation of periosteal cells during fracture healing. J CellPhysiol 2017;232(5):913-21.

122. Zhang X, Awad HA, O'Keefe RJ, et al. A perspective: engineering periosteum for structural bone graft healing. Clin Orthop Relat Res 2008;466(8):1777-87.

123. Tsiridis E, Upadhyay N, Giannoudis P. Molecular aspects of fracture healing: which are the important molecules? Injury 2007;38(1):11-25.

124. Kanczler J, Oreffo R. Osteogenesis and angiogenesis: the potential for engineering bone. Eur Cell Mater 2008;15(2):100-14.

125. Omar O, Elgali I, Dahli C, et al. Barrier membranes: More than the barrier effect? J Clinical Periodontol 2019; 46:103-23.

126. McGovern JA, Griffin M, Hutmacher DW. Animal models for bone tissue

engineering and modelling disease. Dis Mod Mech 2018;11(4):dmm033084.

127. Baldwin JG. Unravelling the mechanisms behind periosteal regeneration and its application in bone tissue engineering. Queensland University of Technology 2017.

128. Lin Z, Fateh A, Salem DM, et al. Periosteum: biology and applications in craniofacial bone regeneration. J Dent Res 2014;93(2):109-16.

129. Roberts SJ, van Gastel N, Carmeliet G, et al. Uncovering the periosteum for skeletal regeneration: the stem cell that lies beneath. Bone 2015;70:10-8.

130. Marsell R, Einhorn TA. The biology of fracture healing. Injury 2011;42(6):551-5.

131. Sambrook P, Schrieber L, Taylor T, et al. The musculoskeletal system (2nd edition). London: Elsevier, 2010.

132. Ueno T, Kagawa N, Mizukawa N, et al. Cellular origin of endochondral ossification from grafted periosteum. Anat Rec 2001;264(4):348-57.

133. Zhang XP, Chao X, Lin ASP, et al. Periosteal progenitor cell fate in segmental cortical bone graft transplantations: implications for functional tissue engineering. J Bone Miner Res 2005;20(12):2124-37.

134. Raab-Cullen DM, Akhter MP, Kimmel DB, et al. Periosteal bone formation stimulated by externally induced bending strains. J Bone Miner Res 1994;9(8):1143-52.

135. Lindhe J, Cecchinato D, Tomasi C, et al. Ridge preservation with the use of deproteinized bovine bone mineral. Clin Oral Impl Res 2014;25:786-90.

136. Corbella S, Taschieri S, Francetti L, et al. Histomorphometric results after postextraction socket healing with different biomaterials: a systematic review of the literature and meta-analysis. Int J Oral Maxillofac Implants 2017;32(5):1001-17.

Clinical cases

Tomás Beca Campoy, DDS
Dentist
Visiting Professor at Master in Oral Surgery and Implantology, Francisco de Vitoria University, Madrid
Private practice, Madrid

Fulvio Bromuri, DDS
Dentist
Private practice, Milan

Marcello Contessi, MD
Surgeon
Postgraduate in Implantology and Oral Surgery, New York University
Private practice, Trieste

Ugo Gambardella, MD
Surgeon, Specialist in Odontostomatology and Pathophysiology
Postgraduate in Periodontology, Royal Dental College of Aarhus, Denmark
Private practice, Seriate (BG)

Edoardo Giacometti, MD
Surgeon
Adjunct Professor, University of Genoa
Postgraduate in Implantology and Oral Surgery, New York University
Private practice, Turin

Henry K.L. Ho, DDS
Dentist
Visiting Professor, University of Frankfurt, University "Titu Maiorescu" of Bucharest, University of Naples "Federico II"
Master in Dental Surgery, National University of Singapore
Member of the Royal College of Surgeons, Edinburgh
Private practice, Singapore

Mauro Libertucci, DDS
Dentist
Visiting Professor of the II level Master in Surgery and Implant Prosthetics, University of Siena
Visiting Professor of the II level Master in Advanced Technologies of Bone Reconstruction, Saint Camillus International University of Health Sciences, Rome
Visiting Professor of the II level Master in Complex Oral Rehabilitation, University of Catania
Private practice, Rome

Elio Minetti, DDS
Dentist
Visiting Professor, University of Milan
Postgraduate in Implantology and Oral Surgery, New York University
Private practice, Milan

Jesus Santillana, DDS
Dentist
Master in Implantology, University of Barcelona
Member of the General Dental Council, Manchester
Private practice, Bilbao

Johannes Schmitz, DDS
Dentist
Visiting Professor Professor, University of Milan (1999-2011)
Research Doctorate (PhD) in Morphological Sciences
Private practice, Milan

Unless otherwise specified in the text, all the cases described have been treated using dentin only.

ALVEOLAR PRESERVATION

Alveolar preservation with membrane

Clinical case 1

E. Minetti, Milan, Italy

50-year-old female reporting bleeding and pain in area 3.6. Physical and radiographic examination shows the fracture of the mesial root of 3.6 with loss of vestibular bone tissue (2nd class). It was decided to carry out an alveolar socket preservation to maintain the volume and ensure an aesthetic appearance of the implant restoration. After cleaning the roots, due to the small size, the presence of endocanalar screws and endodontic filling, the amount of material produced is less than needed. It is then mixed 50% with xenograft material (Bio-Oss, Geistlich biomaterials, Germany).

Alveolar preservation is carried out using a collagen membrane (Bego-Oss, Bego, Germany) to cover the defect. After 4 months, during the osteotomy, a biopsy cylinder is taken. The follow-up was at 54 months. Visio One Cea implant (Cea medical, Swiss) is placed and, upon maturation, a screw-retained stratified zirconia restoration was used.

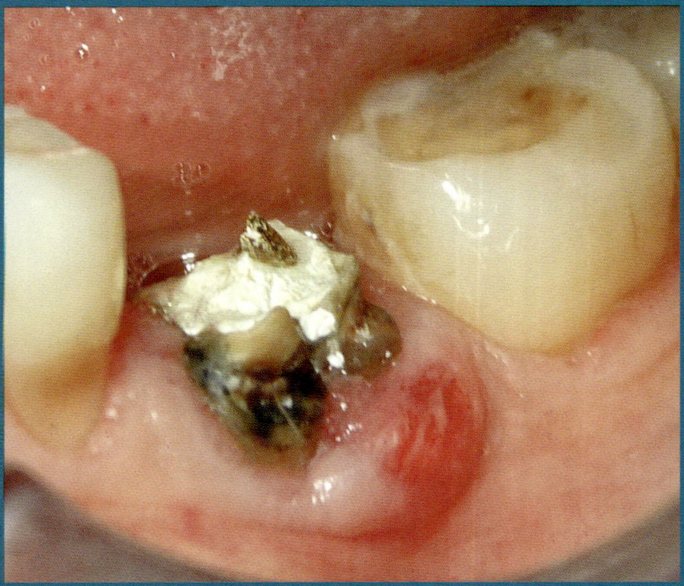

1 Element 3.6 the vertical fracture of the mesial root can be noted.

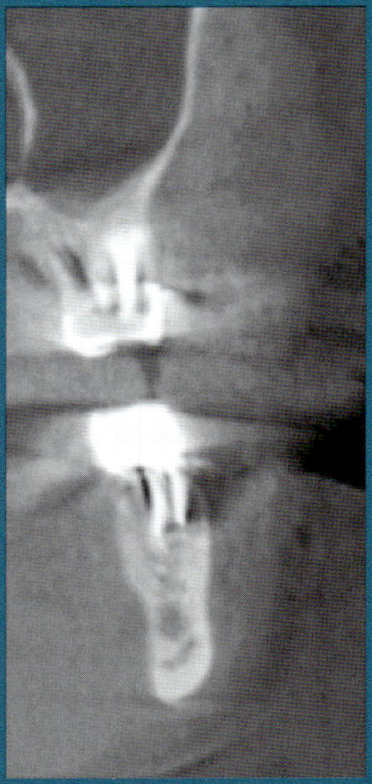

2 Image extracted from CBCT shows loss of buccal bone in mesial area 3.6.

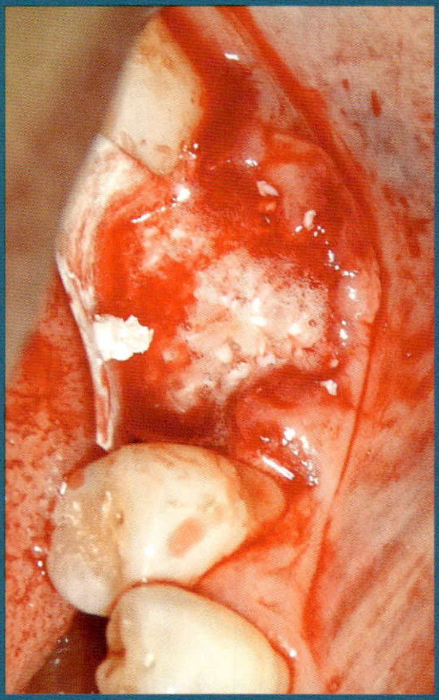

3 Alveolar socket preservation with placement of 50% material derived from the roots of the extracted tooth + 50% xenograft material (Bio-Oss, Geistlich biomaterials) and coverage by the use of a collagen membrane.

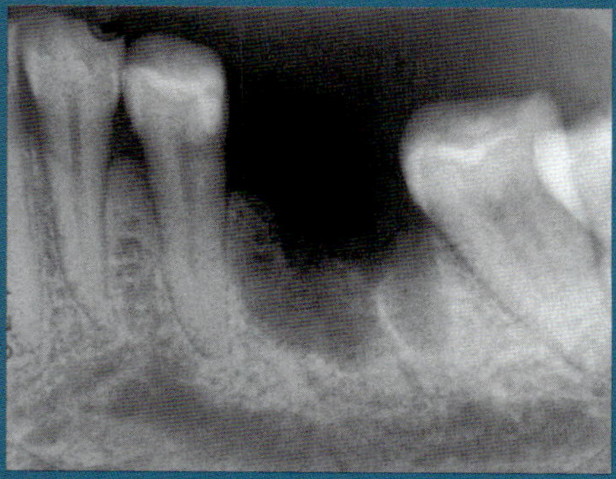

4 Postextraction Rx of 3.6.

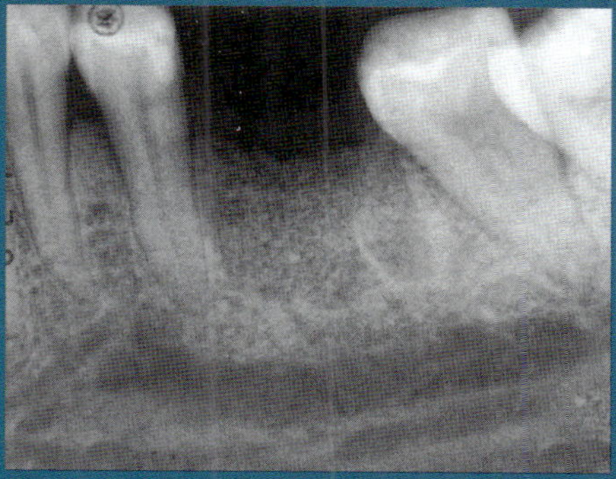

5 Rx at 10 days after alveolar preservation.

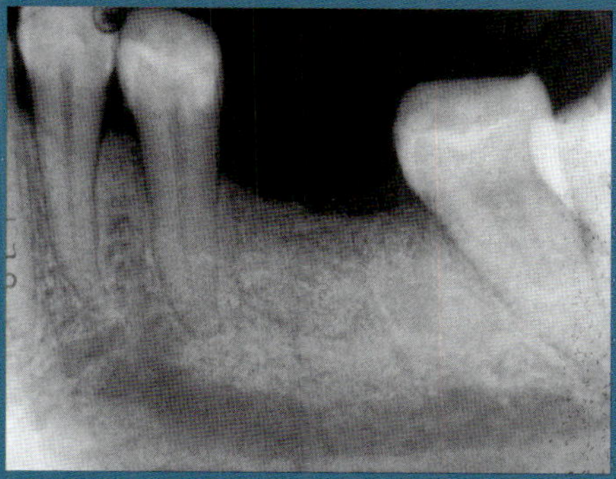

6 Rx at 4 months after alveolar preservation. It can be seen that the graft material is dense and similar to bone tissue.

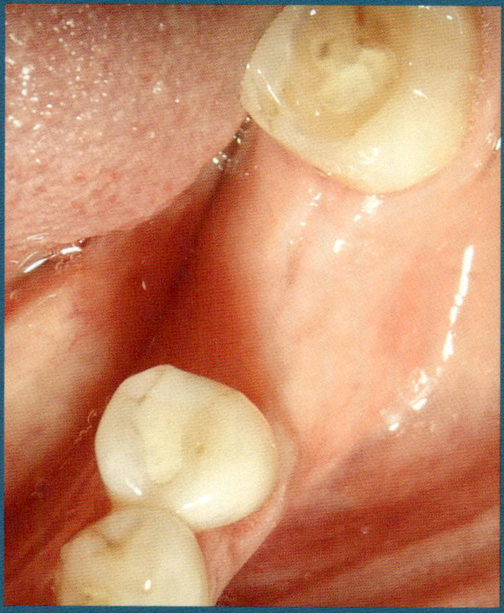

7 Appearance of soft tissues after 4 months.

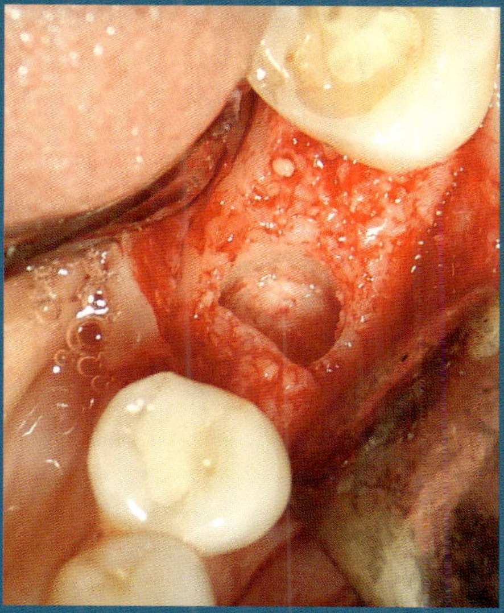

8 Biopsy sampling and implant surgical socket.

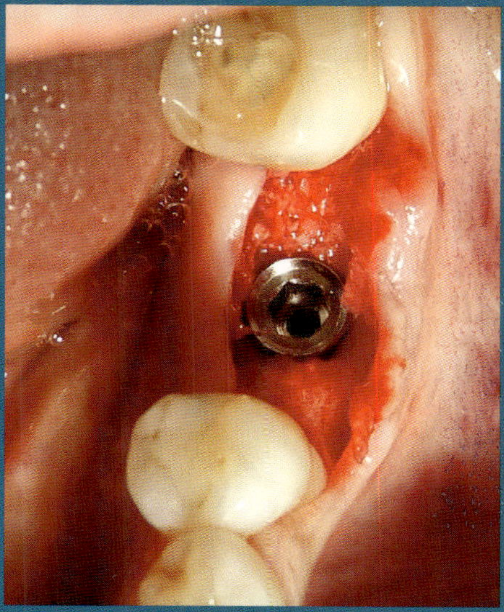

9 Implant in situ.

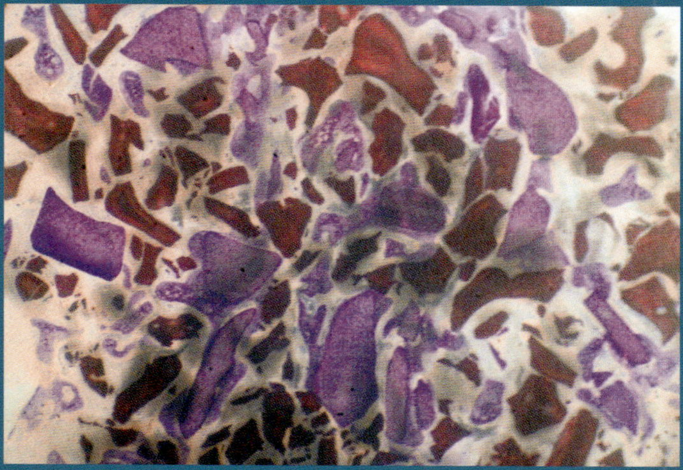

10 Result of histological sampling at 4 months. It can be seen that the dentin granules, in purple, are surrounded and in close contact with newly formed bone. The xenograft granules (Bio-Oss), in red, have no contact with bone tissue.

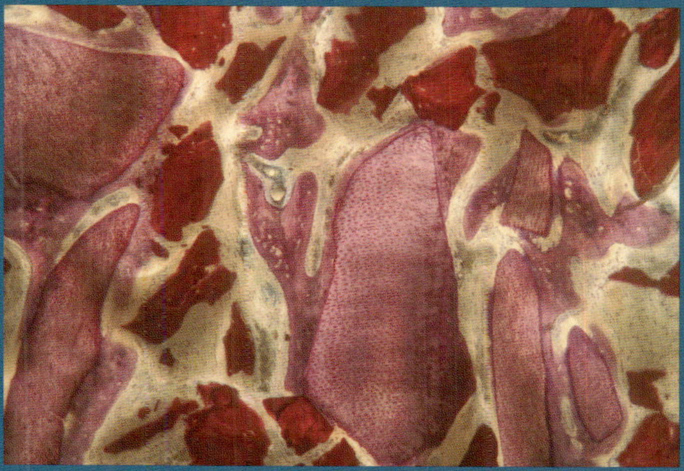

11 Histological image at higher enlargement; in purple, the dentin granules surrounded by bone in formation and, in red, xenograft (Bio-Oss) without bone contact.

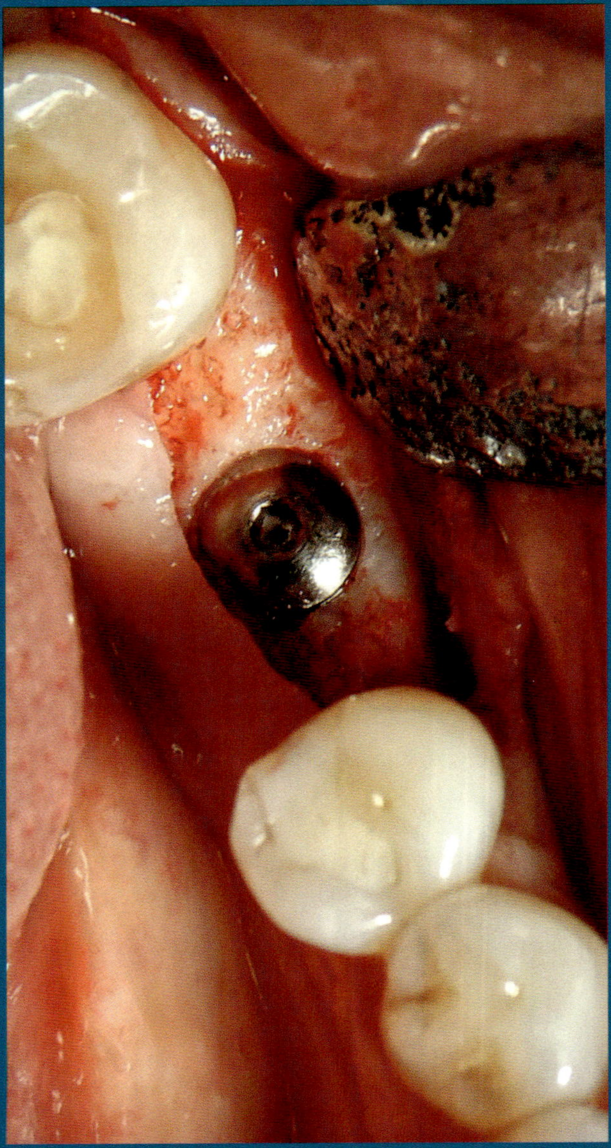

12 Healing 4 months after implantation.

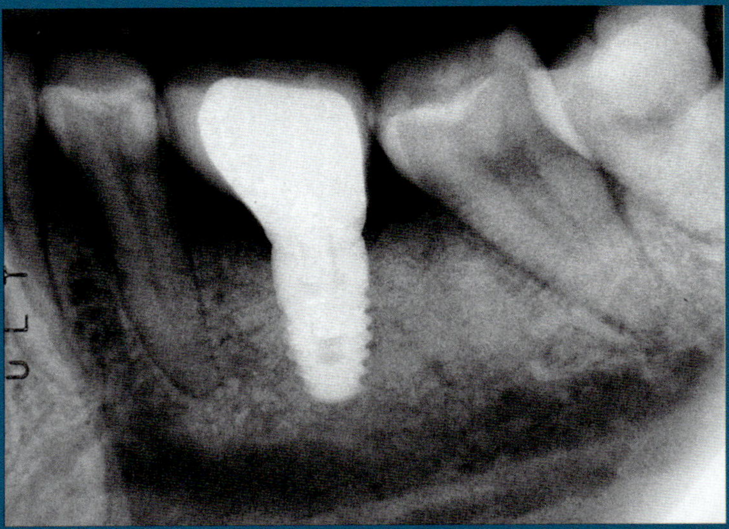

13 Radiographic image 54 months after regeneration.

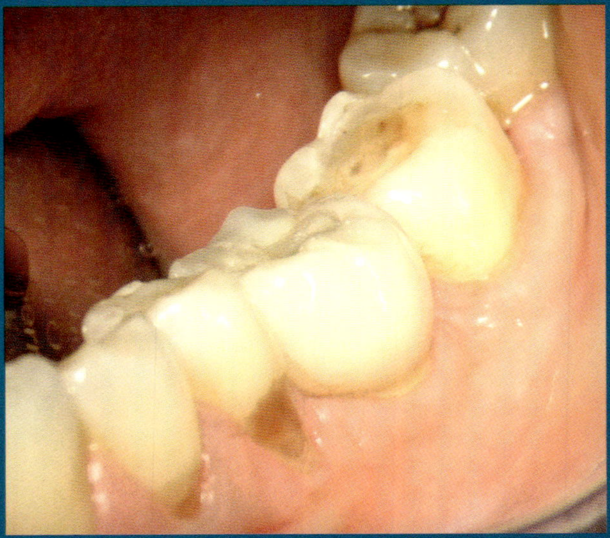

14 Clinical image of the tissues 54 months after regeneration.

Clinical case 2

J. Schmitz, Milan, Italy

63-year-old female patient complaining of pain in the left side of the mouth and complaining of irregular surfaces of the occlusal surface of an upper metal ceramic bridge performed ten years earlier in another practice. Due to exacerbation of pain after bite on a wet cotton roll, the extraction of 3.6 is planned. Given the patient's request to have a fixed prosthesis and to replace the upper bridge, the mesially tilted 3.8 is extracted at the same time in anticipation of the insertion of two implants in area 3.6 and 3.7 (biomet 3i). Once the particulate was obtained, it was placed in the socket and in the supracrestal area at the level of the defect between 3.6 and 3.8, in combination with a resorbable membrane in order to avoid its displacement.

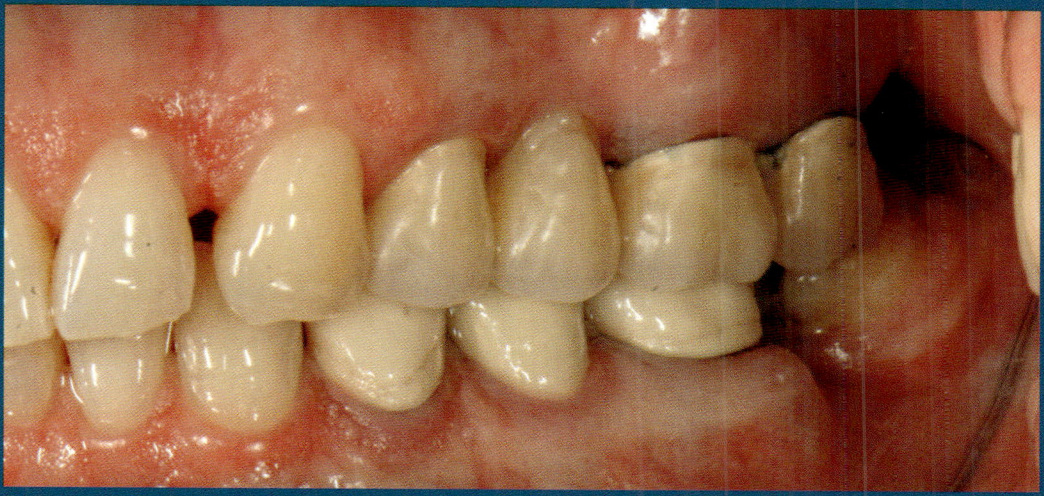

1 Left vestibular view before surgery.

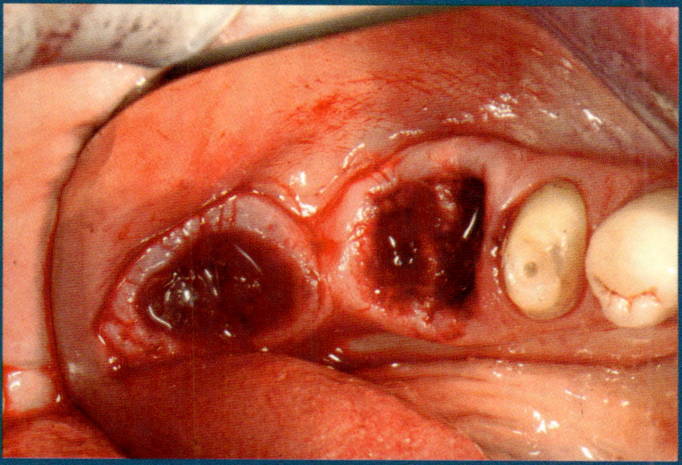

2 The extraction is performed by dissecting the roots and keeping the anatomical structures intact as much as possible.

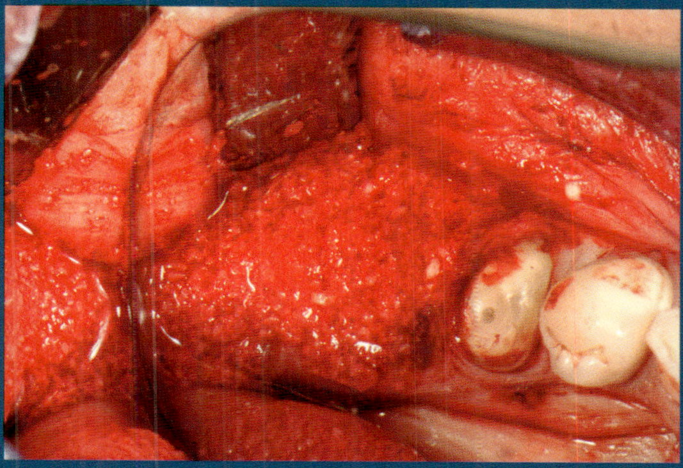

3 The available root and coronal segments are dissected; a ridge preservation technique is chosen for placing the material obtained in the socket and above the bone crest. The particulate is covered with a resorbable membrane.

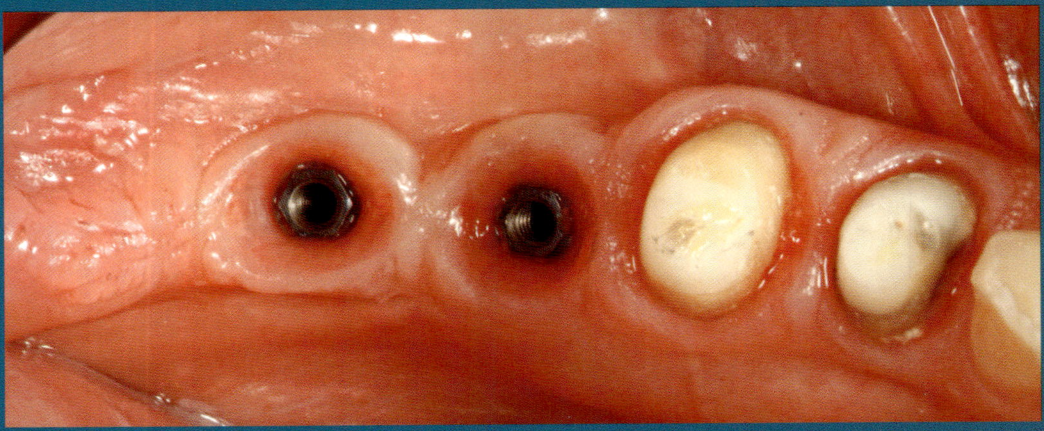

4 Occlusal photo of the implants. After osseointegration, the appearance of the tissues appears satisfactory.

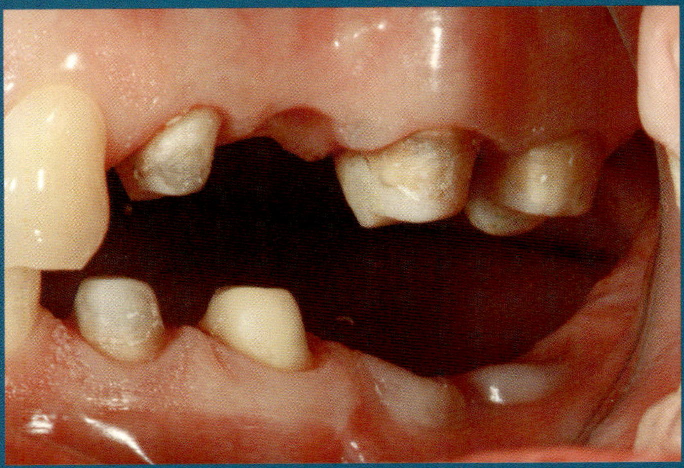

5 Lateral view at the time of taking the impressions for the definitive prostheses (provisional crowns on teeth were previously placed).

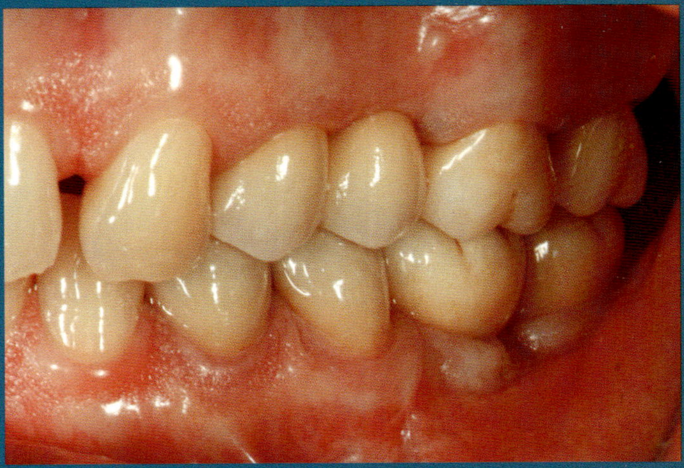

6 Lateral view of the definitive prostheses on teeth and implants made of monolithic zirconia on the molar elements and partially ceramic layered on the premolars.

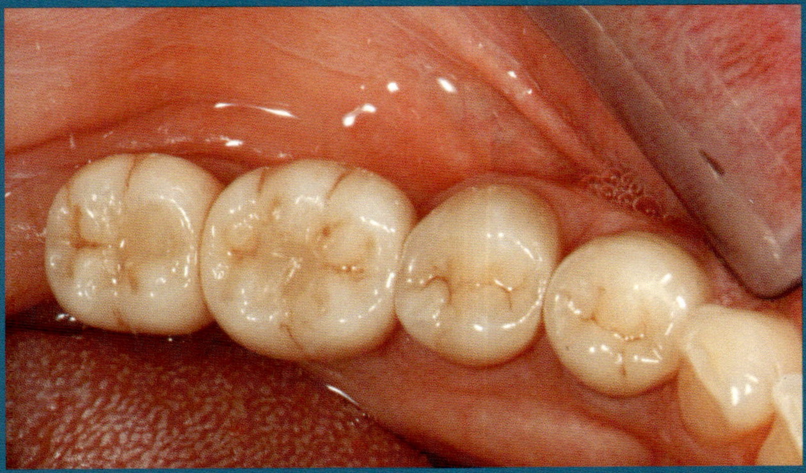

7 Occlusal detail of the restoration made in the third quadrant. The implant-supported restoration is screwed directly and holes have been sealed with composite.

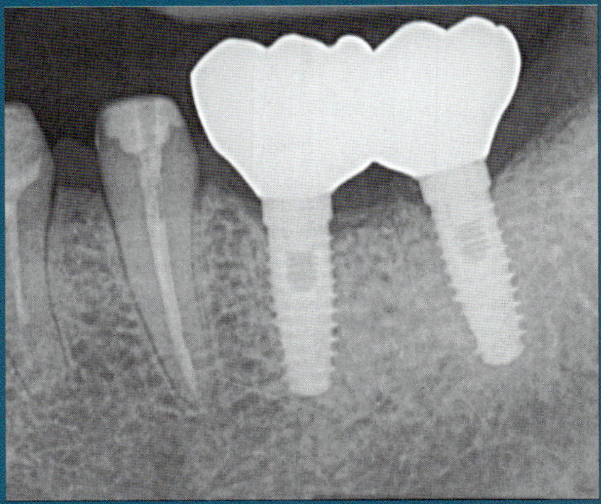

8 Radiographic control 2 months after implant loading confirms the excellent integration of the grafted material.

Alveolar preservation with membrane, platelet derivatives

Clinical case 3

T. Beca Campoy, Madrid, Spain

46-year-old female patient, non-smoker, with no previous pathologies.

The patient comes to the clinic for pain and suppuration in area 4.7-4.8. It is decided to extract the elements and regenerate using Tooth Transformer mixed with CGF. An implant is inserted after 4 months (ETK Naturactis, ETK Spain). Using a trephine drill, biopsy is carried out, which is then analyzed histologically. When the implant is placed, another histological sample is taken and, finally, a ceramic restoration is fit.

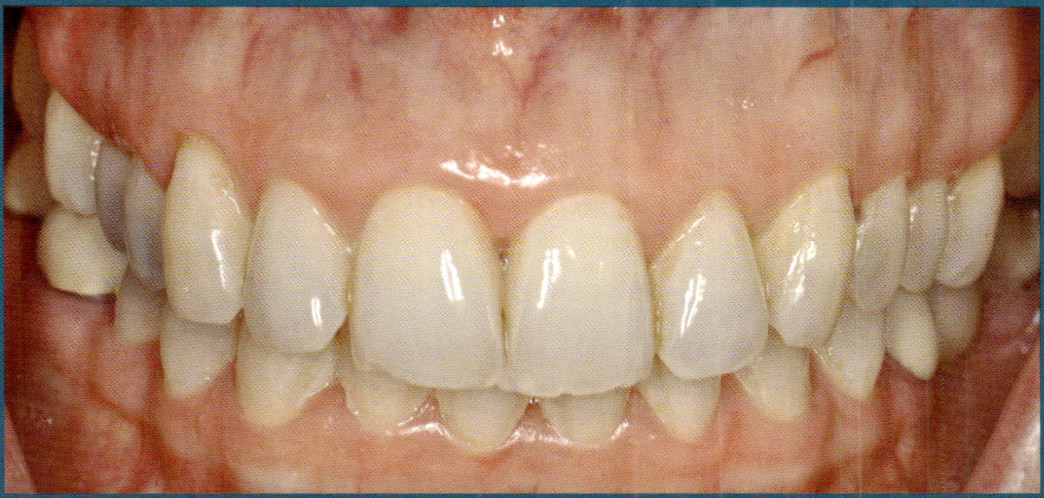

1 Frontal intraoral view.

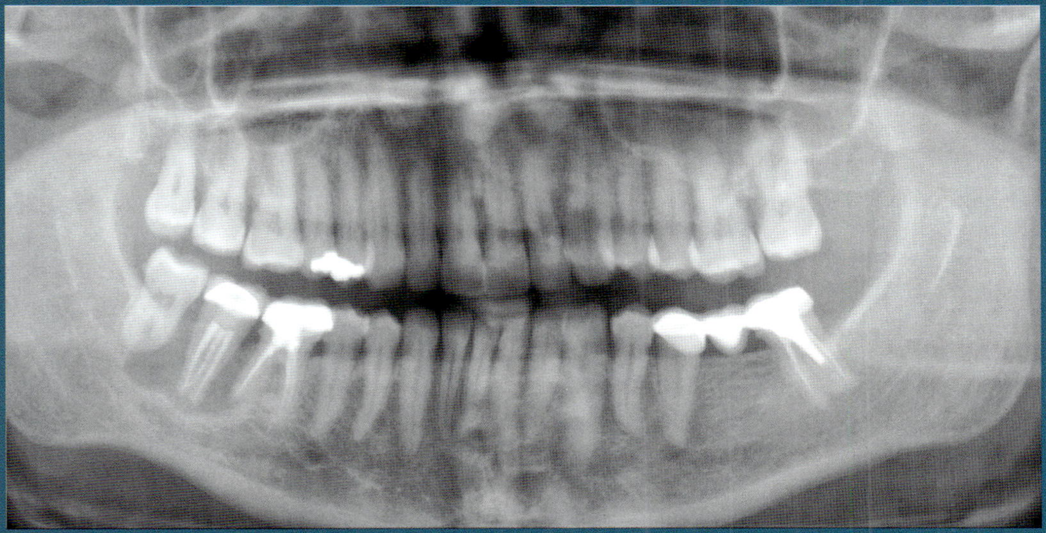

2 Preoperative orthopantomography. The deep lesion can be seen in area 4.7-4.8.

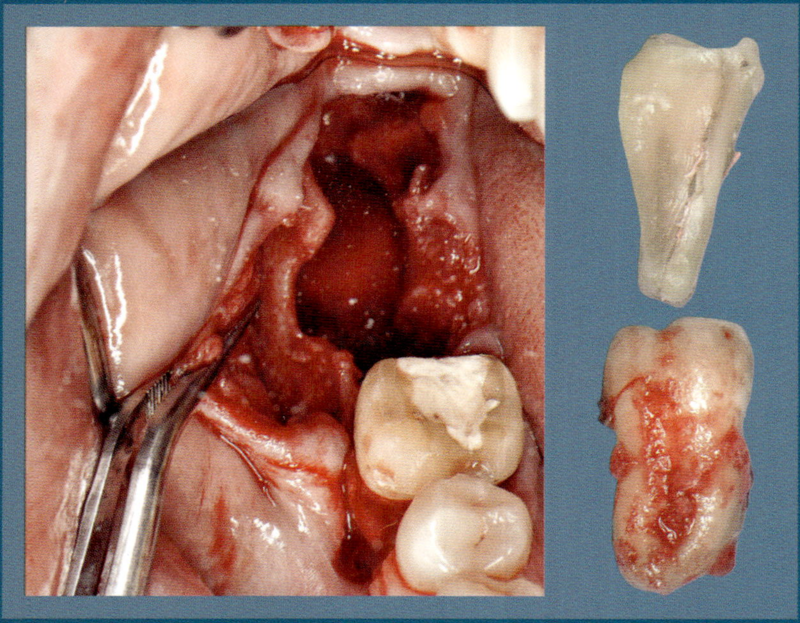

3 Extraction of 4.7-4.8 with vestibular dehiscence. You can see the vertical fracture of the extracted element.

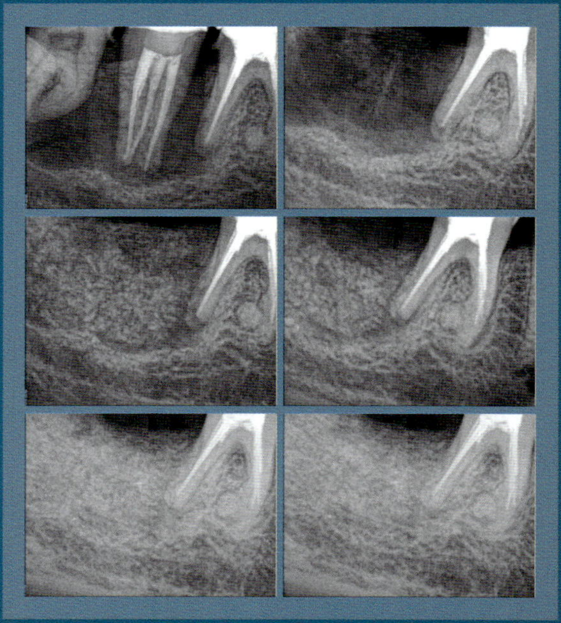

4 Radiographic evolution of the treated area.

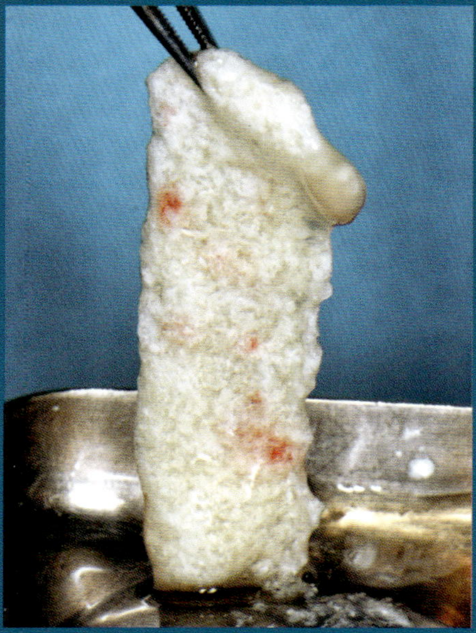

5 Sticky bone prepared using the dentin of the extracted teeth.

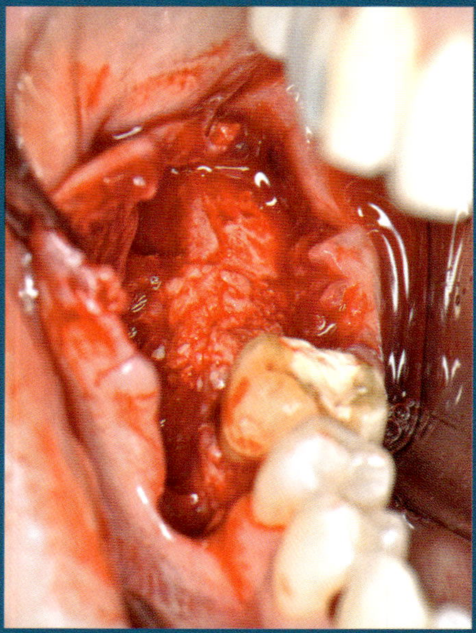

6 Condensed sticky bone to completely fill the bone defect.

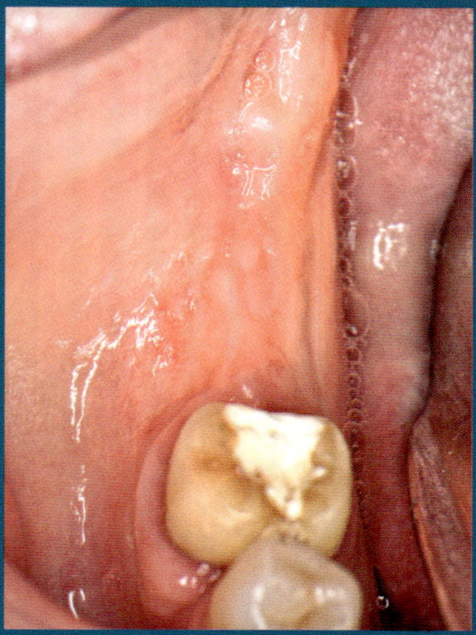

7 Tissue maturation before implant placement.

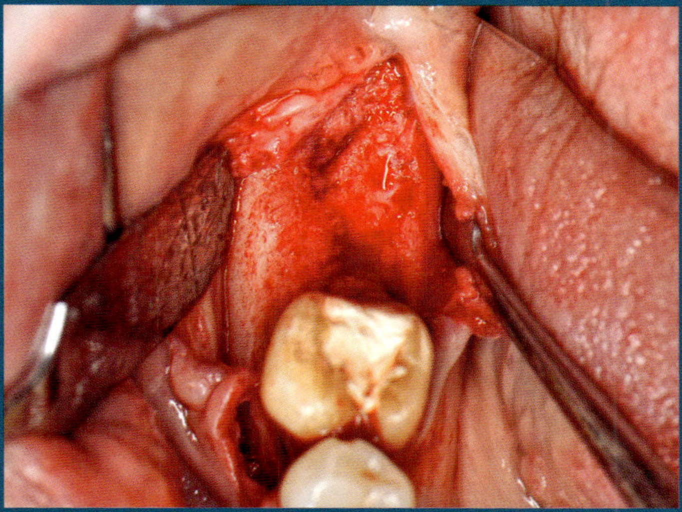

8 Opening of the flap and exposure of the newly formed tissue.

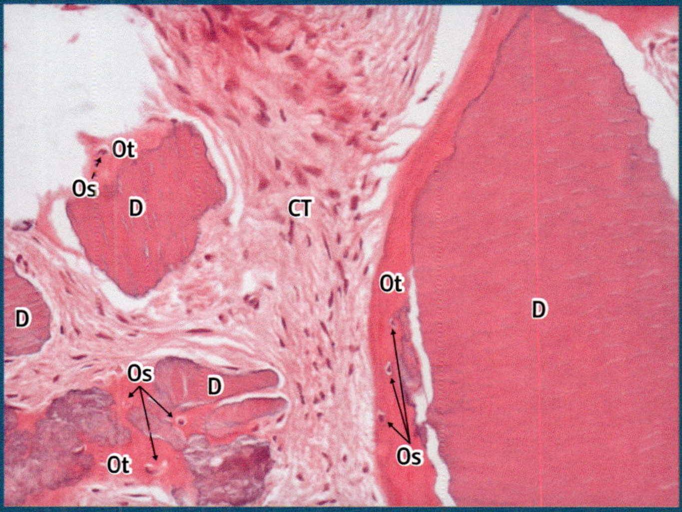

9 First histology performed at 4 months where it is possible to see osteoid tissue and osteocytes together with dentin. D: dentin; CT: connective tissue; Os: osteocytes; Ot: osteoid.

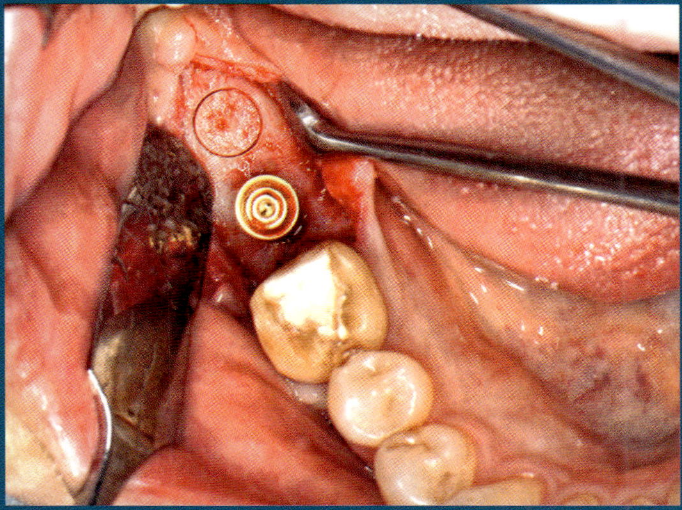

10 At 4 months, placement of the healing cap and second biopsy.

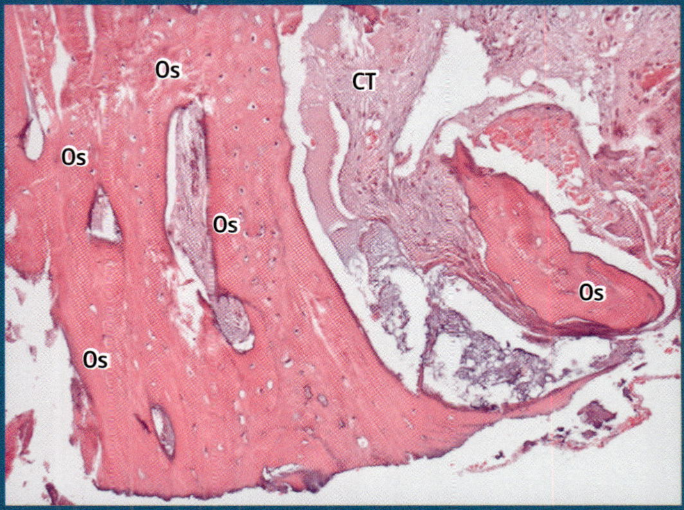

11 Second biopsy performed at 8 months highlights the large amount of bone and osteocytes. D: dentin; CT: connective tissue; Os: osteocytes.

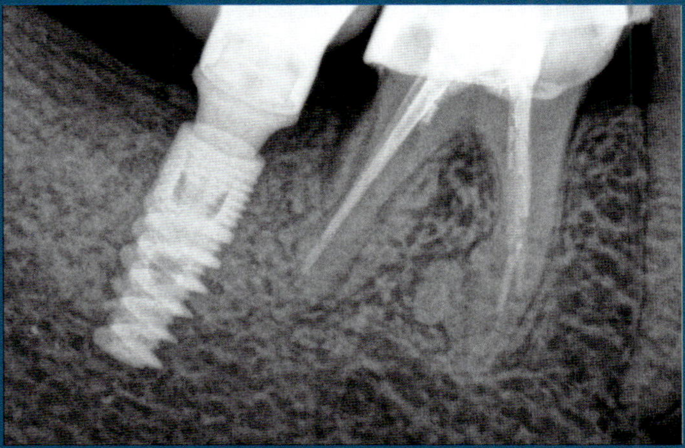

12 Post-op IOPA.

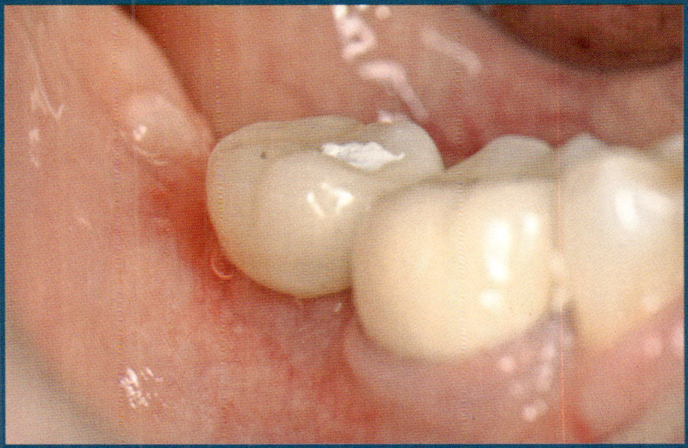

13 Intracral view of the prosthesis and the soft tissues.

Clinical case 4

U. Gambardella, Seriate (BG), Italy

56-year-old female patient suffering from systemic lupus erythematosus, on continuous therapy with steroids and methotrexate. Endo/periodontal lesion on 2.4 already treated with endo surgery. The tooth has a hopeless prognosis. At radiological control with CBCT, loss of the entire vestibular cortex of 2.4 is highlighted. Given the clinical condition of the patient, the minimally invasive treatment is opted for:

- extraction of 2.4, use of the element as a donor for Tooth Transformer treatment;
- GBR with flapless access and use of TT dentin added to plasma rich in PRGF growth factors and fibrin membrane.

After 4 months, the bone regeneration is complete, with horizontal and vertical regeneration (highlighted on CBCT) which allows the placement of the Straumann *SLActive* (Straumann, Swiss) endosseous implant (4.1 mm by 12 mm). The biopsy macroscopically shows a sample of 5 mm × 0.4 mm which histologically presents bone with completely included fragments of dentin.

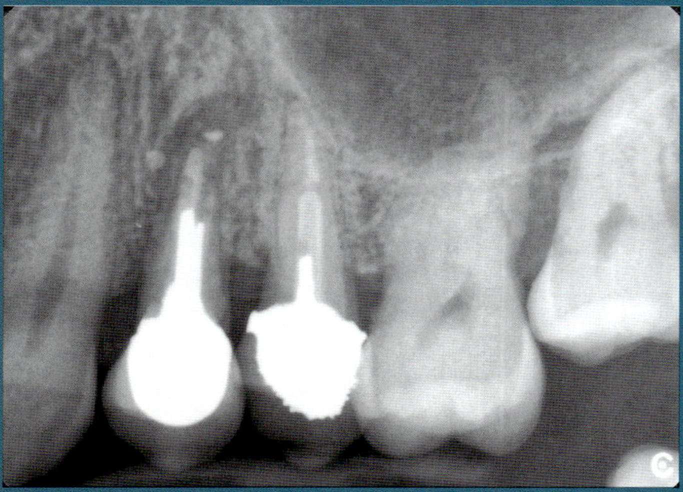

1 IOPA of 2.4.

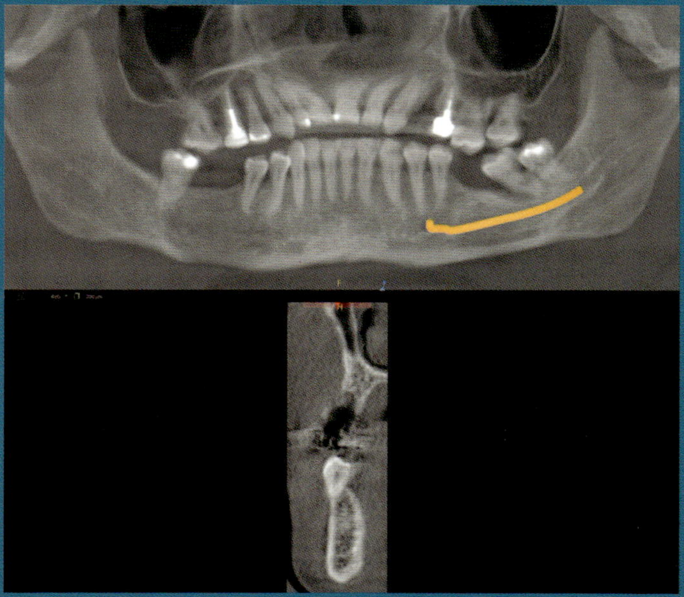

2 CBCT after the extraction of 2.4. The vestibular bone defect can be noted.

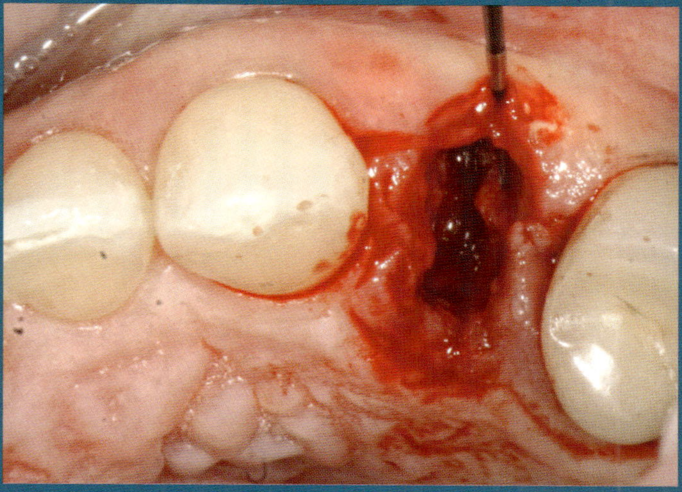

3 Tissues after the XLA. The lack of buccal bone wall may be noted.

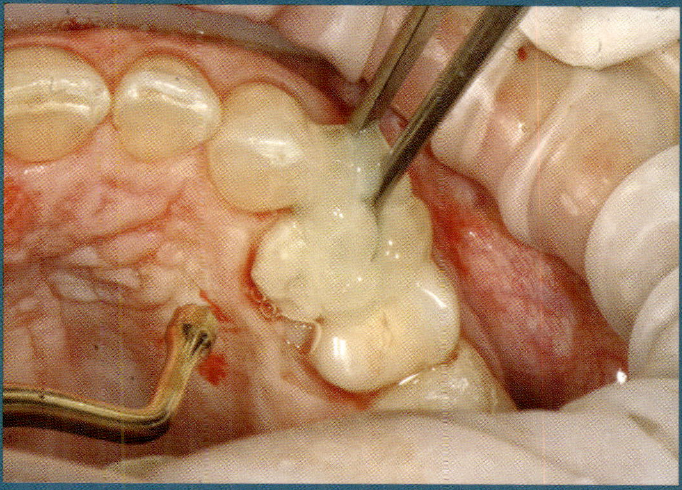

4 Condensation of the PRGF mixed with the dentin granules obtained from the root of the extracted tooth.

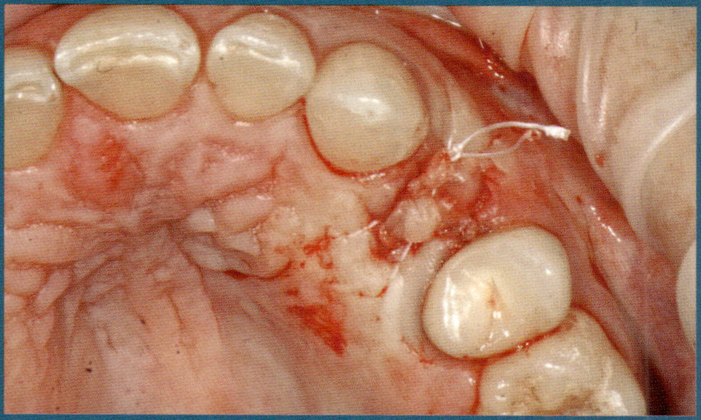

5 Suture and fibrin membrane in situ.

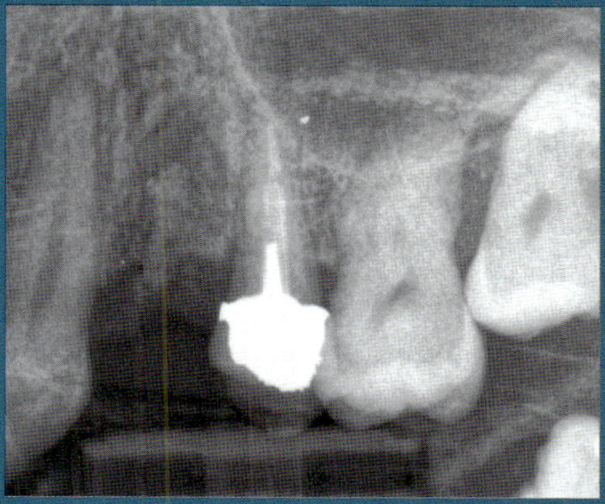

6 Postoperative intraoral X-ray.

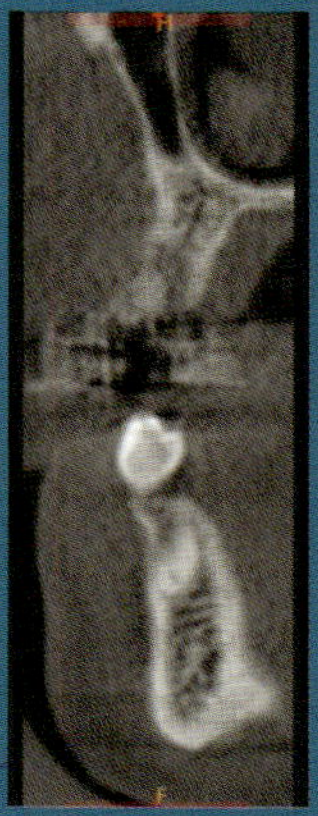

7 Postoperative CBCT.

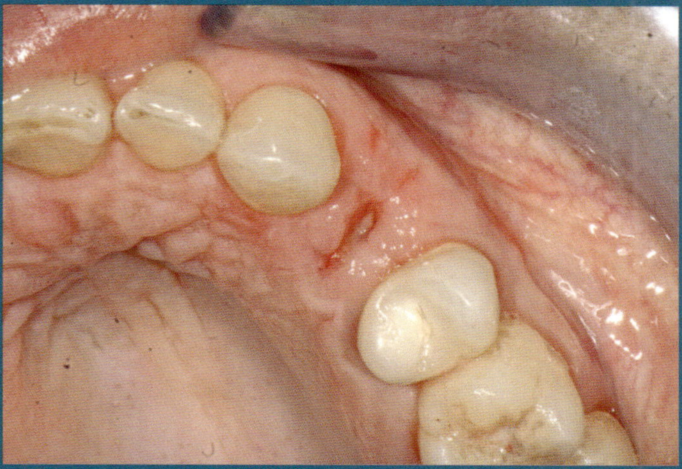

8 Healing after 1 week.

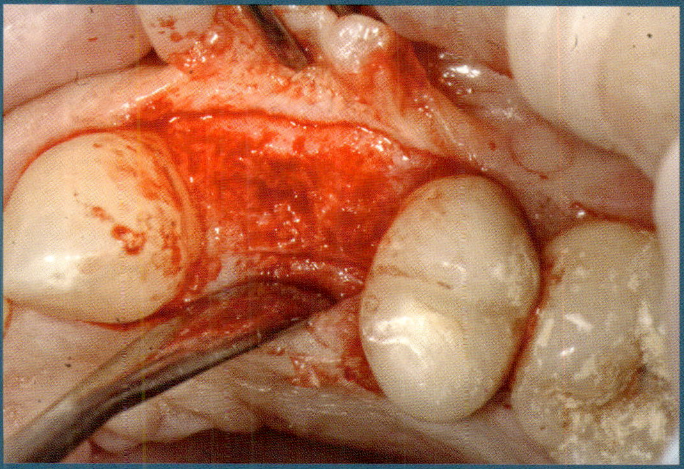

9 Opening at 4 months: the bone appears compact and the cortex is present.

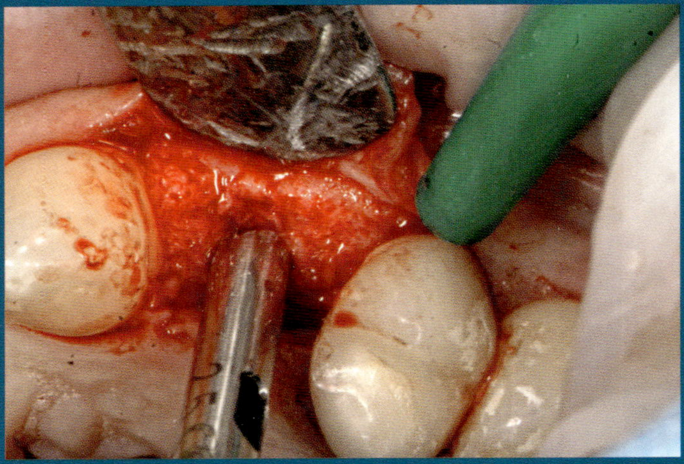

10 Biopsy sampling carried out during the drilling for implant placement.

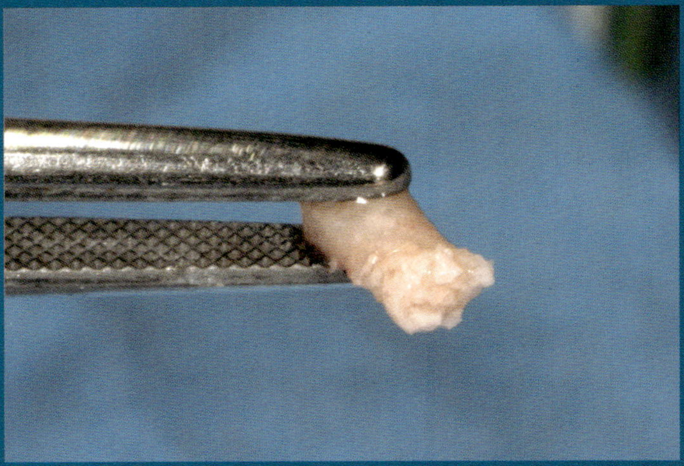

11 Biopsy sampling. Note the firmness of the structure.

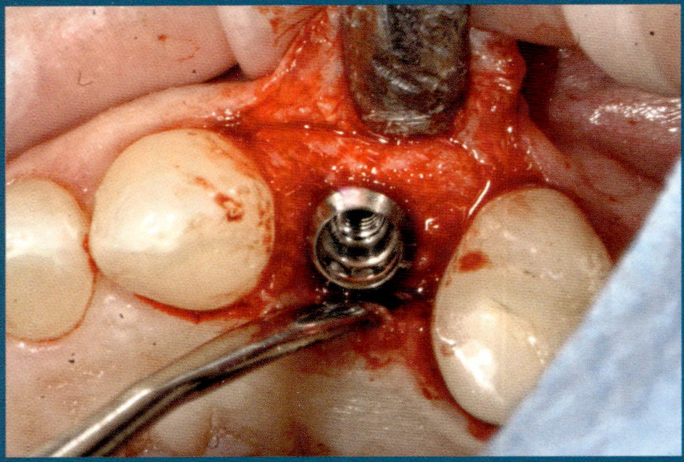

12 Implant positioned. The cortical tissue is visible where, after the extraction it was completely missing.

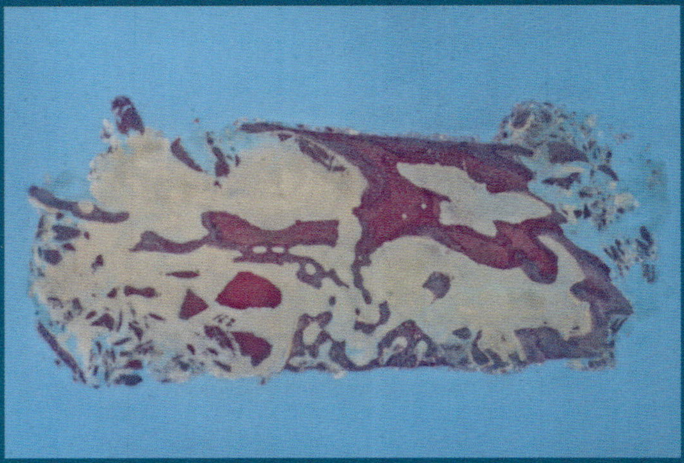

13 Sagittal section of the sample.

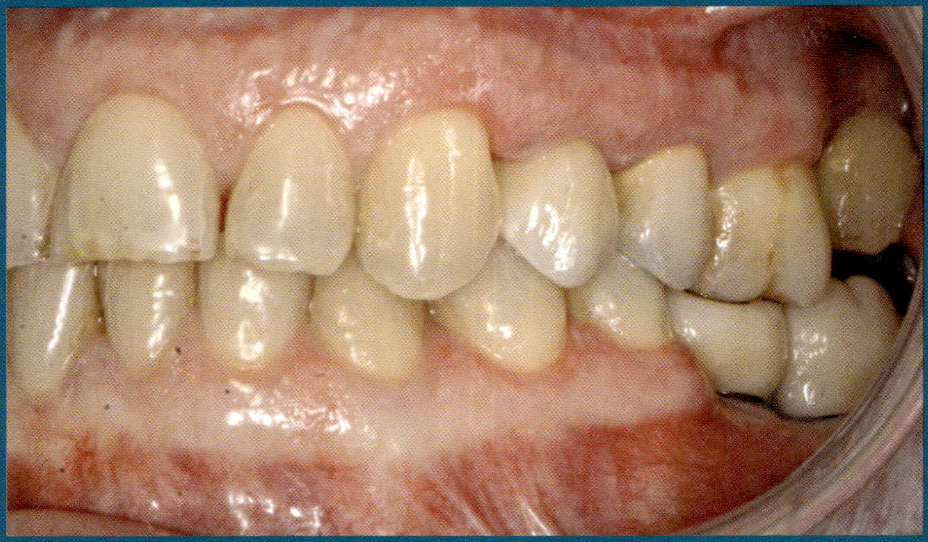

14 Restoration carried out upon integration of the implant.

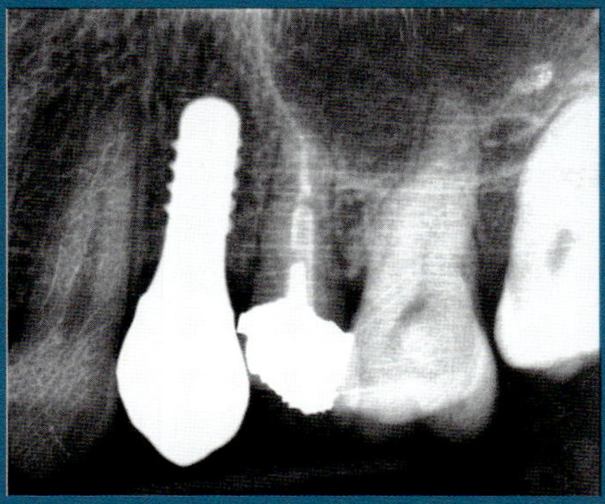

15 Intraoral X-ray 1 year after loading.

Alveolar preservation without membrane

Clinical case 5

E. Minetti, Milan, Italy

47-year-old male patient, non-smoker, and without any pathology. The patient has vestibular root caries with suppuration and probing. The gingival phenotype often allowed for a pocket without recession. At the time of extraction, a H_2O CEA (Cea medical, Swiss) implant is placed in the post-extraction socket by condensing the material derived from the extracted tooth in the vestibular area where there is a collapse of the vestibular wall and containing the material by means of immediate restoration.

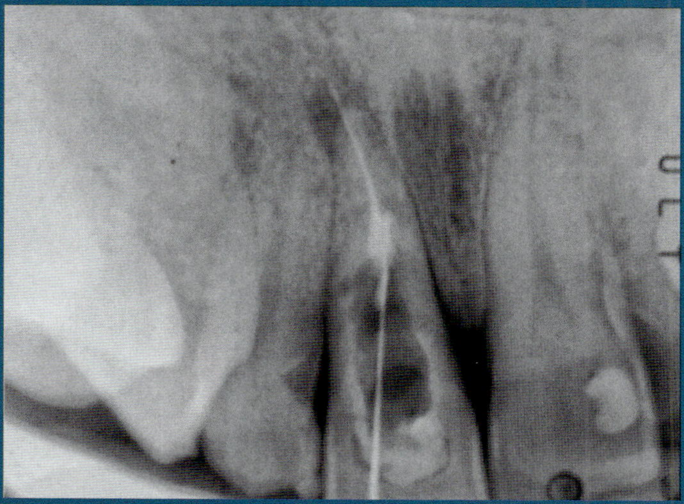

1 Preoperative X-ray.

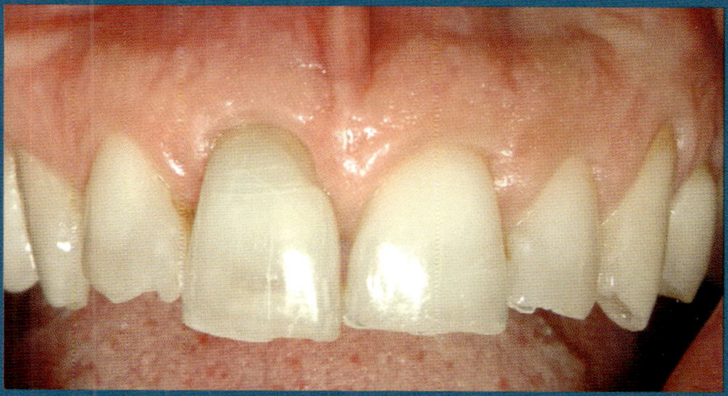

2 Preoperative image.

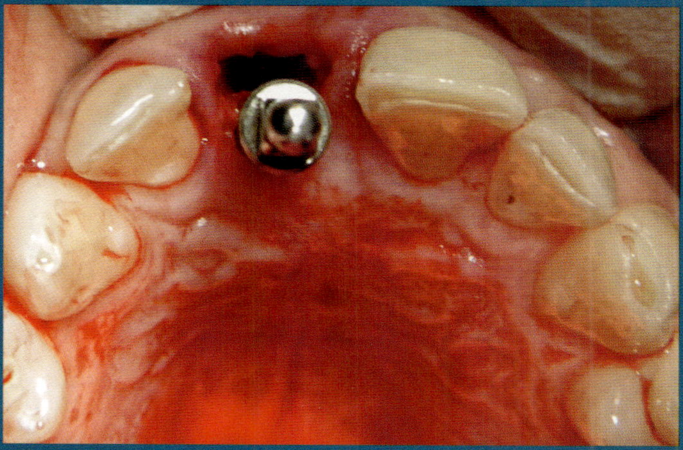

3 Insertion of the implant. Collapse of the vestibular wall can be noted.

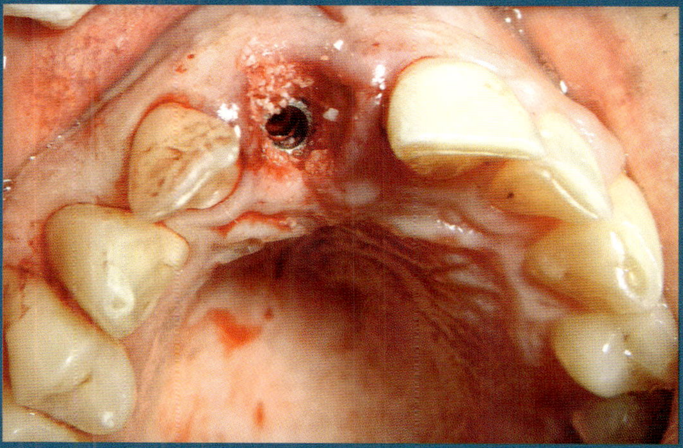

4 Condensation of the dental material graft without membrane positioning.

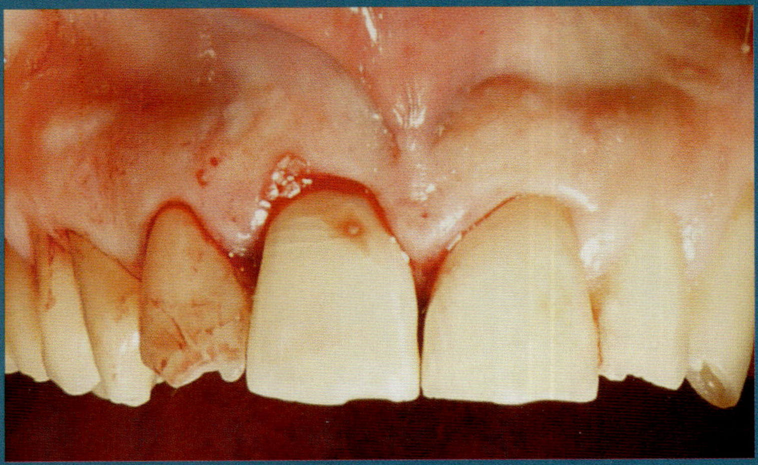

5 Prosthesis containing the grafting material.

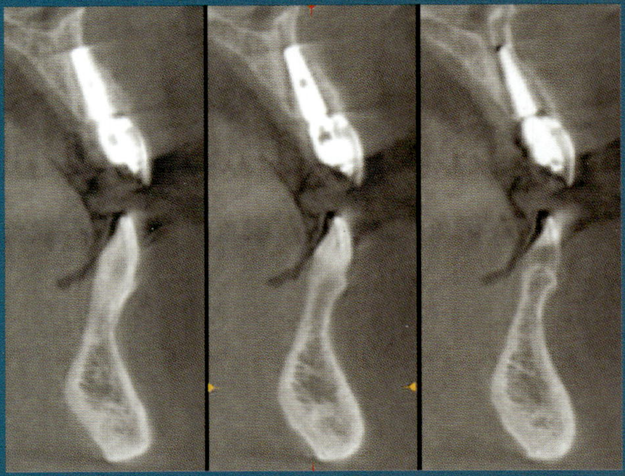

6 CBCT control after 2 months.

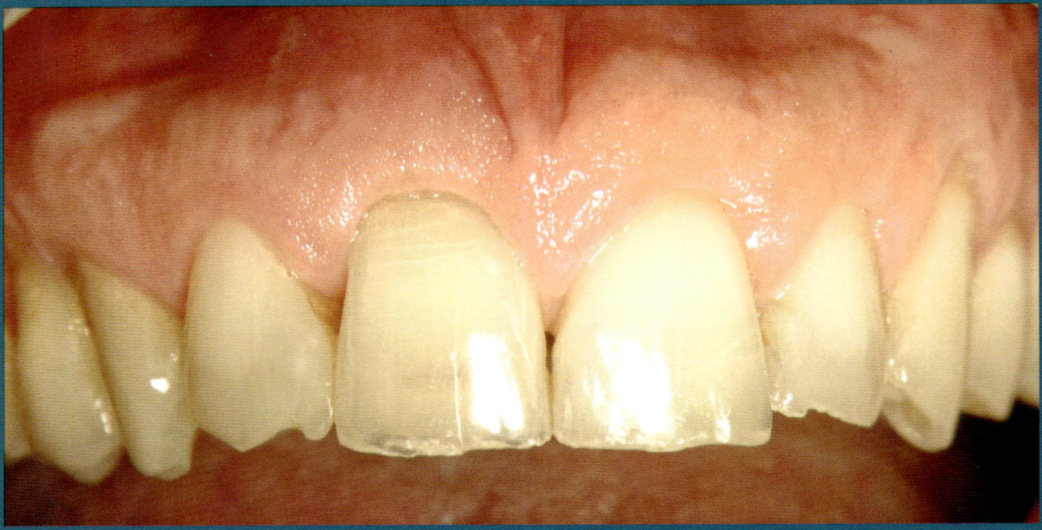

7 Check-up after 1 week.

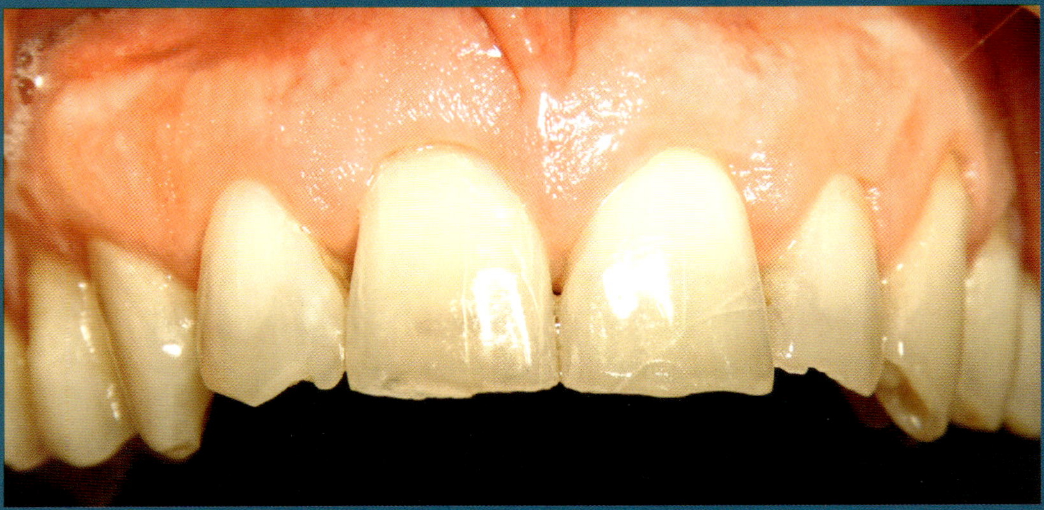

8 Checks on implant healing.

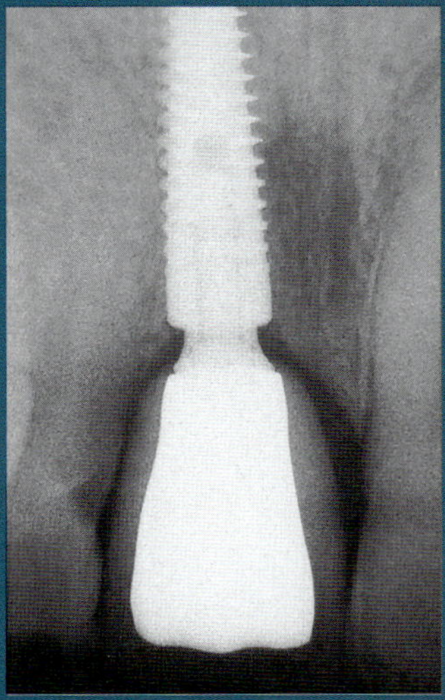

9 Rx 20 months after loading.

Clinical case 6

F. Bromuri, Milan, Italy

Patient ASA 1, man, 45 years old, with 2.3 in non-orthodontically recoverable palatal bone impaction, and persistent 5.3 in the arch. The position of 2.3 does not allow the correct insertion of any implant rehabilitation. Clinically, high mobility of the deciduous element is observed. We proceed with the extraction of 2.3 and 5.3 and contextual insertion of the T3 Biomax 4.3 × 15 mm implant and Tooth Transformer protocol both for the palatal socket of 2.3 and for the peri-implant area. A connective tissue graft is placed to thicken the soft tissues and a temporary Maryland-Bridge with metal reinforcement is placed.

At 6 months we proceed with the 2nd stage by a screw retained temporary crown (Tlink base, Biomax). At 8 months, it is prosthetically treated with a screwed Tissue Angle Biomax and a layered zirconia crown.

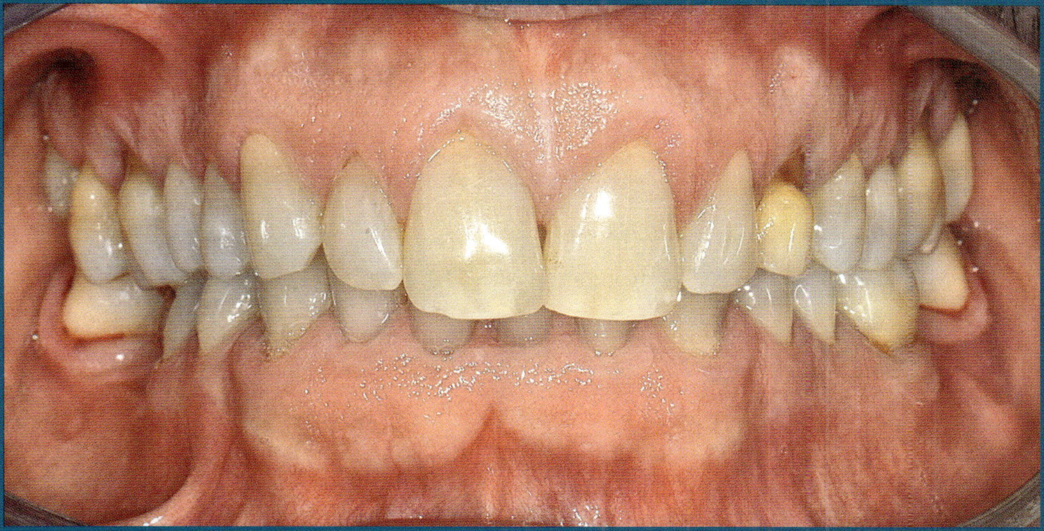

1 Preoperative image.

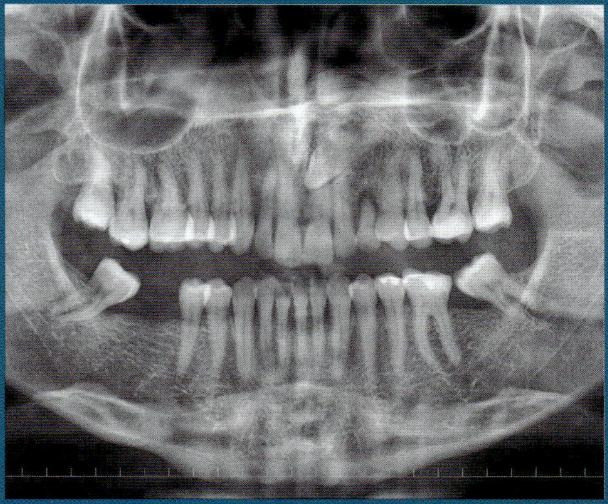

2 Preoperative OPG.

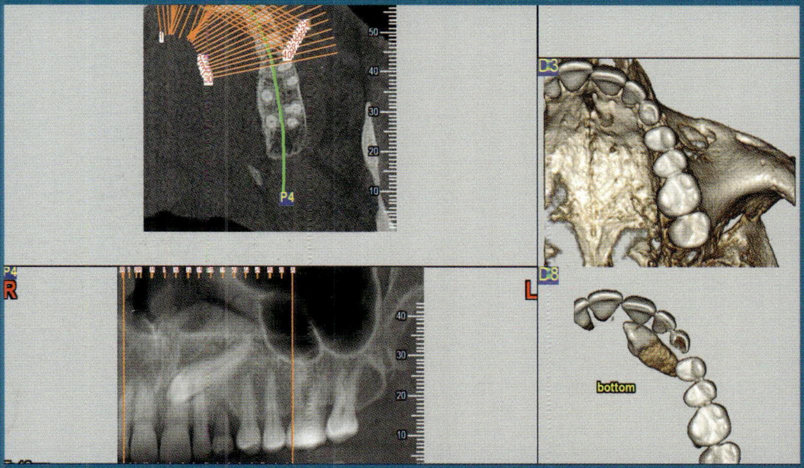

3 Preoperative CBCT.

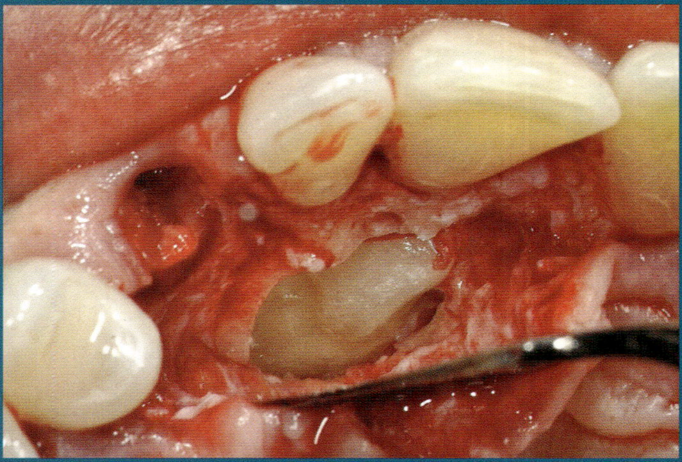

4 Palatine flap for the extraction of impacted 2.3. The section of the root allows to keep the cortical tissue intact.

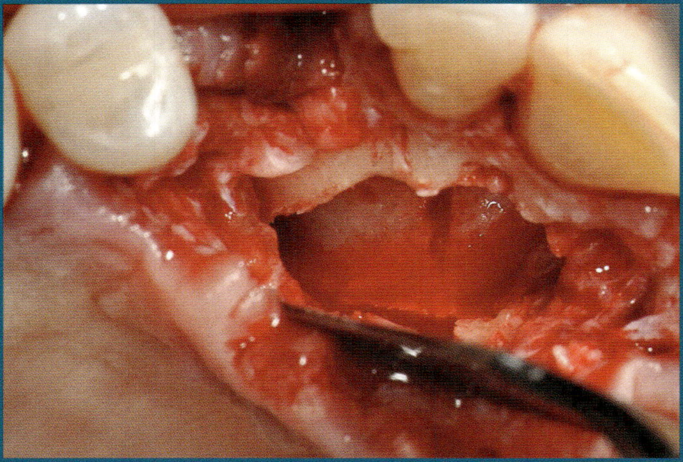

5 Residual cavity after the extraction of 2.3.

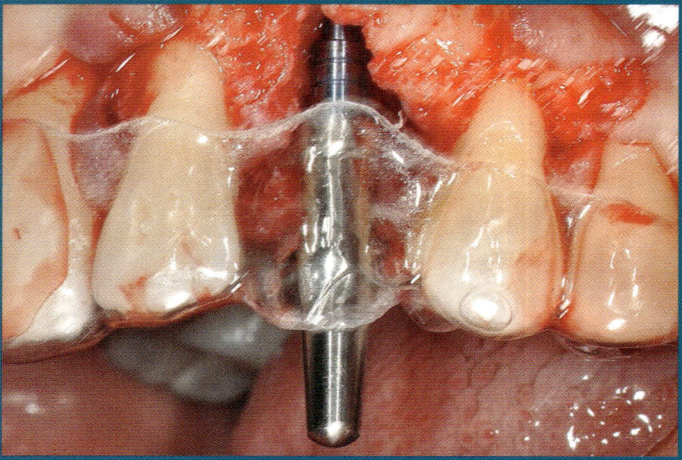

6 Surgical guide for correct implant positioning.

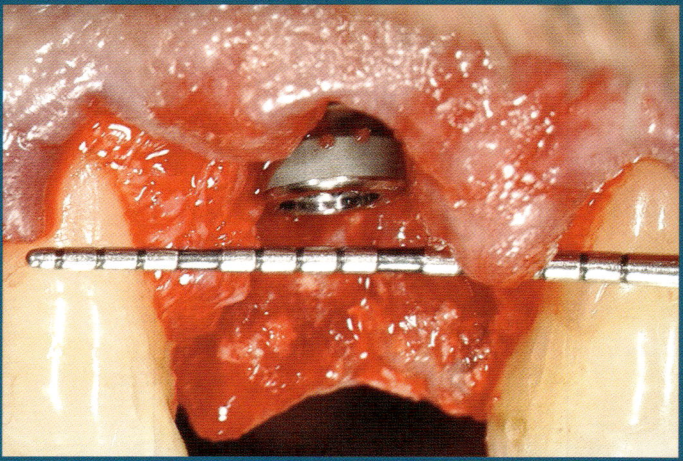

7 Correct positioning of the implant in the apical-coronal direction (3 mm beyond the CEJ of the adjacent teeth).

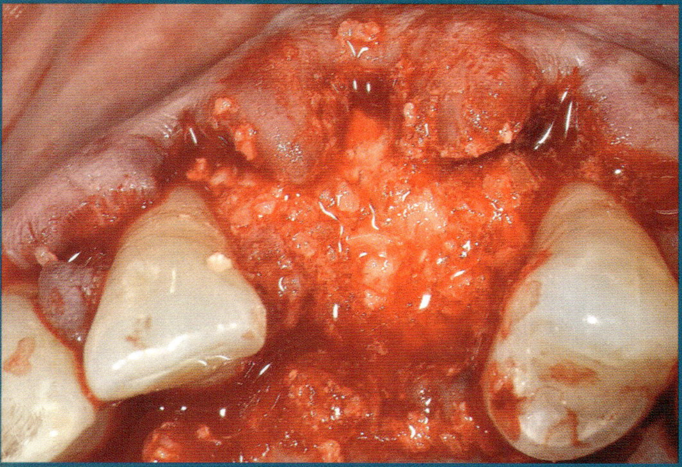

8 Dentin grafting. The socket of the impacted tooth was also filled before the palatal suture.

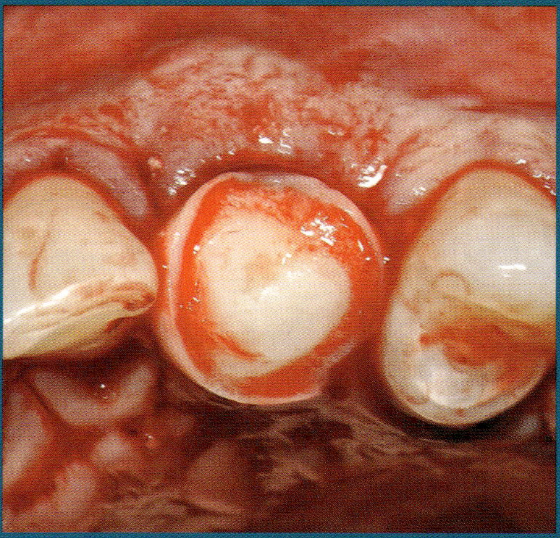

9 Connective epithelium graft taken from the palate.

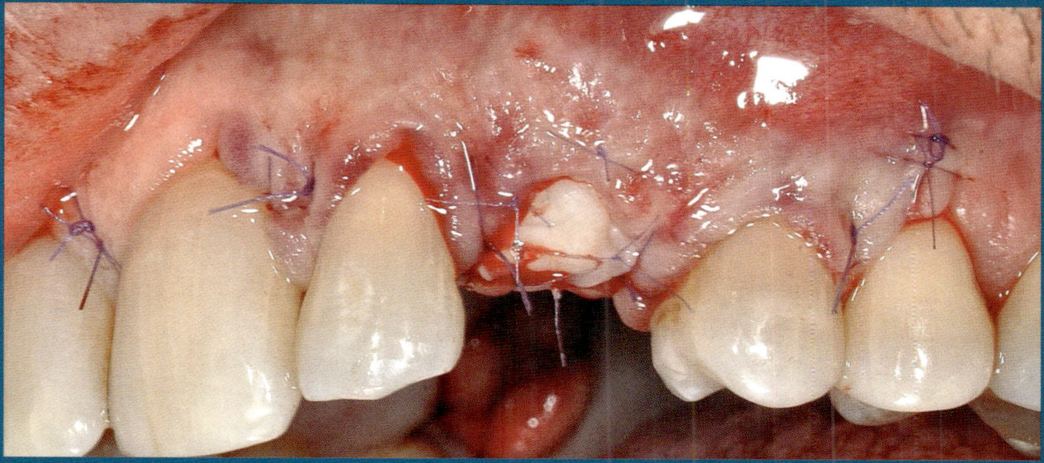

10 Suture 6-0 PGA.

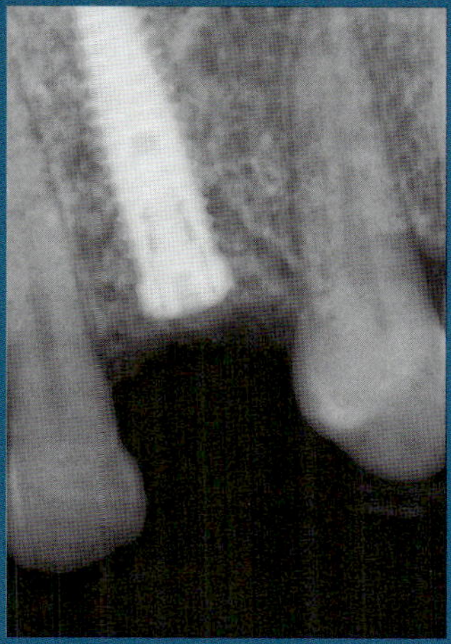

11 RVG of the grafted site. Note how the dentin graft has the same chromatic density as the surrounding alveolar bone of the patient.

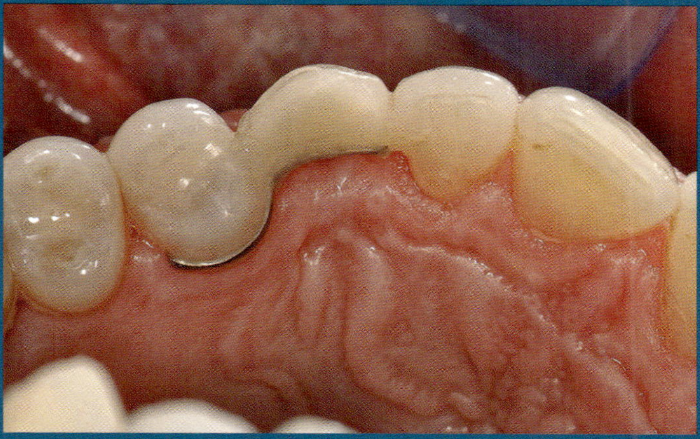

12 Adhesive temporary Maryland bridge with metal reinforcement.

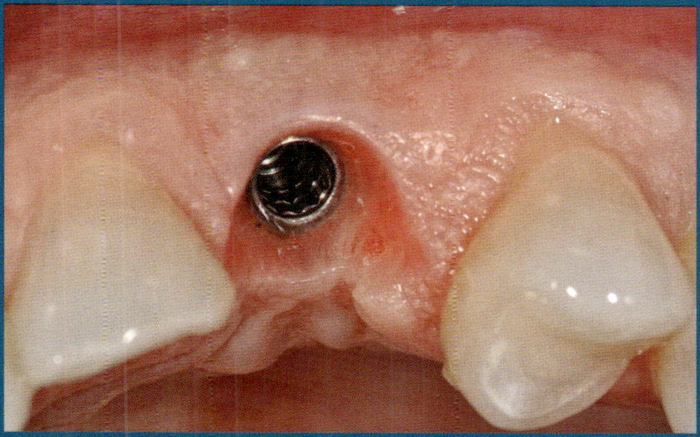

13 Healing of the papillae.

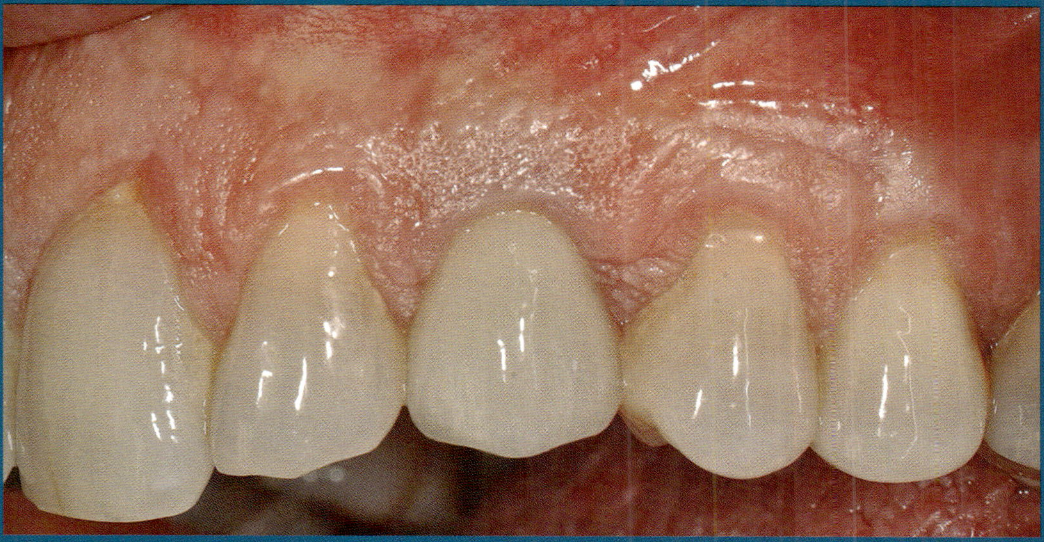

14 Crown in place. The maturation of the papillae is almost complete. Note the excellent response of the graft.

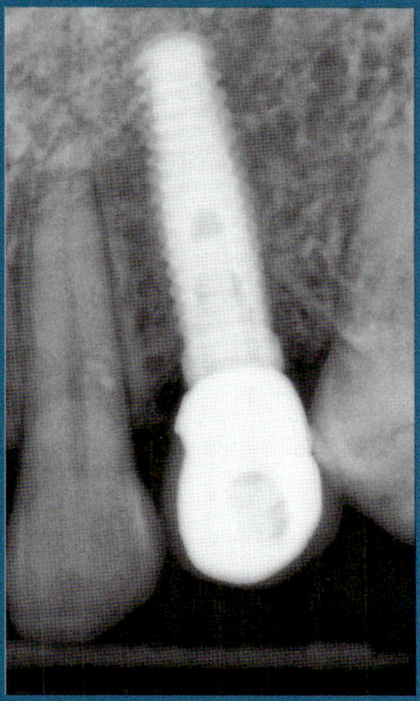

15 Intraoral X-ray 1 year after loading.

CREST PRESERVATION

Ridge preservation with membrane

Clinical case 7

E. Minetti, Milan, Italy

44-year-old female patient, no medical pathology, non-smoker, suffering from severe periodontal lesions. In zone 3.5-3.6 the patient complains of severe pain, mobility and suppuration with bone defects of 10-15 mm in depth and grade III mobility for both elements. Once the extraction has been performed, a GBR is performed using the extracted teeth together with the turning the apical inflammatory tissue occlusally in order to avoid any periosteal incisions. The graft material is then covered with a collagen membrane (overturning of Bego, Germany). Two Visio One Cea implants (Cea medical, Swiss) are then inserted and ceramic restorations applied.

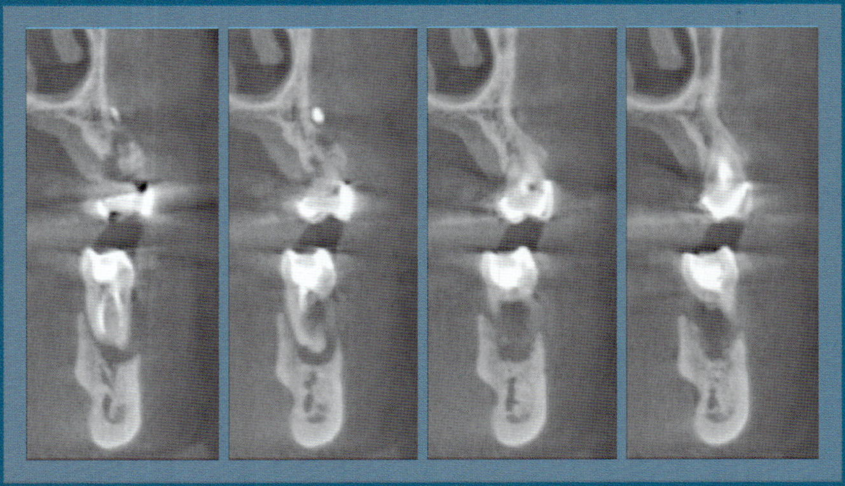

1 Preintervention CBCT. The extensive loss of bone tissue can be noted.

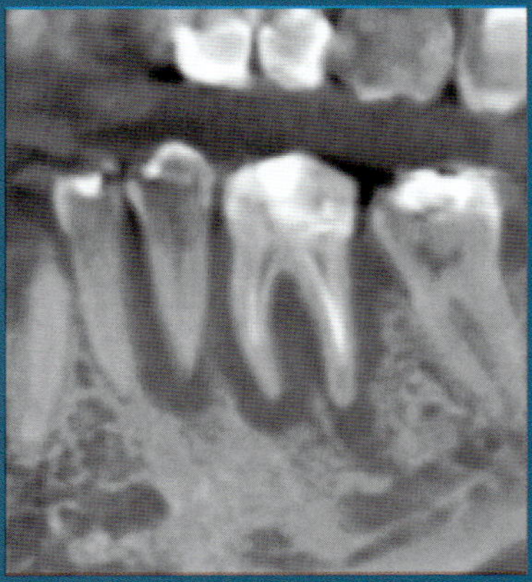

2 Elements 3.5-3.6 preavulsion.

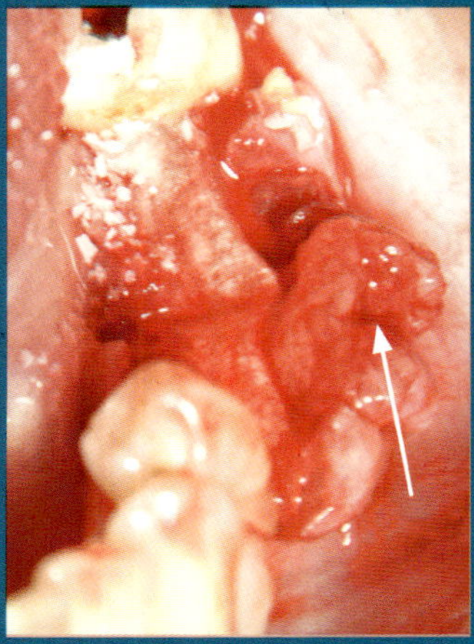

3 Closing phase of the regeneration. You can see the collagen membrane and the overturned pedicle to facilitate closure without tension.

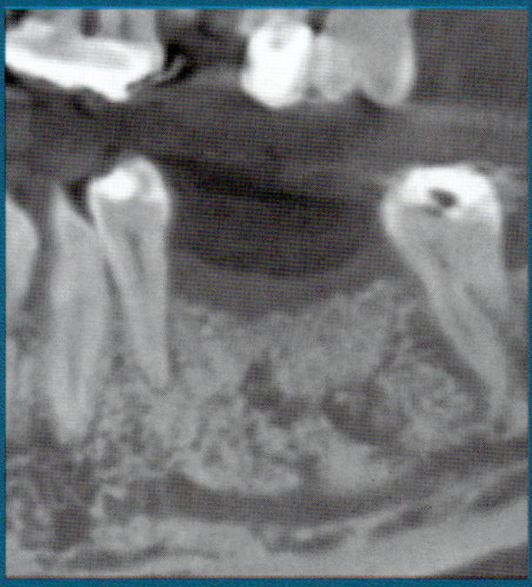

4 Rx 3 months after GBR.

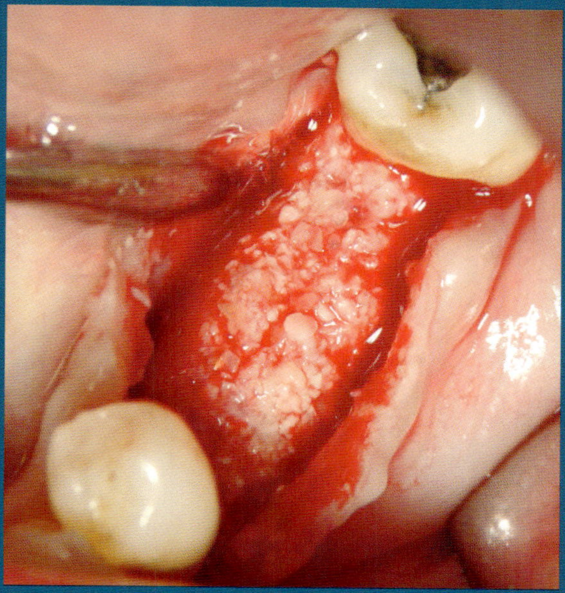

5 Flap opening to insert implants.

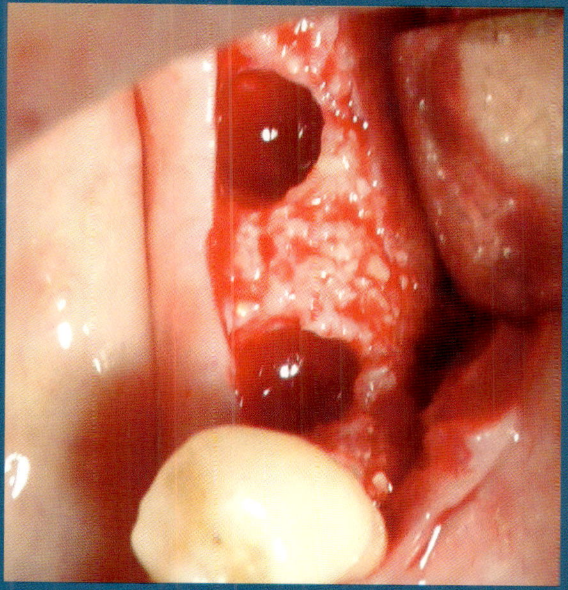

6 Surgical ostetomies performed in regenerated tissue. Note the compactness of the tissue after only 3 months.

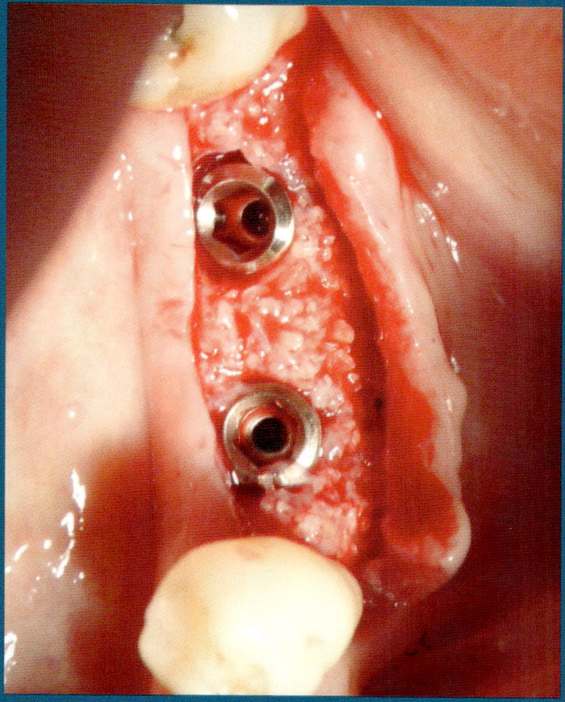

7 Implants placed in the regenerated tissue.

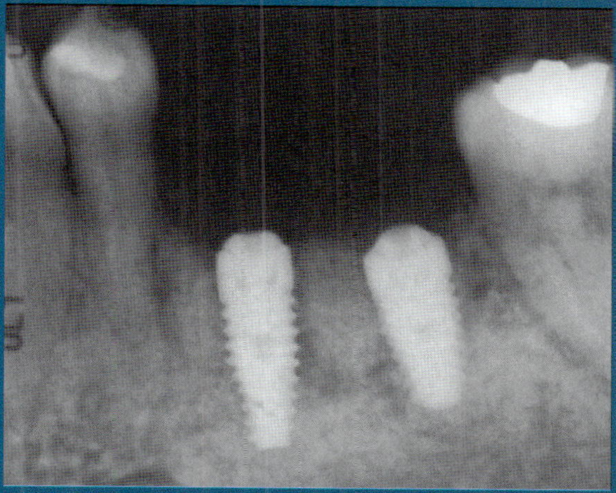

8 Rx after implant placement.

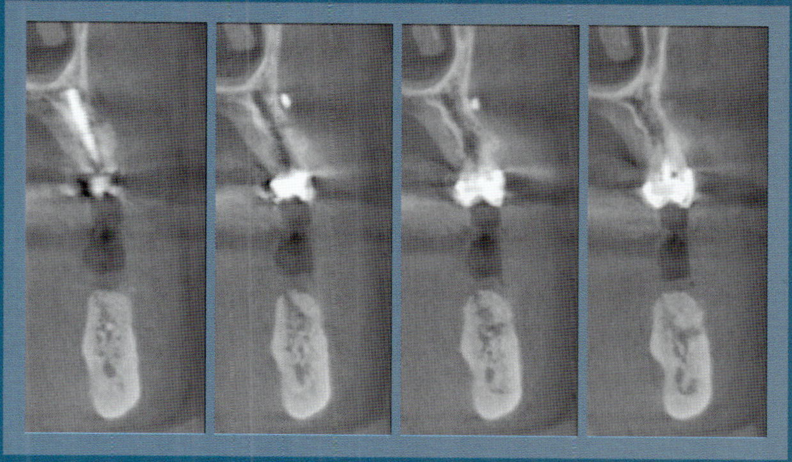

9 CBCT before implant placement.

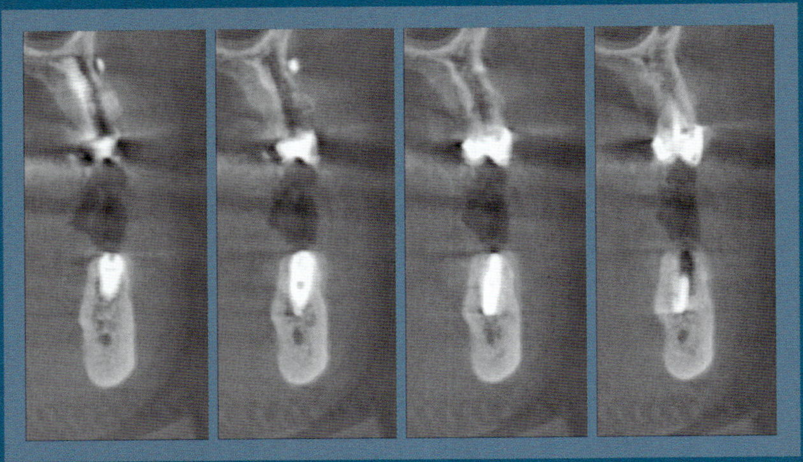

10 CBCT after implant placement.

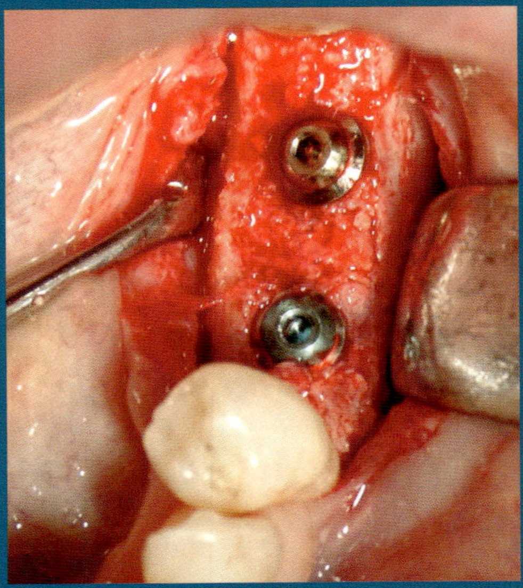

11 Implant healing and implant recovery. Note the compactness of the tissues and the new cortex where there was a defect of 10/15 mm in depth.

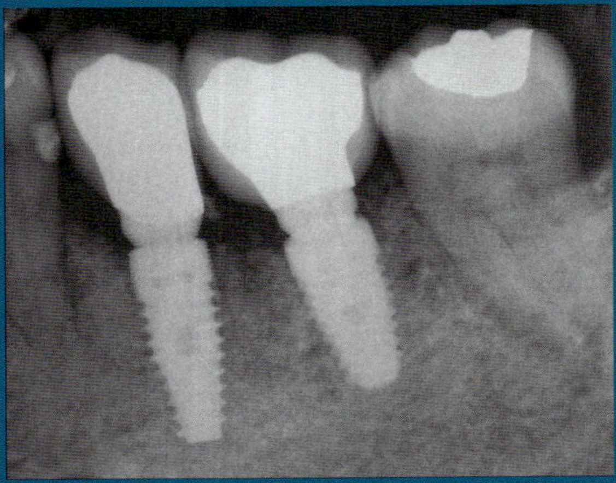

12 Rx at 1 year follow-up.

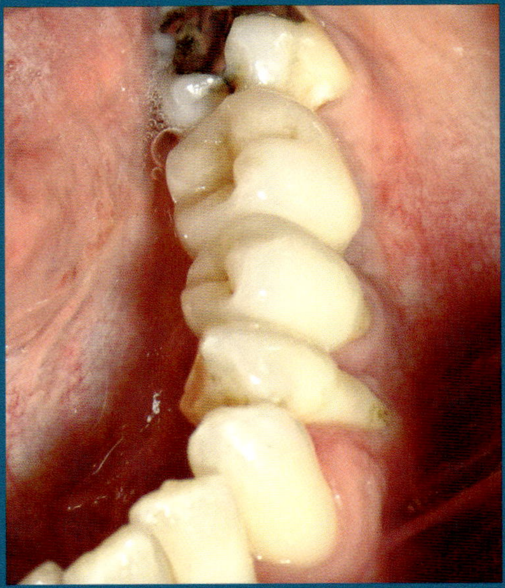

13 Result at 44 month follow-up.

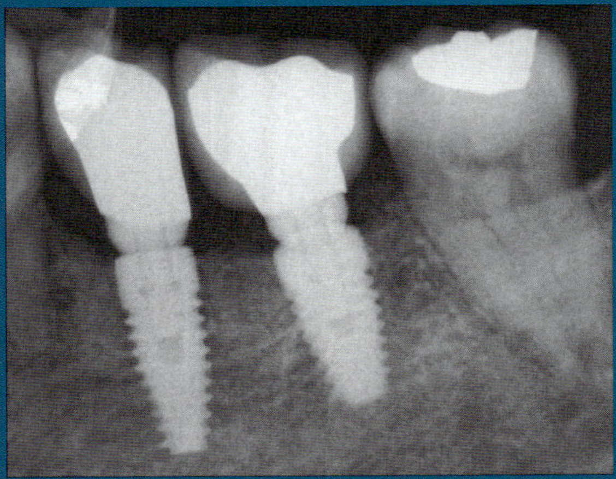

14 Rx at 44-month follow-up.

Clinical case 8

E. Minetti, Milan, Italy

Female patient 46 years old, no medical pathology, non-smoker.

Implant placed about 10 years earlier with evident peri-implantitis and pain on percussion. It is decided to remove the implant and made a regeneration using material derived from the tooth extracted due to a root fracture in area 4.5. The extracted element 4.5 is replaced with an immediate implant. After extracting the implant, contiguous to the lower alveolar canal (0.67 mm), there is an opening of the upper cortex of the canal. Regeneration is then carried out by placing a collagen membrane to cover the communication with the canal to avoid the possible fall of granules and a membrane (Bego-Oss, Bego Germany) to cover the graft. Five months later, a Visio One Cea implant (Cea medical, Swiss) was inserted and a biopsy was taken of the newly formed tissue showing a corticalized and very dense appearance. The prosthetic finalization is carried out using full ceramic crowns.

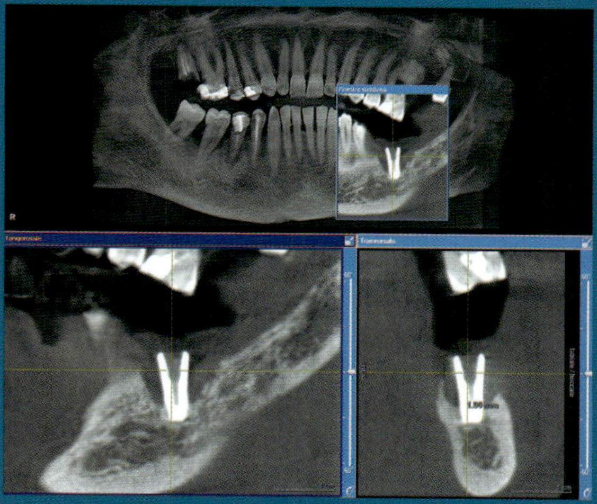

1 Preoperative CBCT. The large loss of peri-implant bone tissue can be noted.

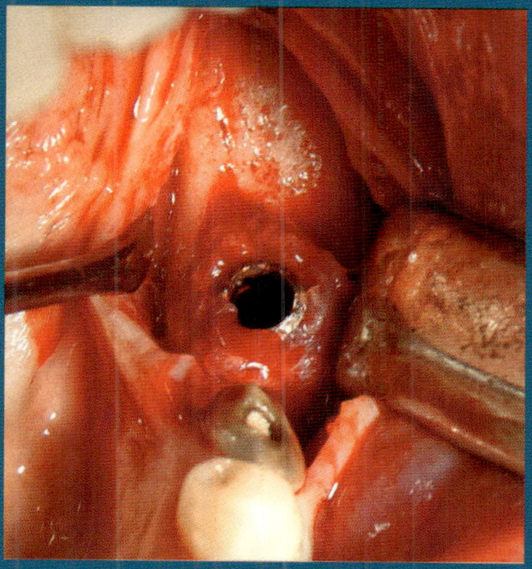

2 Opening of the flap and highlighting of the peri-implant fibrous tissue.

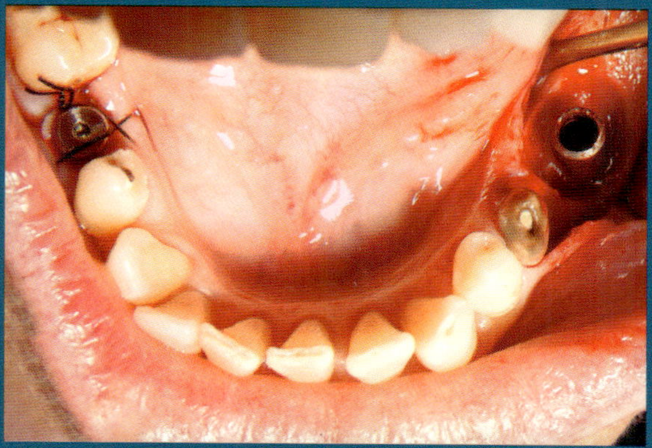

3 You can see in zone 4.5 the immediate implant placed after the extraction of 4.5 used for bone regeneration and in the area of 3.5, the crater caused by peri-implantitis.

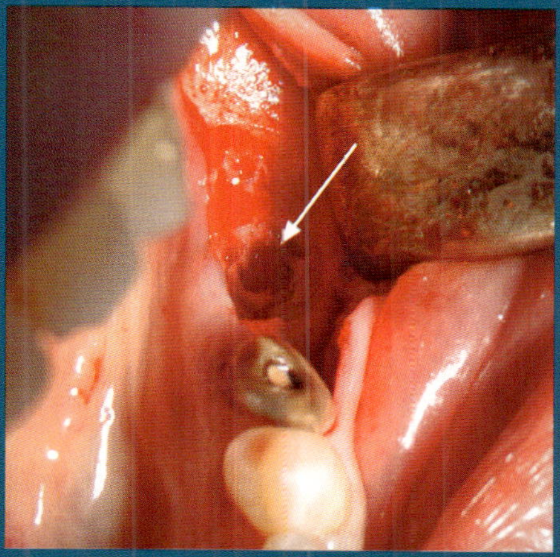

4 Communication with the inferior alveolar verve canal.

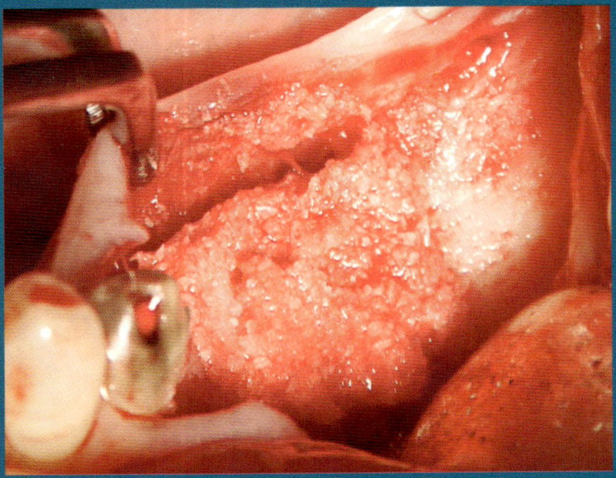

5 Condensation of the graft material.

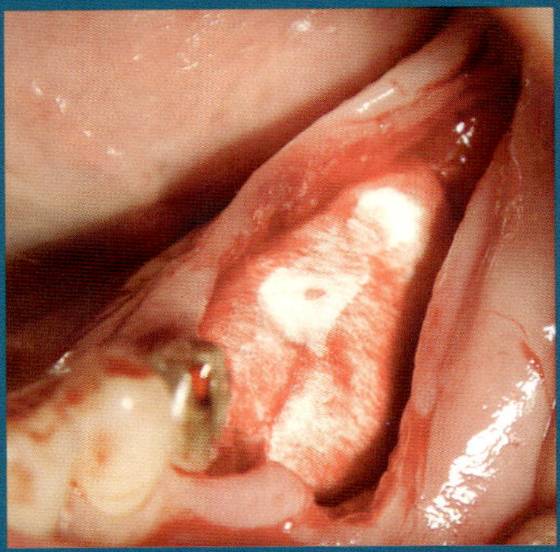

6 Collagen membrane covering the graft material.

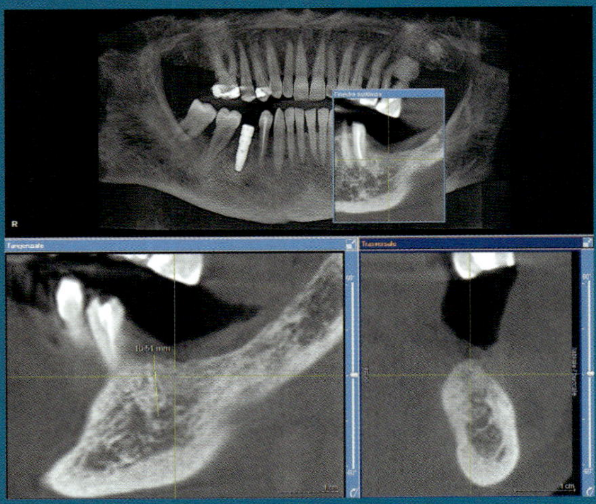

7 CBCT with assessment of bone volume and quality after 5 months.

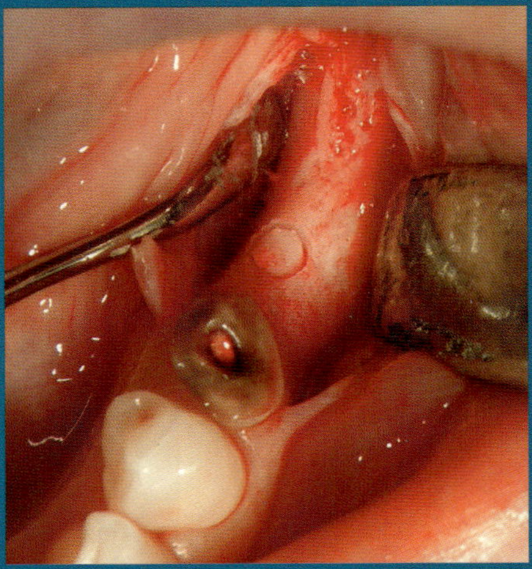

8 Bone volume present at the time of implant placement. A histological sample was taken during the trephine drilling phase.

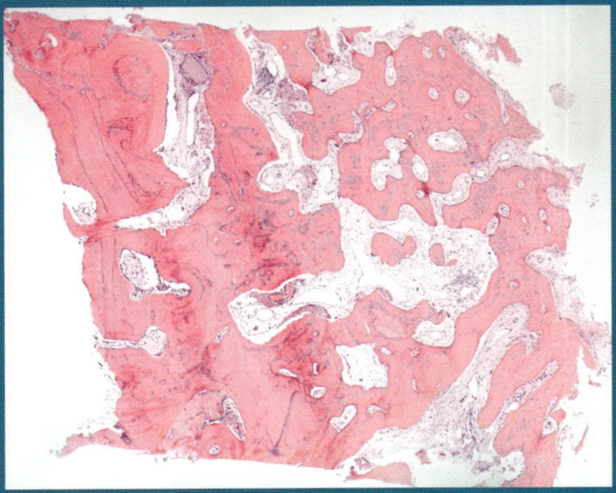

9 Histological sampling.

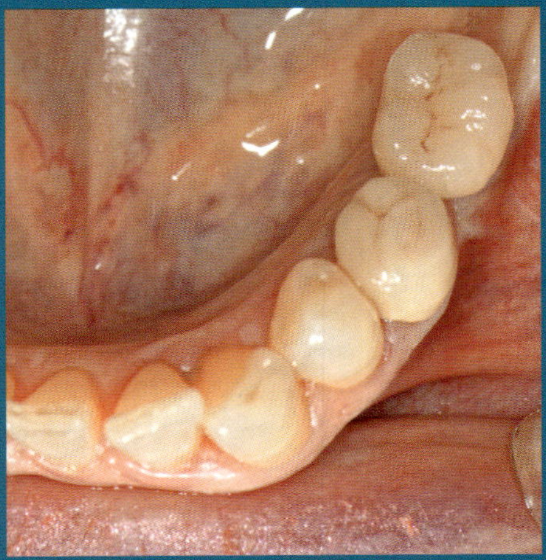

10 Implant restoration.

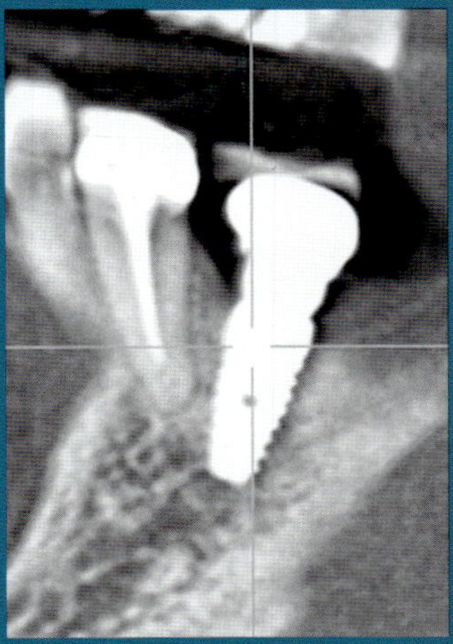

11 X-ray image in CBCT section 8 months after loading

Clinical case 9

E. Minetti, Milan, Italy

26-year-old female patient, no pathology, non-smoker.

She has an apical cyst of elements 3.1 and 4.1 that cannot be treated endodontically which has caused the complete resorption of the lingual wall. Both teeth are not usable for regeneration. The patient is asked to be able to extract 48, but she denies permission. The next day, the patient comes to the office with a plastic box containing all the deciduous teeth kept by her mother. She then decided to carry out the extraction of elements 3.1-4.1 and, at the same time, a GBR using the deciduous teeth as graft material and placing a collagen membrane (Bego-Oss, Bego, Germany) to contain the granulate. After 5 months, two Visio One Cea implants (Cea medical, Swiss) are placed and a histological sample is taken during the drilling phase.

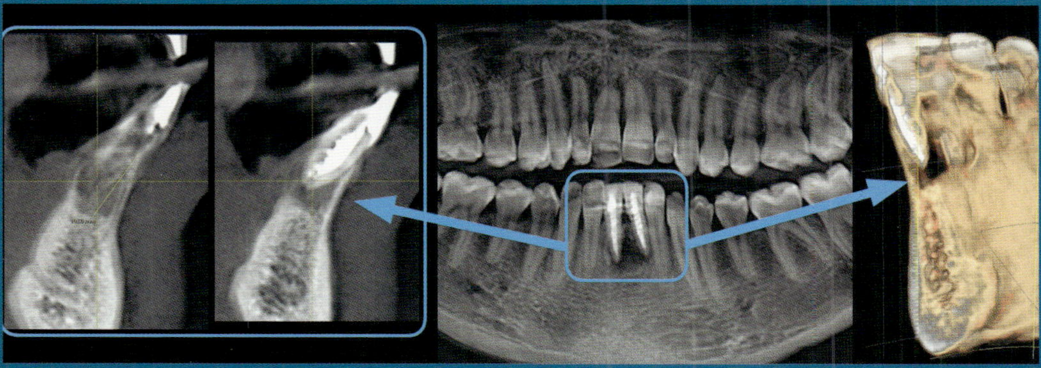

1 Initial situation.

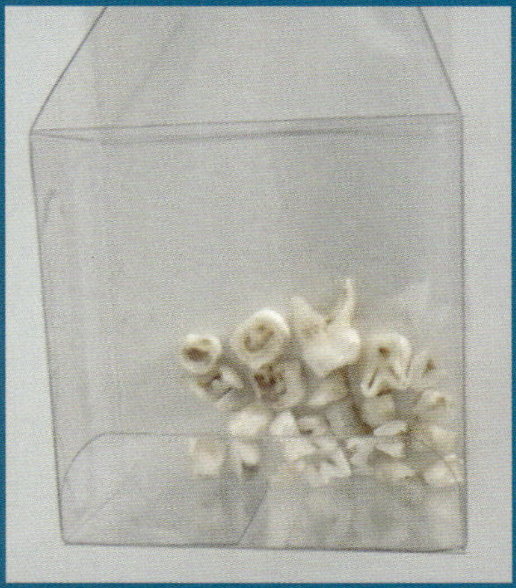

2 Plastic box containing the patient's deciduous teeth extracted 15-20 years earlier and kept by the mother.

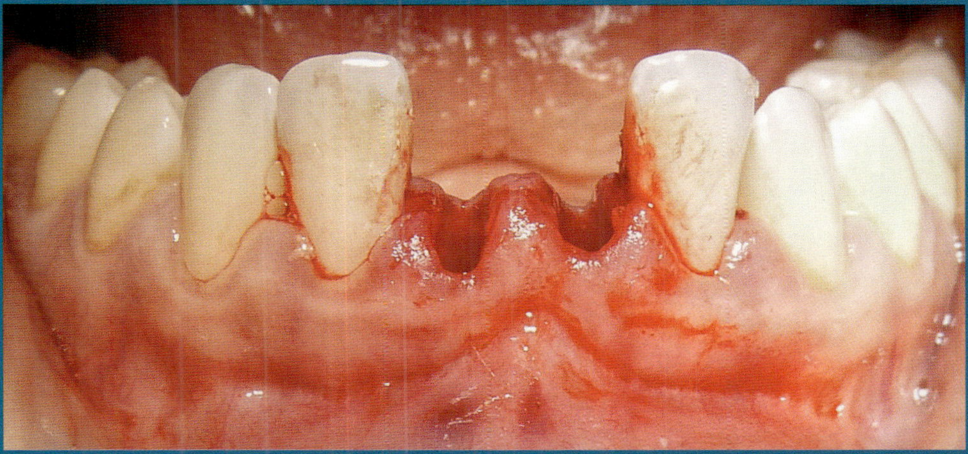

3 Extraction of 3.1-4.1.

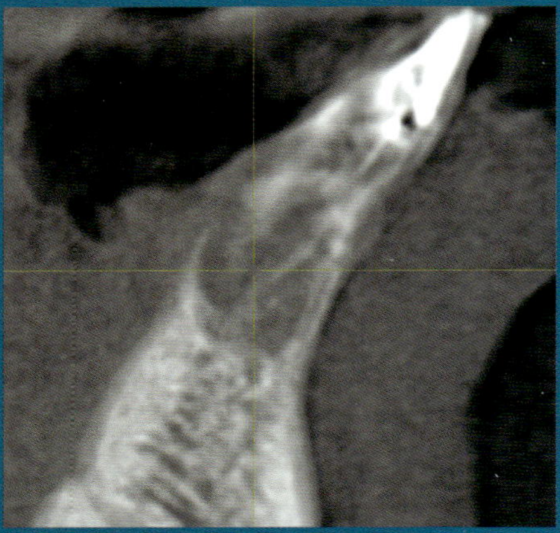

4 CBCT of the area before surgery.

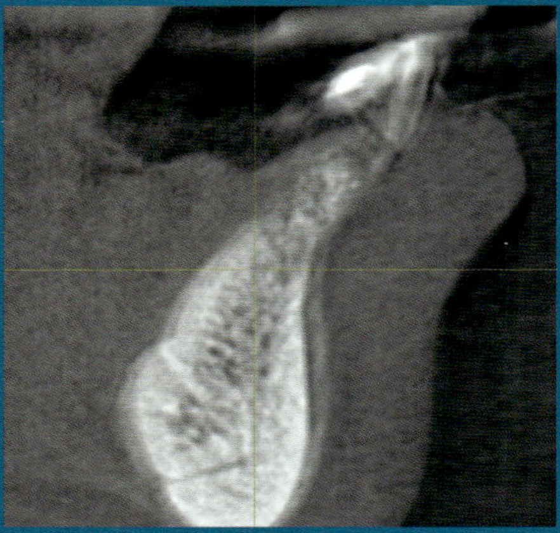

5 CBCT 3 months after regeneration.

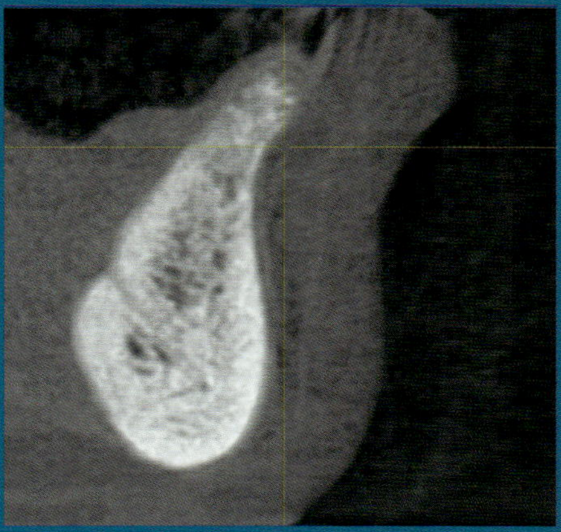

6 CBCT 5 months after regeneration. A marked thickening of the regenerated tissue can be noted.

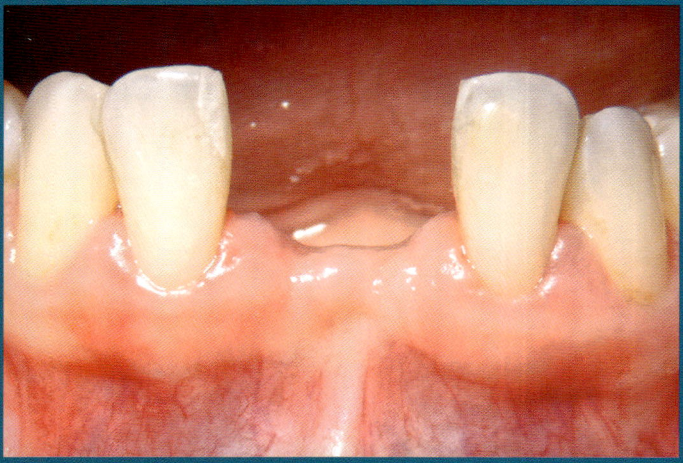

7 Implant preoperative tissues 5 months after GBR.

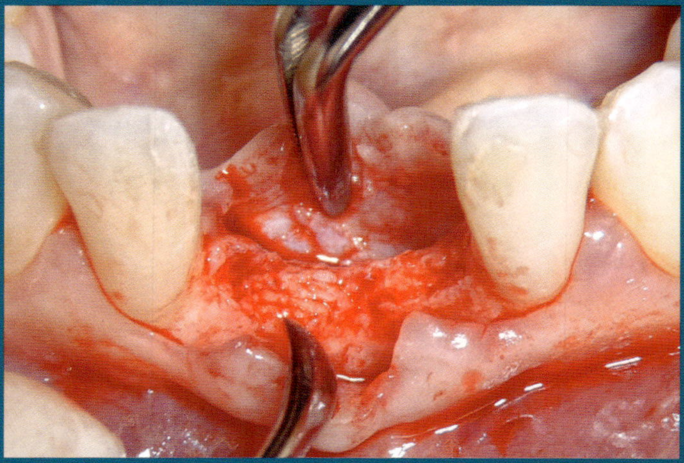

8 Regenerated bone tissue after 5 months.

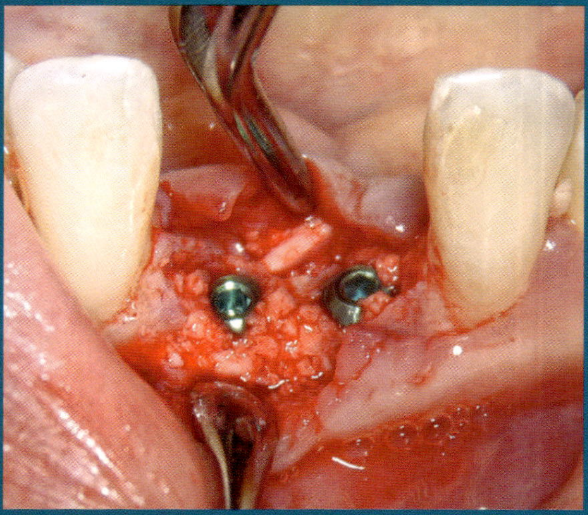

9 Implants inserted.

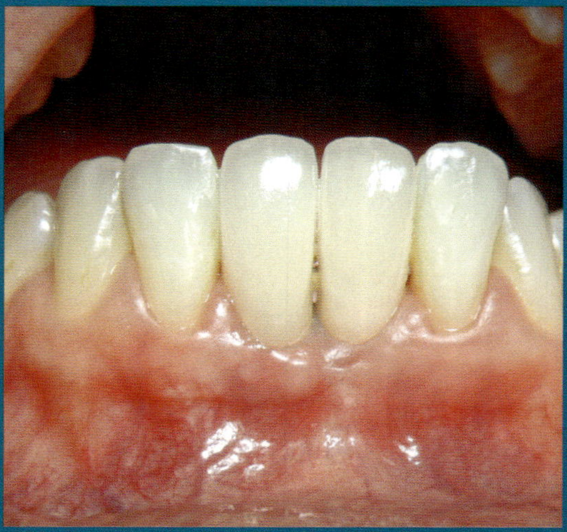

10 Full ceramic final restoration.

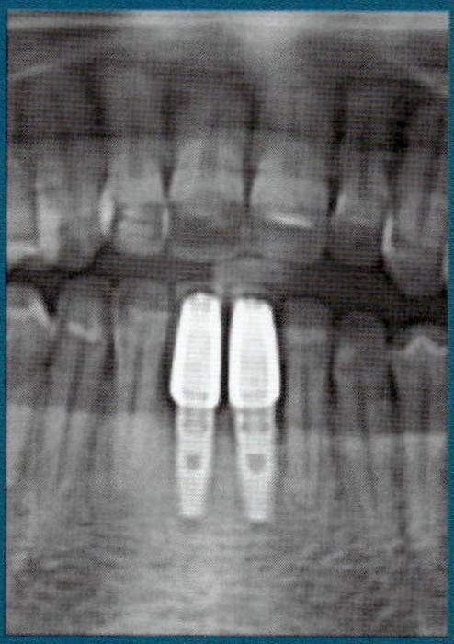

11 Detail from OPT 18 months after loading.

Clinical case 10

E. Minetti, Milan, Italy

64-year-old female patient, non-smoker, allergic to amoxicillin, presents with a vertical fracture of the mesial root of 4.6. Once the extraction has been carried out, the tooth is used for an alveolar preservation on the residual root socket and for a ridge preservation with a horizontal increase in zone 4.5 in order to recreate a sufficient thickness for the placement of two implants. The material derived from the tooth is covered with a collagen membrane (Bego-Oss, Bego, Germany).

After 4 months, two Visio One Cea implants (Cea medical, Swiss) are placed and the related restoration is fit.

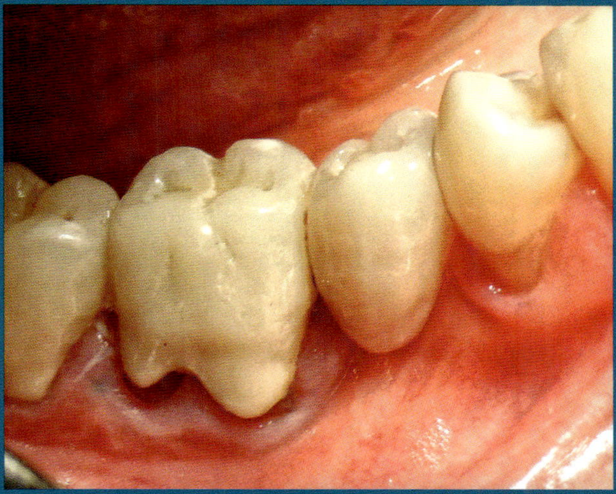

1 Initial situation.

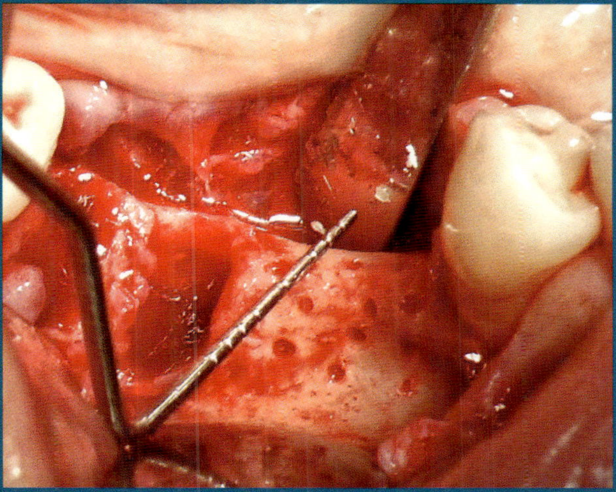

2 Perforations of the cortex in zone 4.5 with a thin crest.

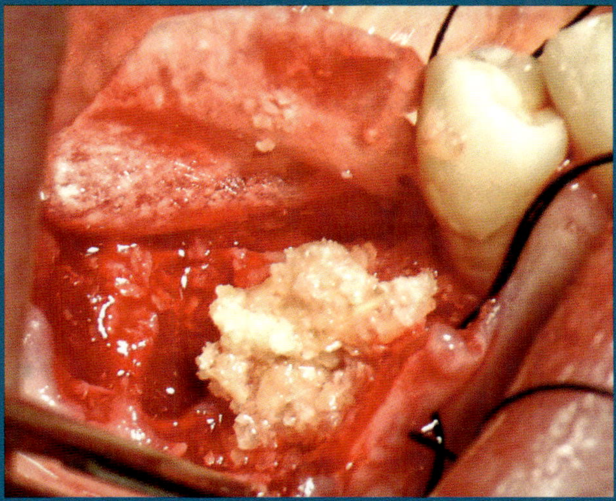

3 Dental material just placed on the site 4.5.

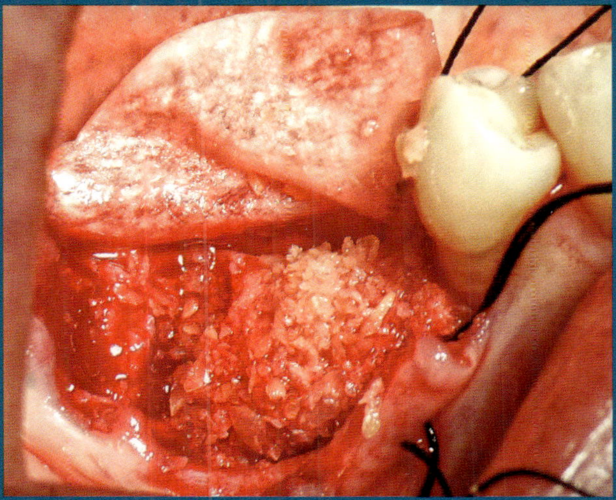

4 The high wettability of the material of dental origin allows the material, after few seconds from positioning, to soak up the blood.

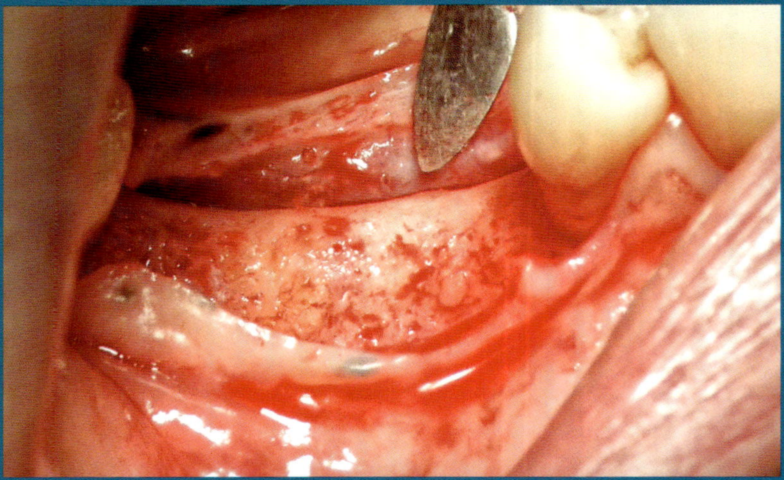

5 The surgical site 4 months after regeneration. The quality of the bone tissue and the three-dimensional reconstruction of the defect can be noted.

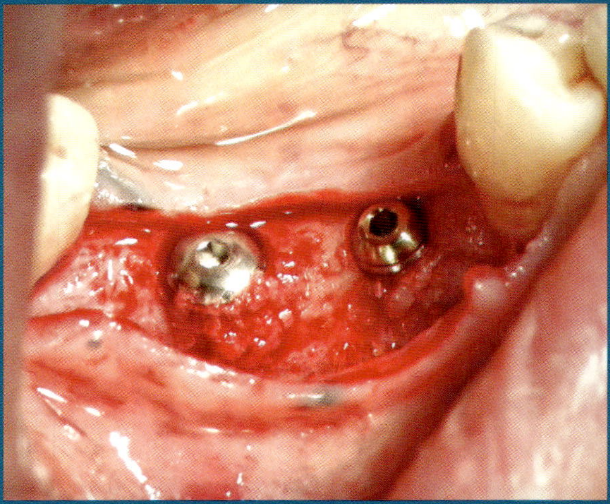

6 Implants in situ.

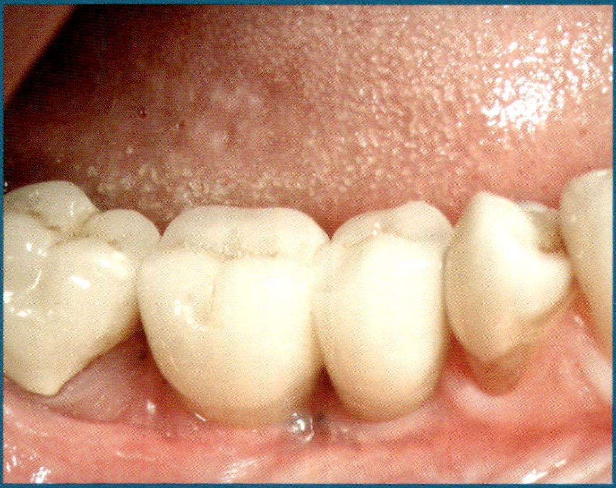

7 Metal-ceramic restorations on implants 20 months after.

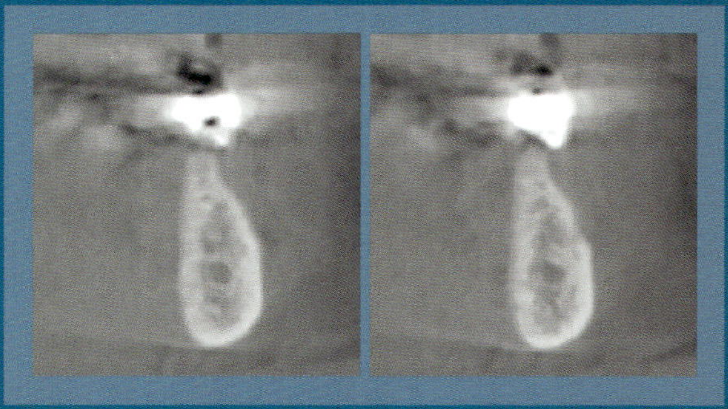

8 Preintervention CBCT view of regeneration in zone 4.5.

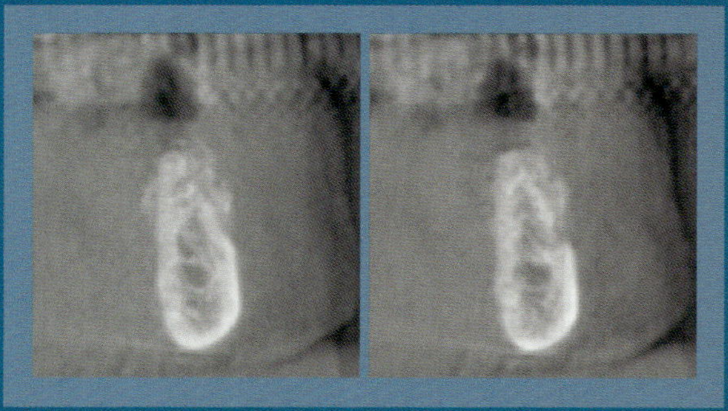

9 CBCT 1 month after GBR in zone 4.5.

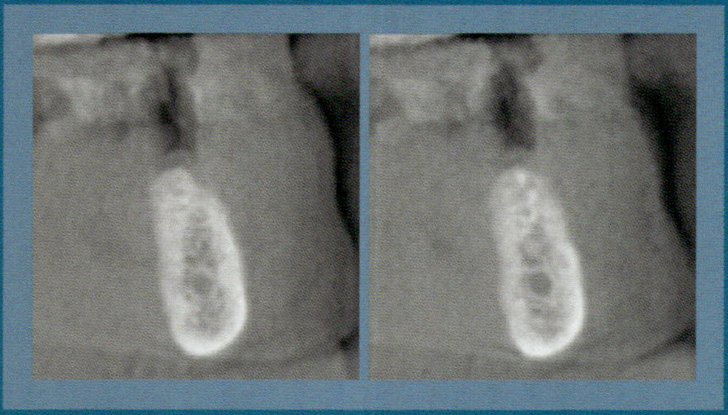

10 CBCT 4 months after GBR in zone 4.5.

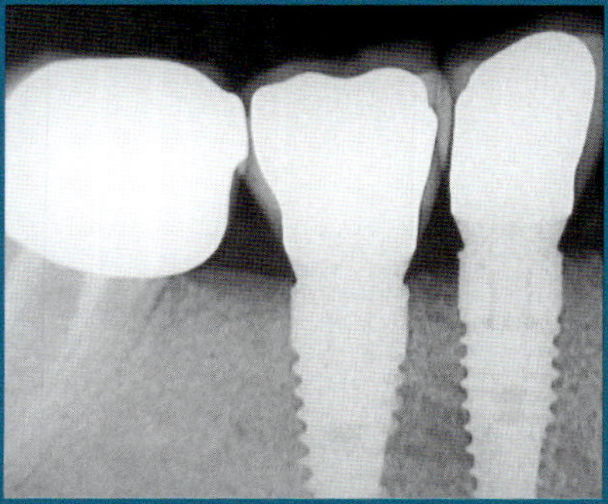

11 Rx 22 months after loading.

Clinical case 11

J. Santillana, Bilbao, Spain

42-year-old female patient, smoker, with no previous pathologies. Element 1.4 has a large cavity and an apical abscess. Much of the vestibular bone wall has been lost due to several infections. Element 1.4 has two roots, which implies the impossibility of correctly positioning the implant during the tooth extraction phase. It was decided to carry out two separate procedures, the first for regeneration using Tooth Transformer and the second for positioning the Dentium implant (Dentium, Seoul, Korea).

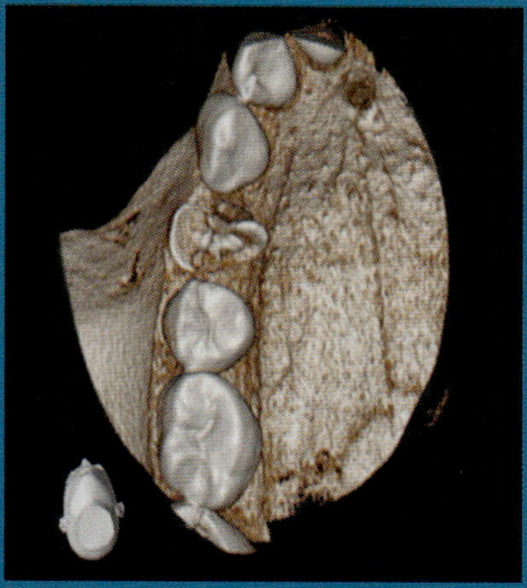

1 Preoperative 3d CBCT, occlusal view.

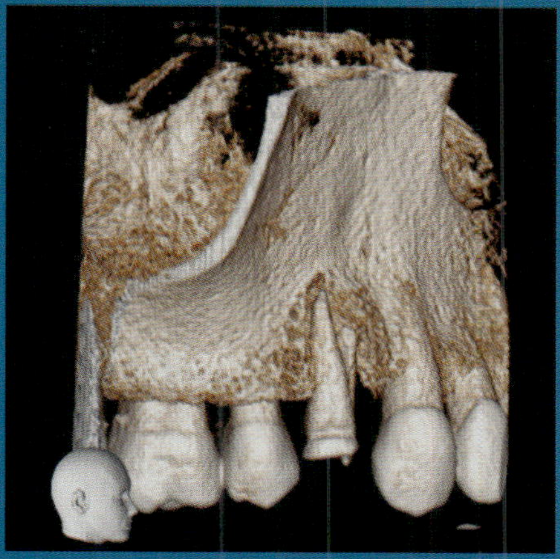

2 Preoperative 3d CBCT, vestibular view.

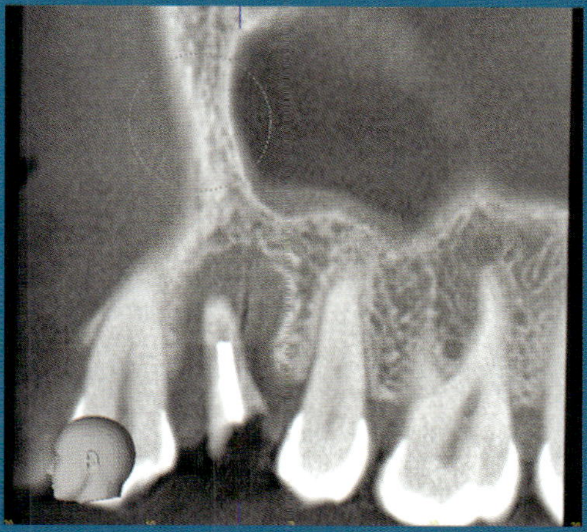

3 CBCT, section of 14. Note the extent of the bone lesion.

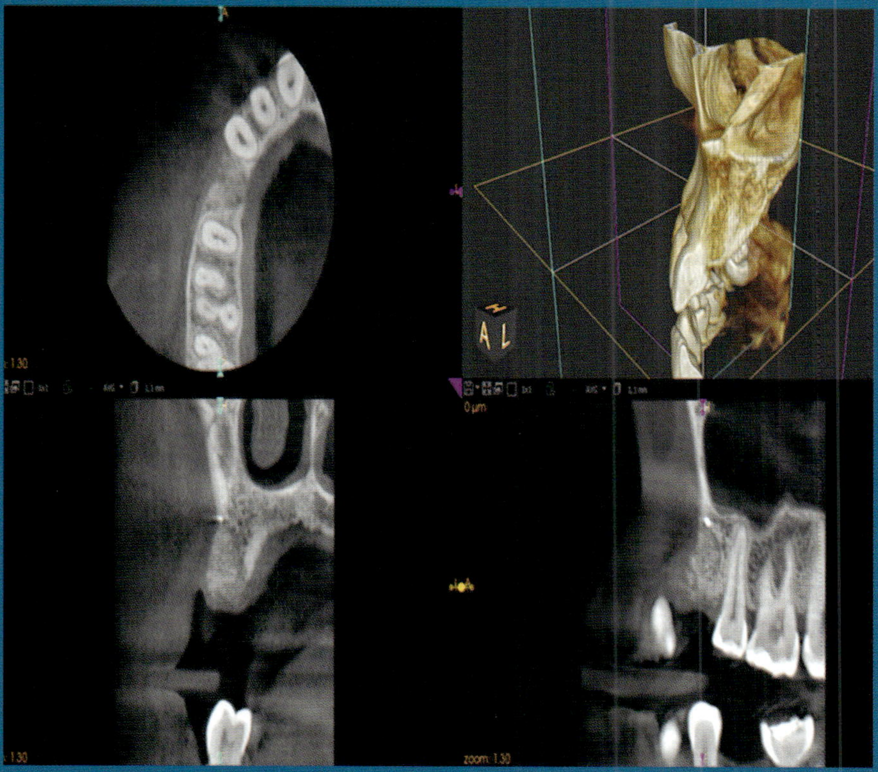

4 CBCT 3 months after placement of the material derived from the extracted tooth.

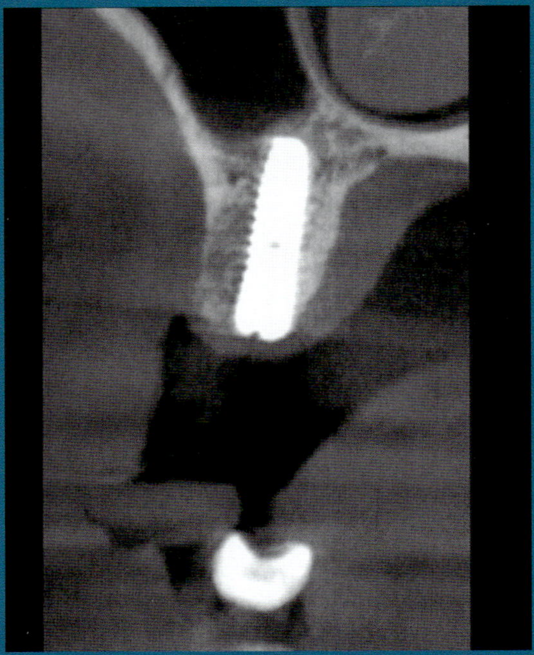

5 CBCT 3 months after implant placement and 6 months after GBR.

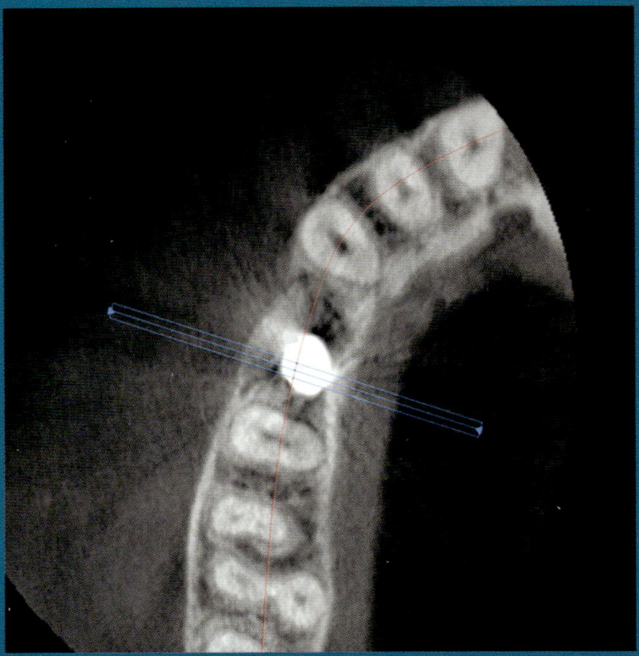

6 CBCT in cross section 3 months after implant placement and 6 months after GBR.

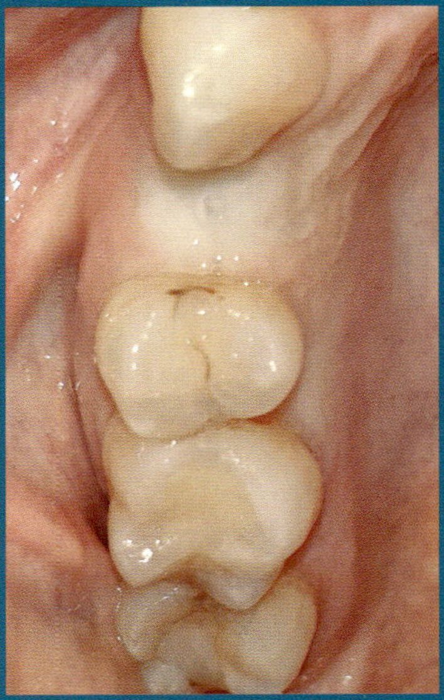

7 Fabrics at the facility meeting point.

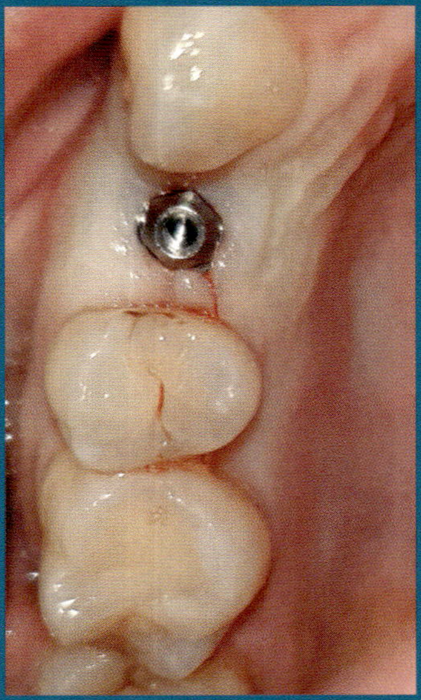

8 Multi-unit positioned stump.

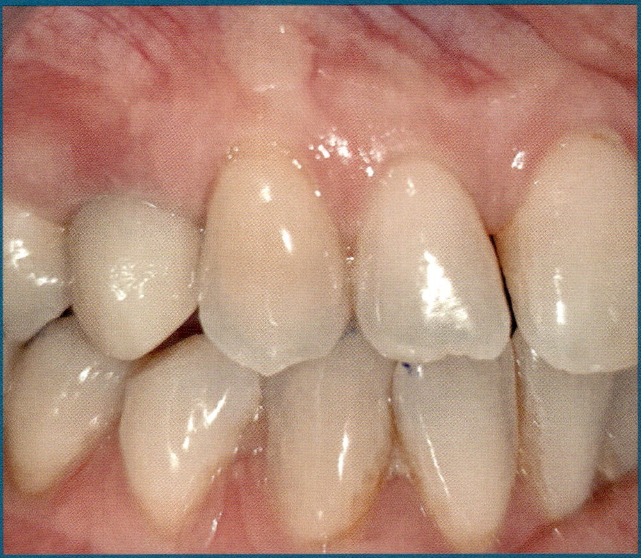

9 Ceramic restoration in situ.

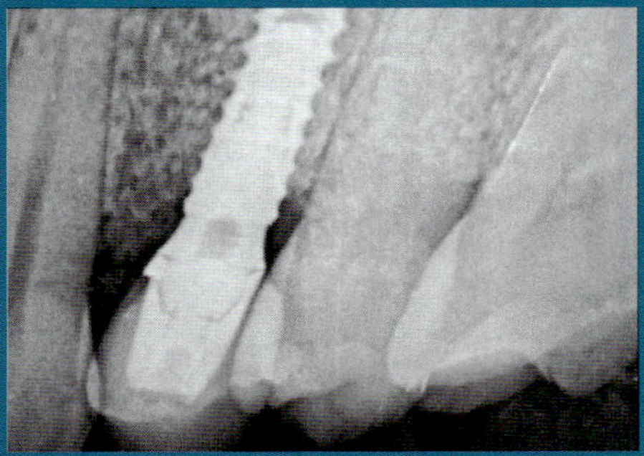

10 Intraoral X-rays 12 months after loading.

Clinical case 12

E. Giacometti, Turin, Italy

82-year-old male patient, non-smoker, without pathologies that constitute a contraindication to bone regeneration surgery. The patient presents with pain and hypermobility of the elements 3.3-3.4, with probing pocket greater than 12 mm. The CBCT examination shows a severe and extensive bone defect with the maintenance of soft tissues (type 2 defect Tarnow's classification). GBR of the defect is performed with the subsequent insertion of 2 implants.

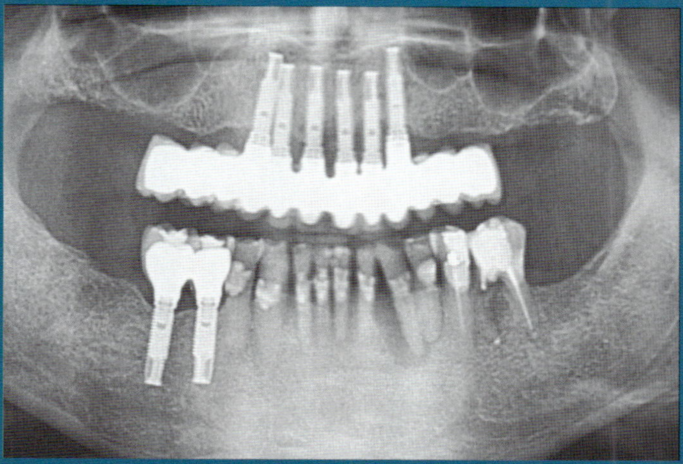

1 Preoperative OPG.

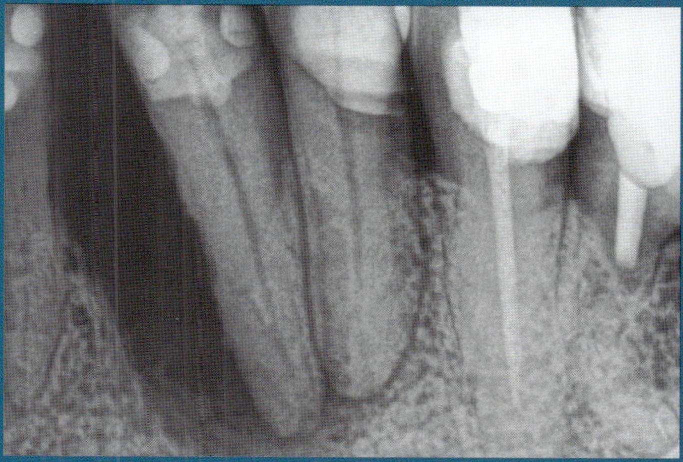

2 Preoperative intraoral X-ray.

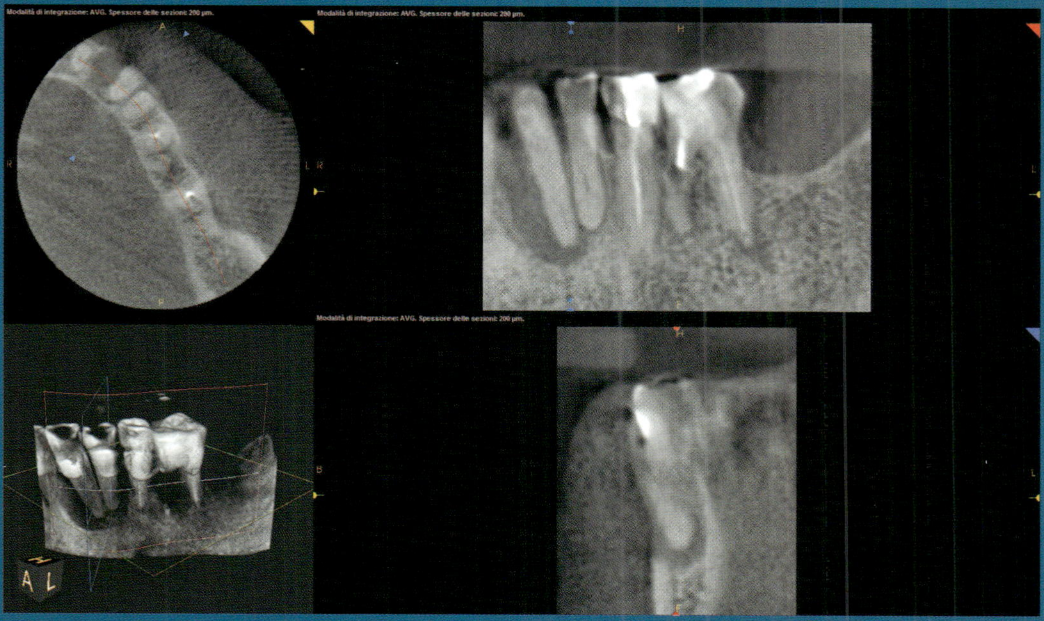

3 Preoperative cone bean CT.

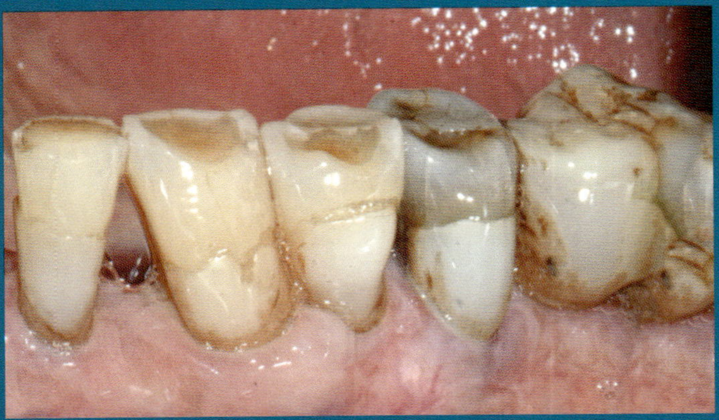

4 Preoperative clinical aspect.

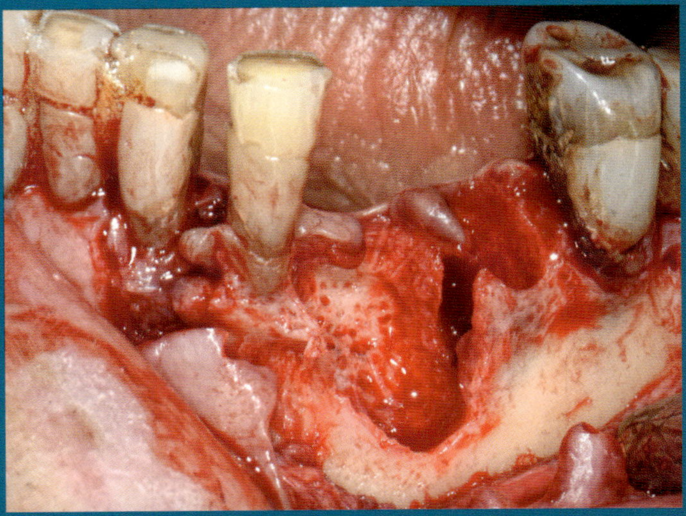

5 Surgical opening and the lesion after extractions have been performed.

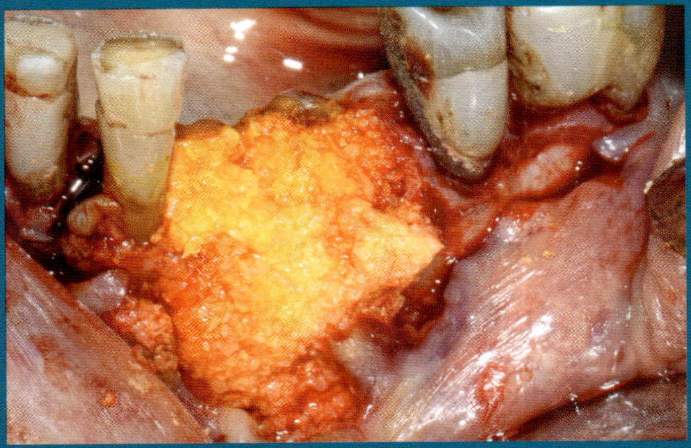

6 Graft of demineralized dentin using the extracted teeth.

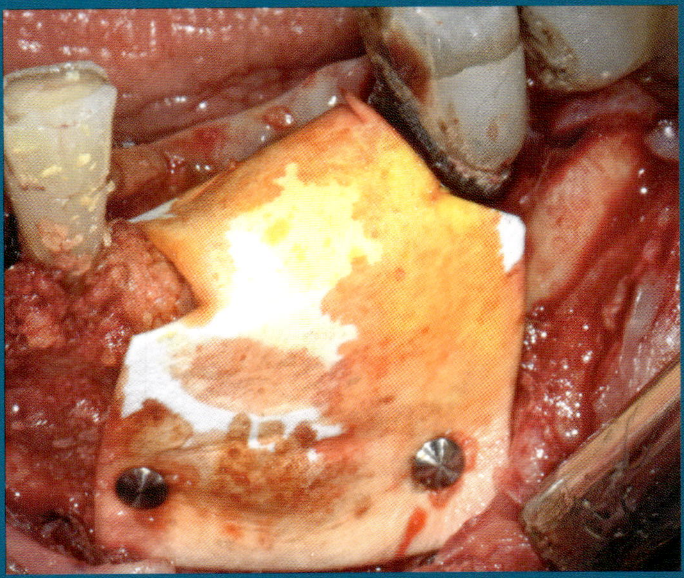

7 Positioning of the cross-linked resorbable membrane (Osseo guard) stabilized with titanium pins.

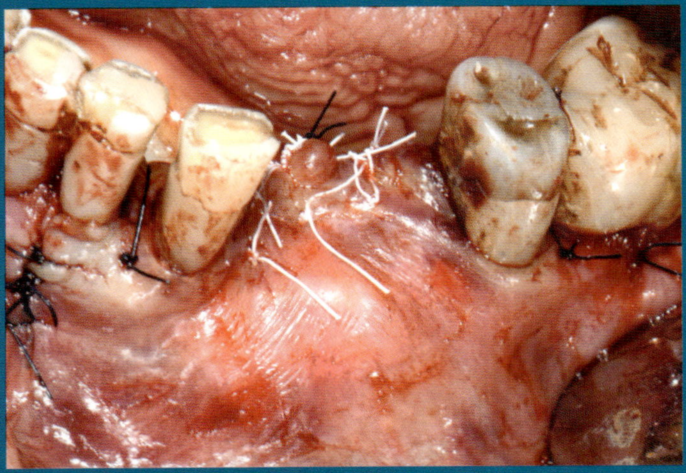

8 Coronal positioning of the flap and PTFE suture.

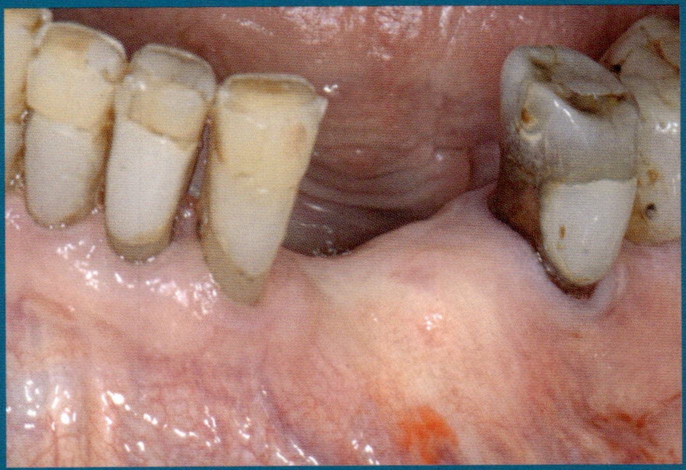

9 Clinical appearance 4 months after surgery.

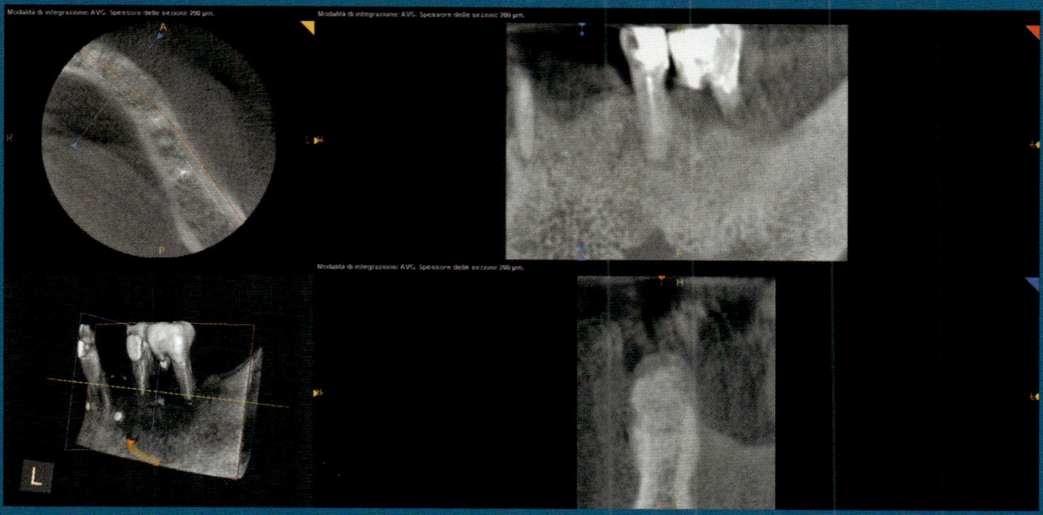

10 CBCT at 4 months.

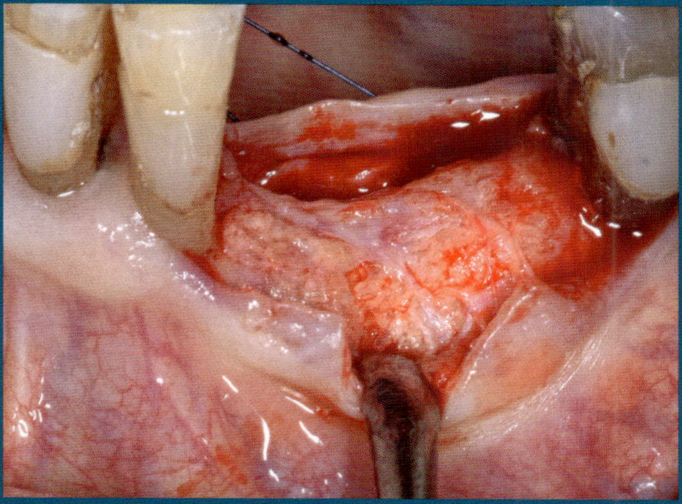

11 Reopening after 4 months.

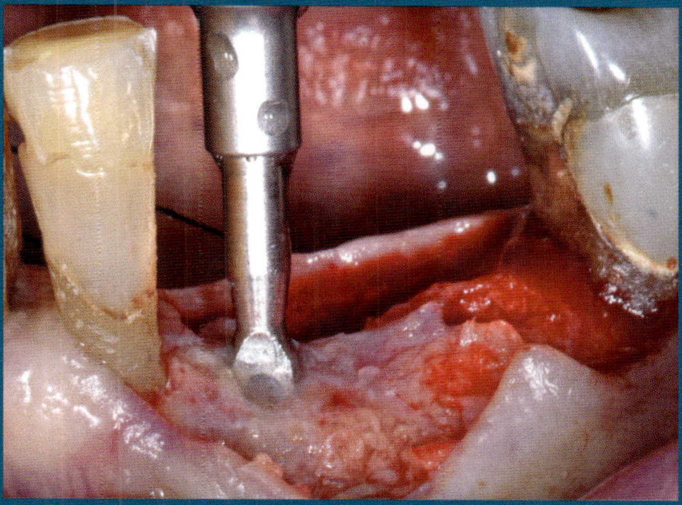

12 Implant placement.

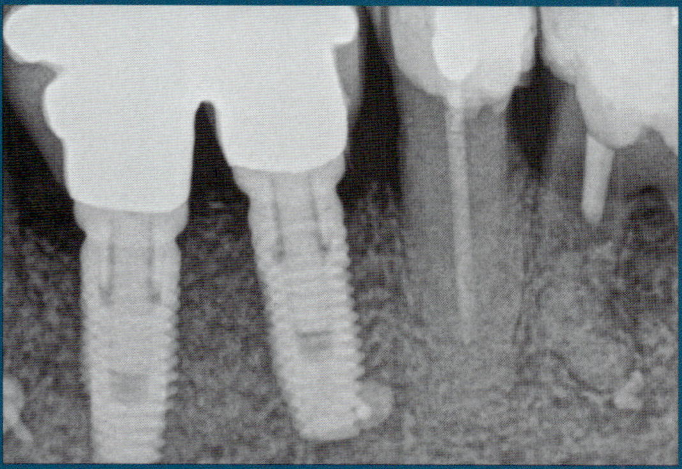

13 Intraoral X-ray after loading.

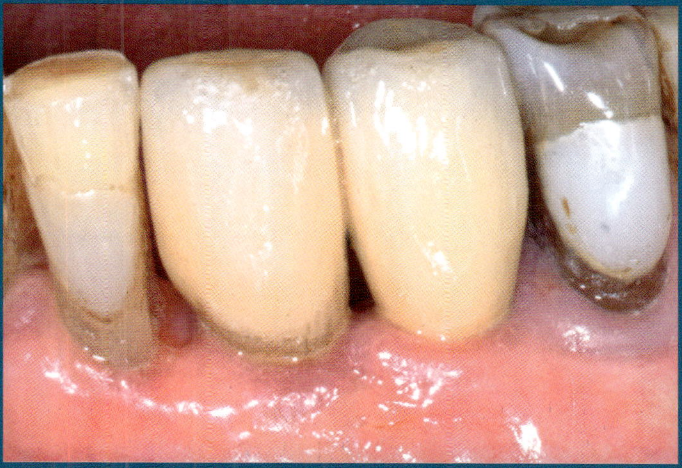

14 Completed restoration.

Ridge preservation with membrane, platelet derivatives

Clinical case 13

H.K.L. Ho, Singapore

The patient, a 36-year-old Asian male, has missing lower incisors with loss of width. By elevating the flap, labial atrophy and the strongly cortical nature of the labial plate can be noted. To facilitate and maintain space, the tent screw was placed evenly at the recipient site. No attempt was made to perforate the cortical plate. The allograft was mixed with CGF concentrated growth factors (Medifuge, Silfradent, Italy), positioned in the recipient site and covered with two layers of CGF membranes. No periosteal release was performed and the wound was closed with slight tension. After 4 months, the graft shows good bone consolidation. The implants were placed with good primary stability.

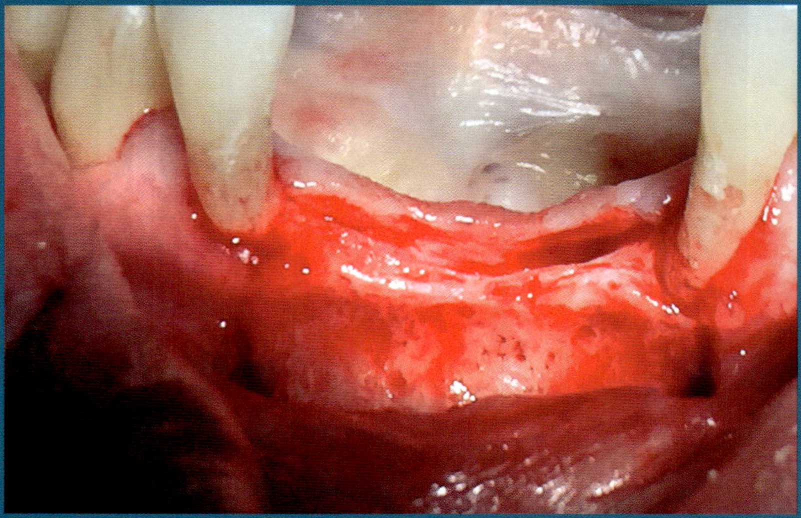

1 Initial situation.

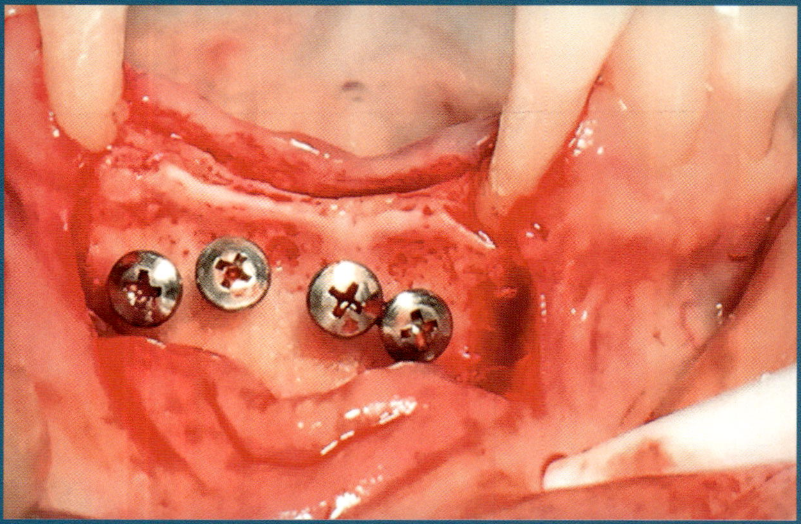

2 Creation of a curtain effect using fixation screws.

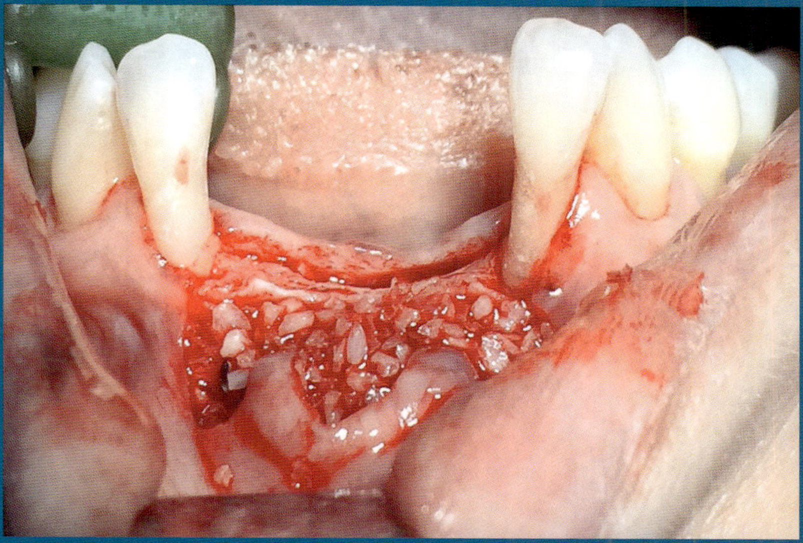

3 Positioning of the grafting material.

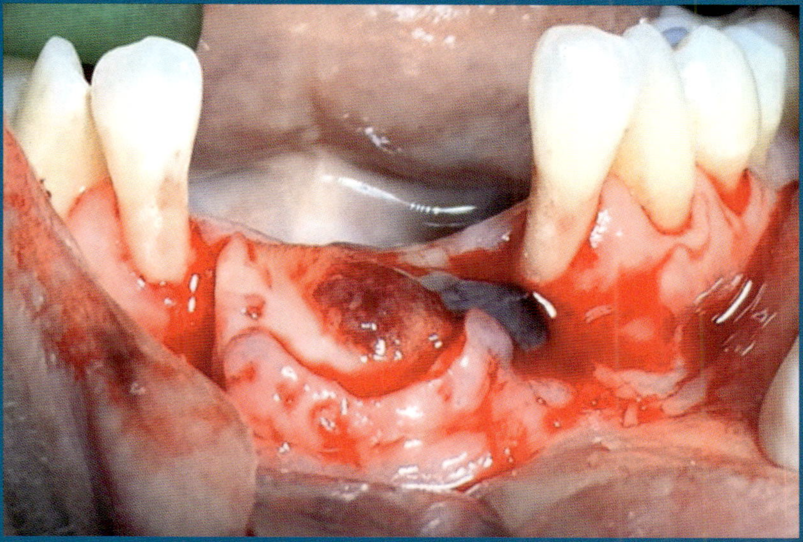

4 Graft coverage with CGF membrane.

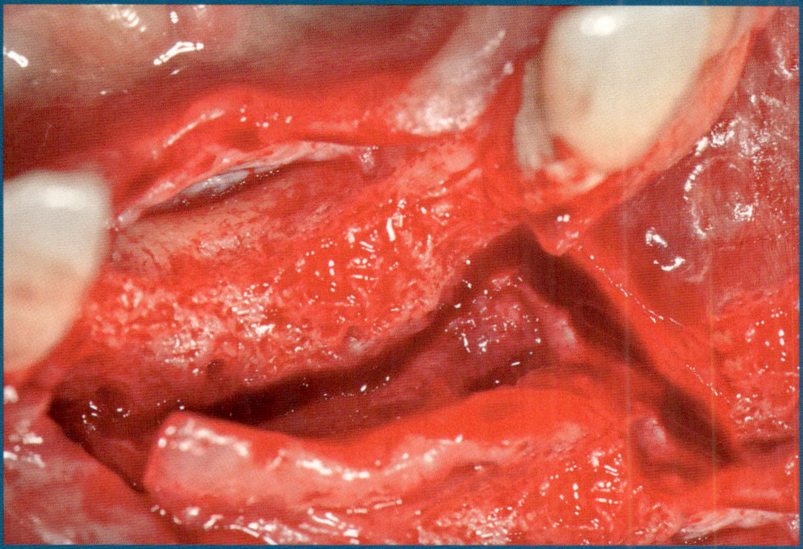

5 Graft is well consolidated. The fixation screw holes are clearly visible.

Clinical case 14

M. Contessi, Trieste, Italy

46-year-old female patient; she has a loss of circumferential attachment at tooth 4.5, endo-perio lesion with chronic flare up suppurative infection. The extracted tooth is processed by Tooth Transformer, and two membranes of autologous fibrin were obtained from 20 cc of the patient's blood using Dr. Choukroun method (A-PRF). An implant was placed in zone 4.6 3i BNST and at the same time a GBR for the defect by mixing bone chips, taken from the bone perforation of the implant, with dentin, covered with equine pericardium collagen membrane (Bioteck, Italy) and autologous fibrin membranes A-PRF. After 4 months, the tissue is compact with an advanced corticalization phase. Two further 3i BNST implants are then inserted into the regenerated bone and finally, when the implants have healed, restored with a screw retained bridge.

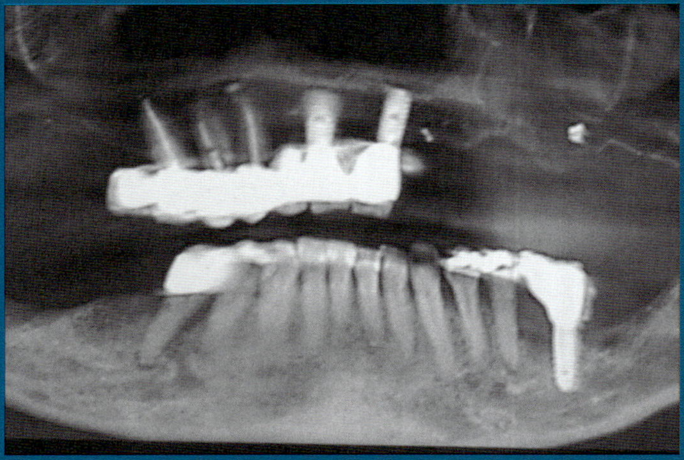

1 Stratigram at the start of treatment. We can guess the profound loss of circumferential attachment to the 4.5.

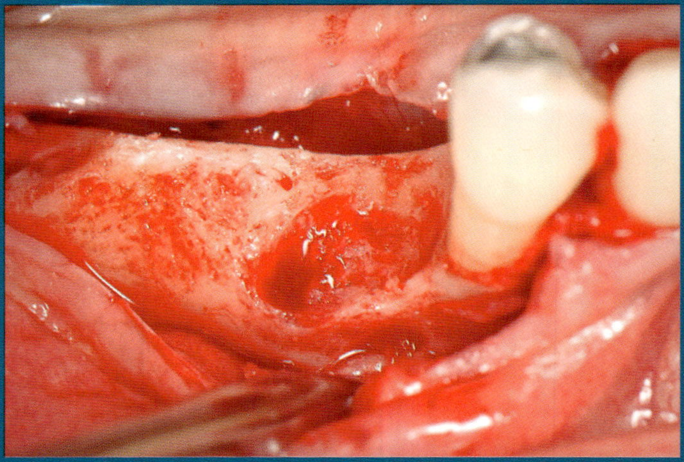

2 The horizontal and vertical component of the crater-like lesion caused by chronic suppuration and the emergence of the NAI below are evident.

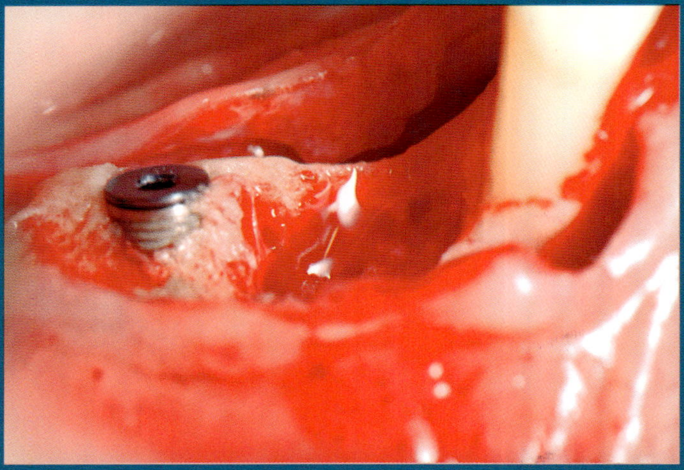

3 Thorough cleaning of the granulomatous tissue in the entire lesion. Perforations of the cortex are fundamental to elicit bleeding from the medullary spaces.

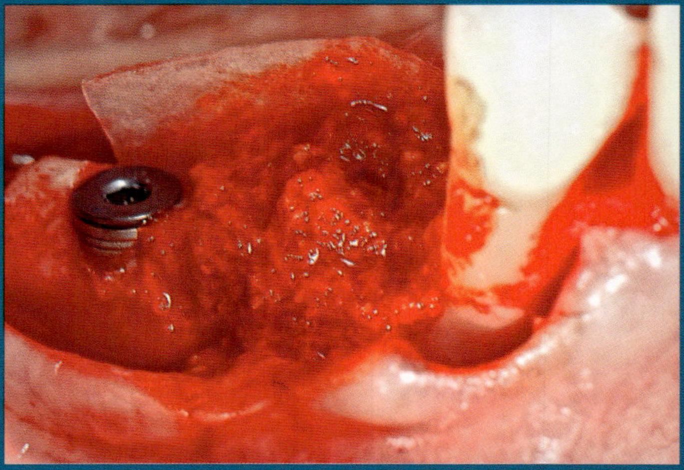

4 The autologous dentinal graft mixed with the local clot is placed under a membrane of equine pericardium. It stays in place and is easily modeled.

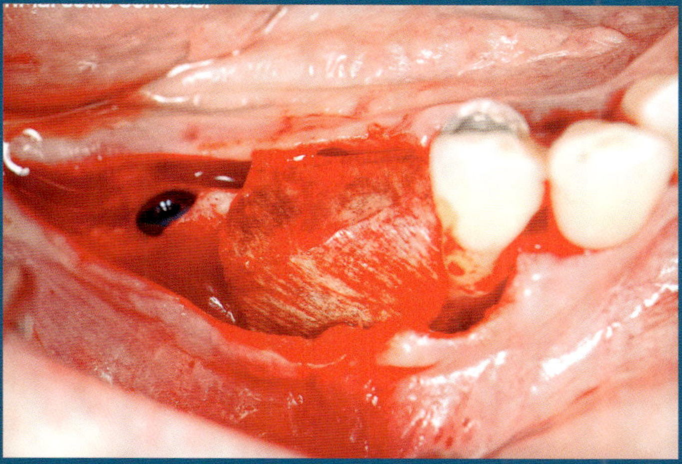

5 The membrane is turned over to cover the graft, then further softened with saline. It is not fixed with mini-screws in this case.

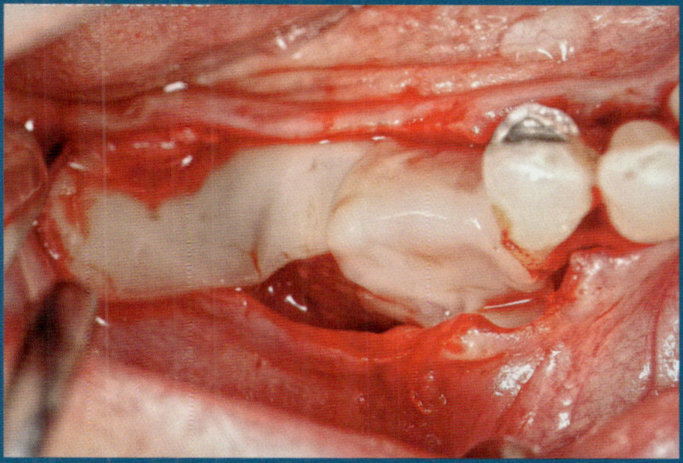

6 The two autologous fibrin membranes, obtained from autologous plasma, are positioned above the collagen membrane and under the surgical flaps.

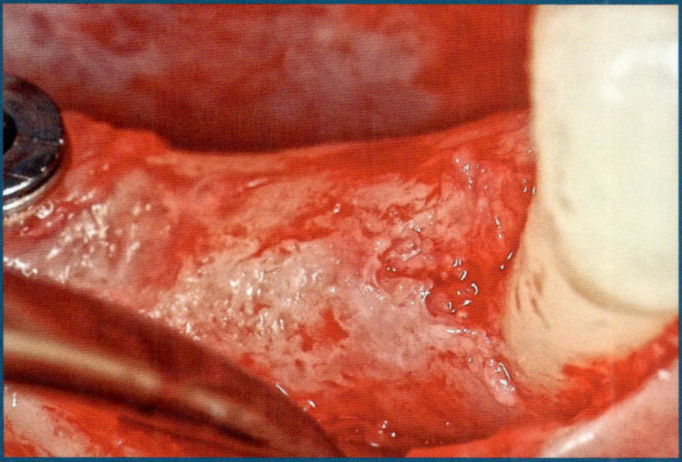

7 16 weeks after, the defect appears completely filled with new-bone of excellent macroscopic quality.

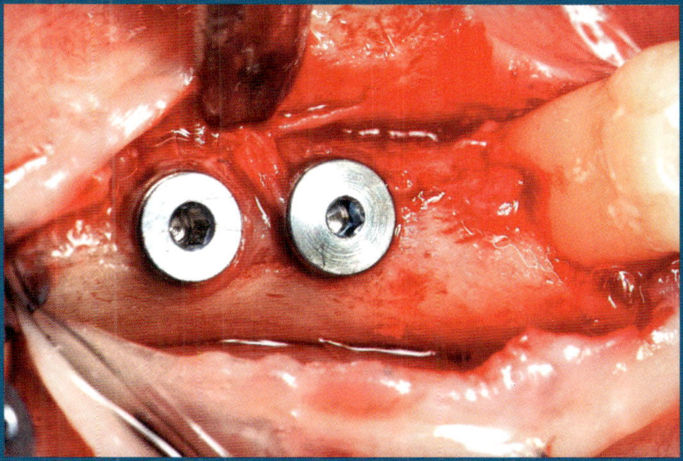

8 Occlusal view of the 3 implants, the most mesial one in regenerated bone.

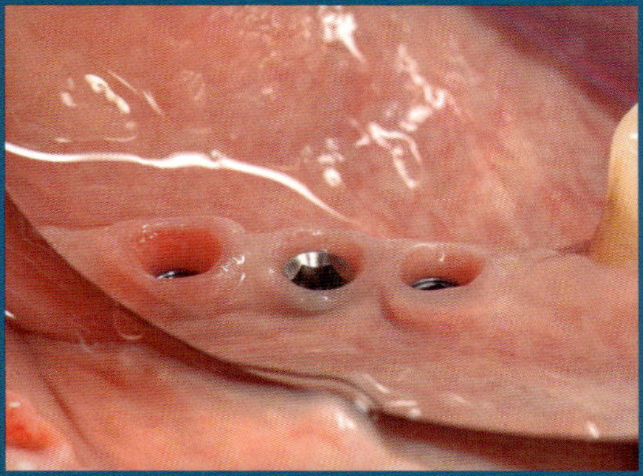

9 Good soft tissue healing after 8 weeks of soft tissue maturation with healing caps.

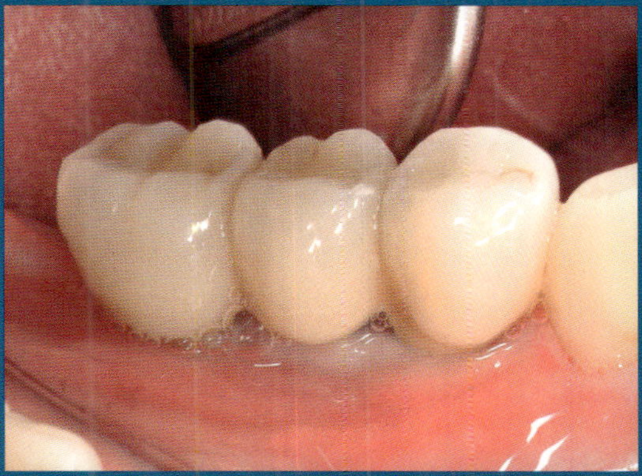

10 Final implant-supported bridge (screw-retained solution).

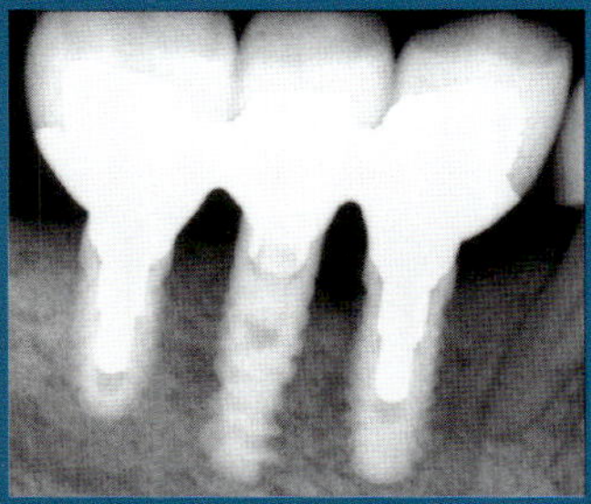

11 Intraoral X-ray 16 months after loading.

Clinical case 15

M. Libertucci, Rome, Italy

The patient, a 69-year-old man, smoker, has some questionable prognosis elements to be extracted and asks to replace the missing teeth in the posterior sectors with a removable prosthesis but anchored on implants, in order not to overload the existing anterior elements that have a reduced bone support due to previous periodontal problems.

The extracted teeth are used to produce osteoinductive dental particles in order to vertically regenerate the ridges for the future insertion of two implants in area 1.4 and 2.4. In this case, the dental particulate is mixed with CGF (Concentrate Grow Factor; Medifuge, Silfradent, Italy) in a liquid form obtained by centrifuging the patient's blood in a silicone-coated tube to prevent coagulation. Four months later, two Biomet 3i implants are placed and an overdenture with implant support is delivered.

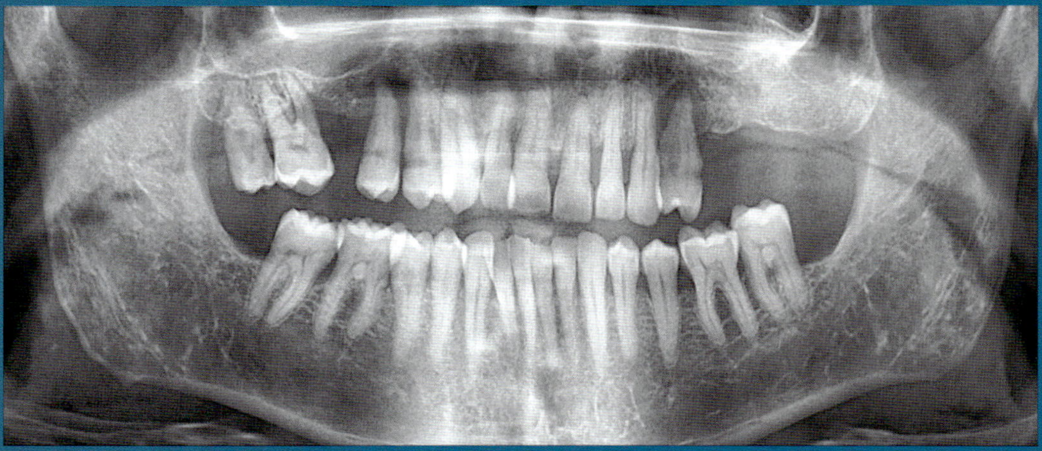

1 Initial OPG.

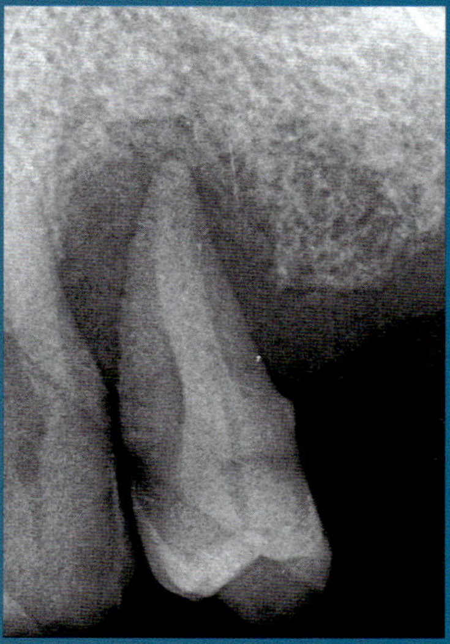

2 Periapical zone 2.4.

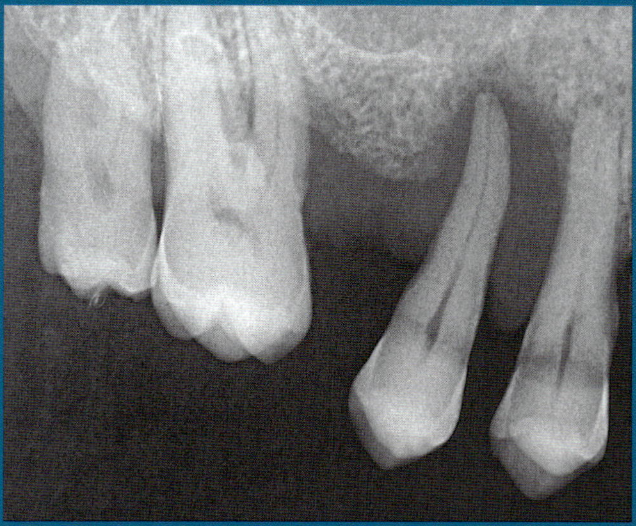

3 Periapical zone 1.4.

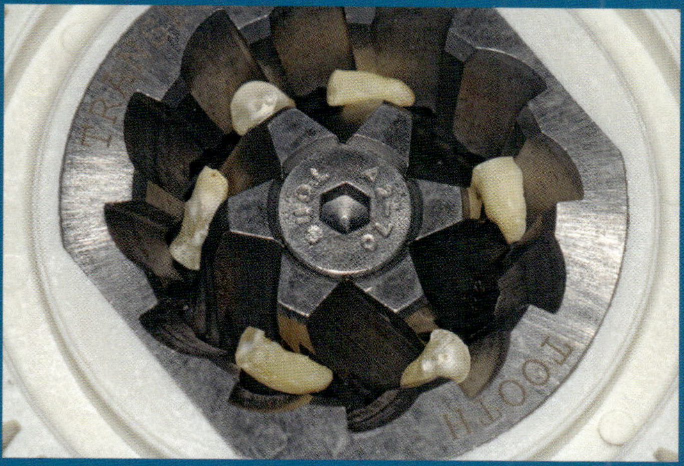

4 Elements 1.4 and 2.4 sectioned and placed in the grinder.

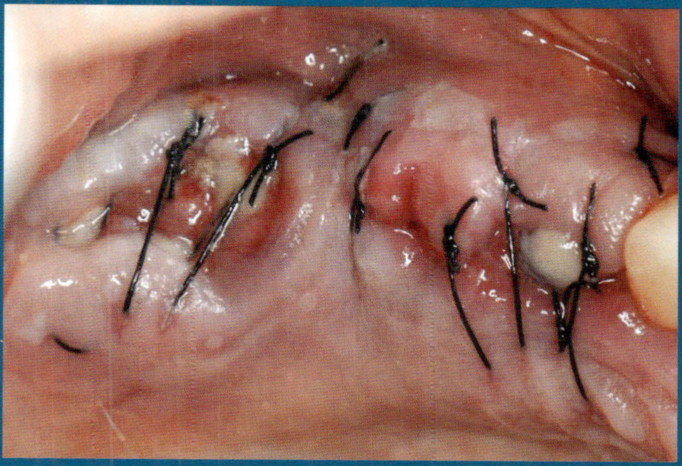

5 Postextraction site with vertical GBR with tooth graft, liquid platelet concentrates and collagen membrane covering the graft in area 1.4 after 1 week.

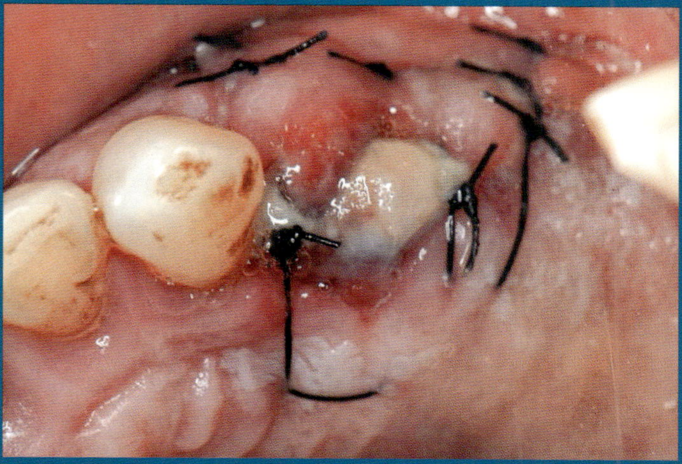

6 Postextraction site with vertical GBR with tooth graft, liquid platelet concentrates and collagen membrane covering the graft in area 2.4 after 1 week.

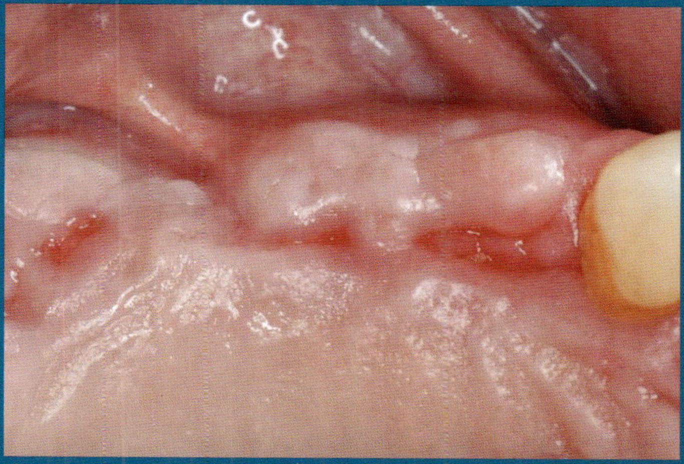

7 Healing of tissues after 2 months in area 1.4.

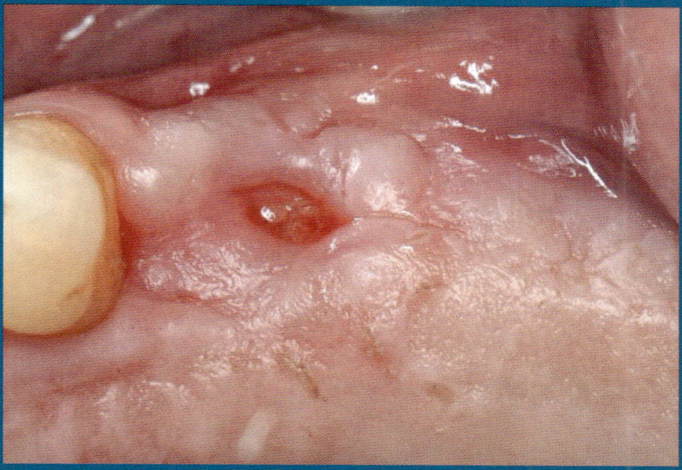

8 Healing of tissues after 2 months in area 2.4.

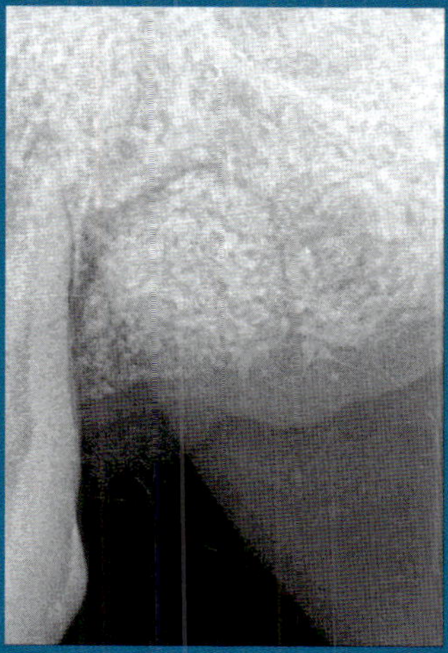

9 Postoperative intraoral X-ray of element 2.4.

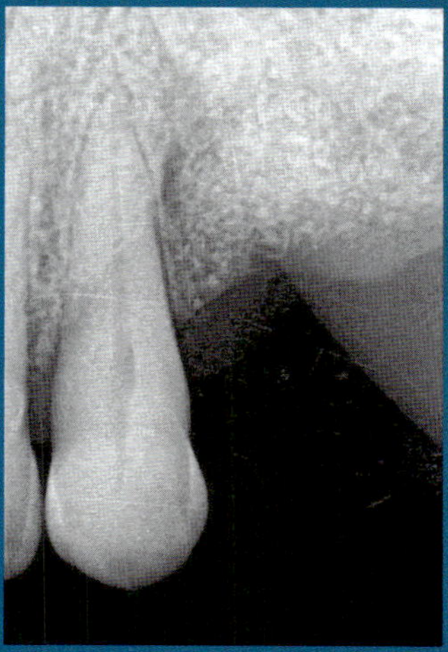

10 Intraoral X-ray of 2.4 after 4 months.

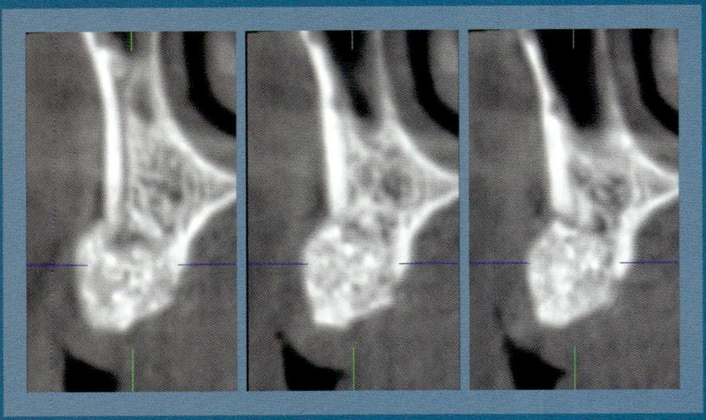

11 Postoperative CBCT of element 1.4.

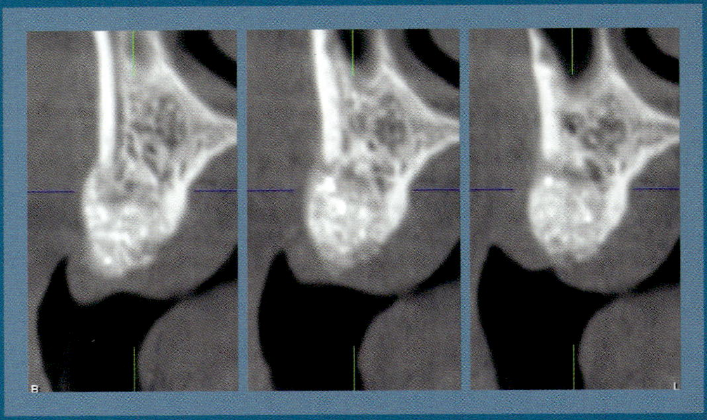

12 CBCT of element 1.4 after 4 months.

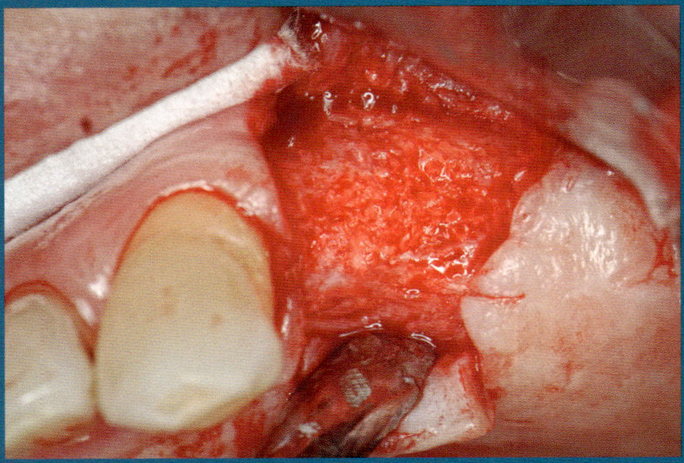

13 Reopening at 4 months and 20 days. Note the quality and quantity of newly formed bone.

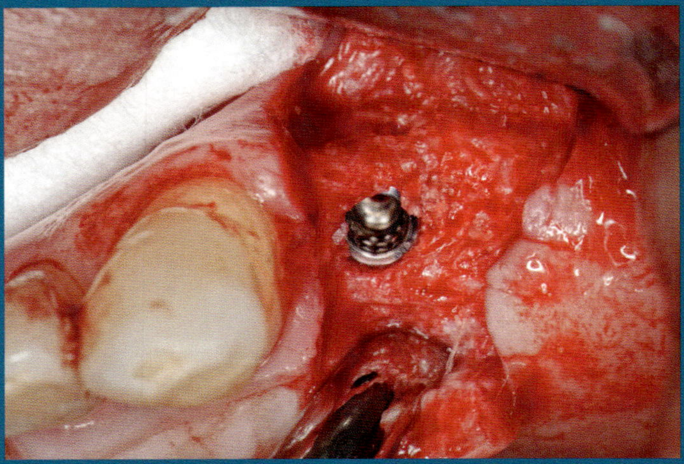

14 Implant insertion - diameter 3.25 and length 15 mm (7.22 mm in regenerated bone).

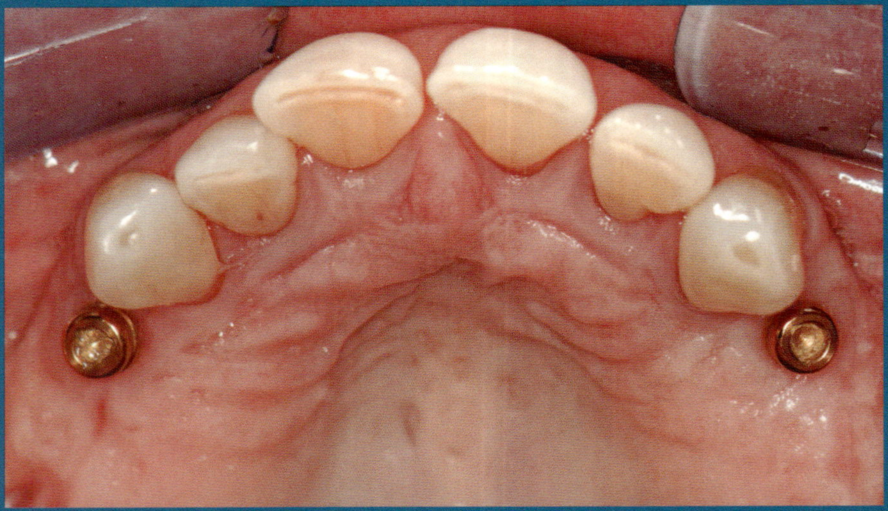

15 Clinical view of of the removable overdenture supported by implants (to avoid excessive loads on the canines already periodontally compromised) 1 and a half years from loading.

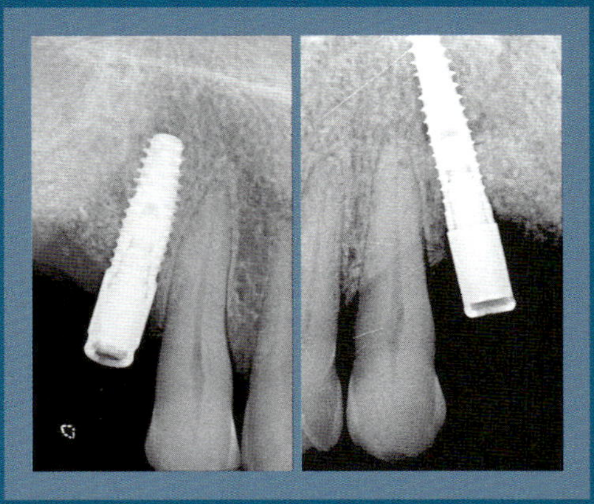

16 Intraoral X-rays 18 months after loading.

SINUS LIFT

Clinical case 16

E. Minetti, Milan, Italy

52-year-old female patient, non-smoker, no previous pathology.

Following the extraction of elements 1.5 and 1.6, a sinus lift is required. For the graft material it was decided to use the impacted element 1.8 which had already caused repeated inflammation. Once the full thickness flap is elevated, the Schneiderian membrane is elevated to allow the extraction of 1.8 without creating perforations. At the same time, two Visio One Cea implants (Cea medical, Swiss) are inserted and the vestibular hole is closed with a resorbable collagen membrane (Bego-Oss, Bego, Germany).

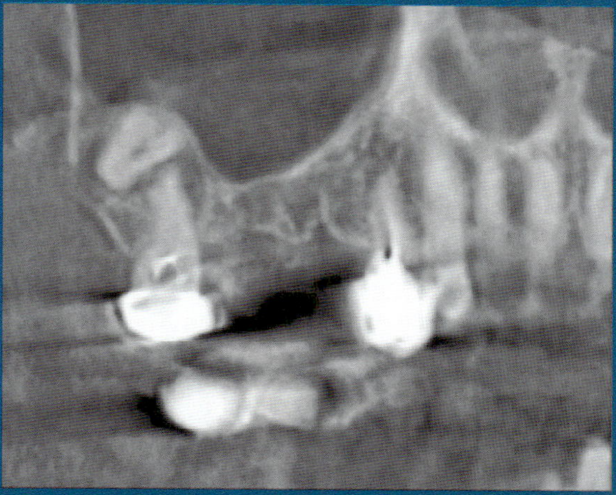

1 Preoperative CBCT. Note element 1.8 impacted apically to 1.7.

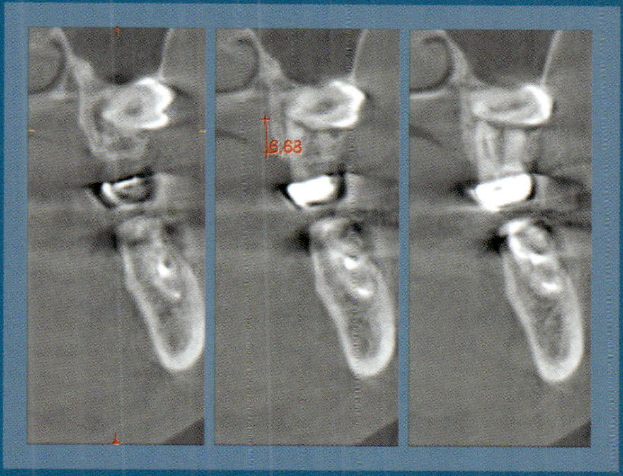

2 Preoperative CBCT of 1.8-1.7.

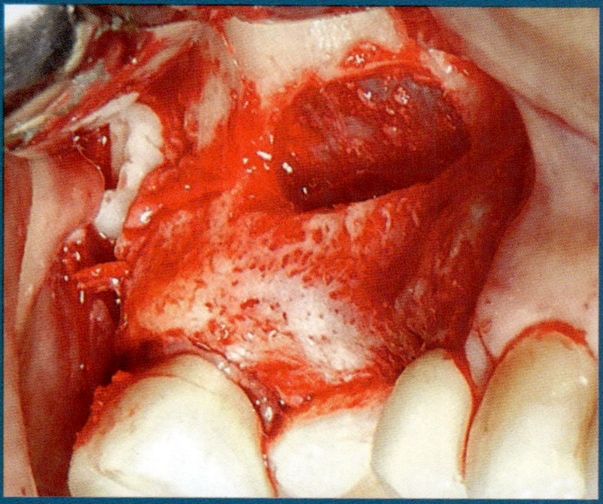

3 Elevation of the vestibular flap and visualization of the crown of 1.8.

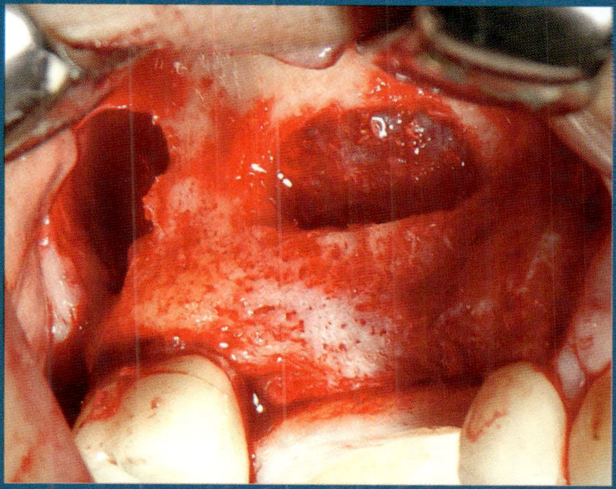

4 Elevation of the membrane and extraction of the element 1.8.

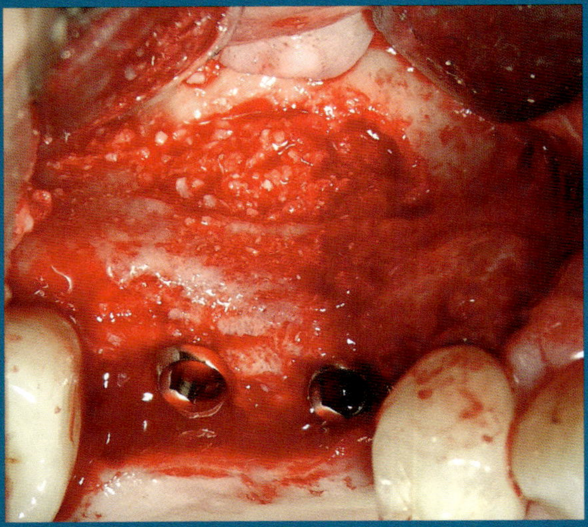

5 Filling of the residual cavity using the material derived from the extracted tooth and implants in position 1.5–1.6.

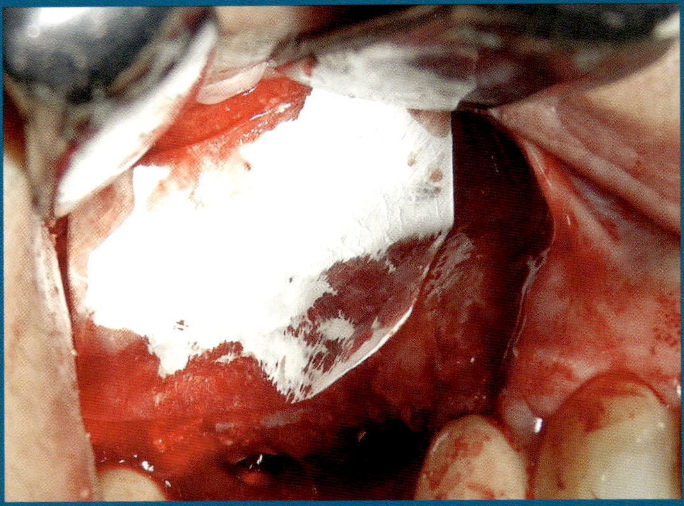

6 Resorbable collagen membrane covering the grafted material.

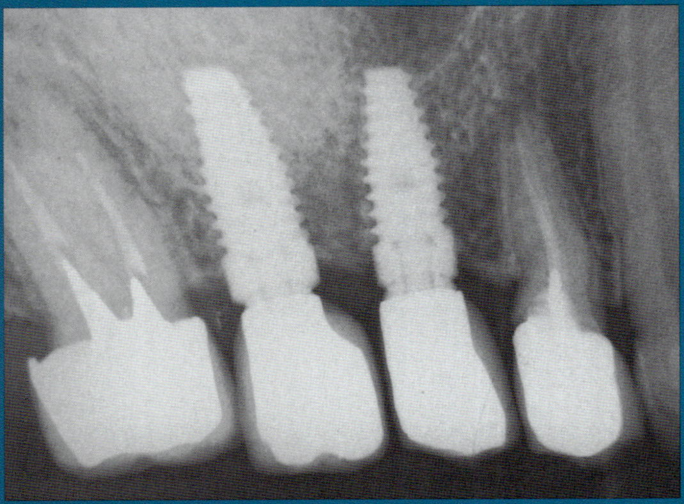

7 Intraoral X-ray at 1 year.

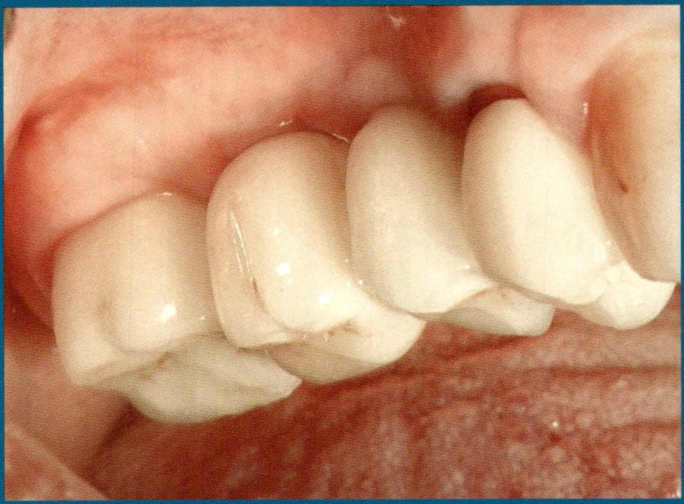

8 Restoration after 1 year.

Clinical case 17

E. Minetti, Milan, Italy

47-year-old male patient, smoker.

The patient needs a prosthetic rehabilitation of 2.6 by a combined sinus lifting and grafting and implant placement. To produce the material necessary for the grafting, one of the three wisdom teeth that the patient had extracted at the age of 20 and that he had kept in a cardboard container is used. Four months after the first surgical phase, a Visio One Cea implant (Cea medical, Swiss) is placed using a trephine drill to create the surgical socket with the aim of taking a tissue to be histologically analyzed. When the implant heals, a full ceramic restoration is produced.

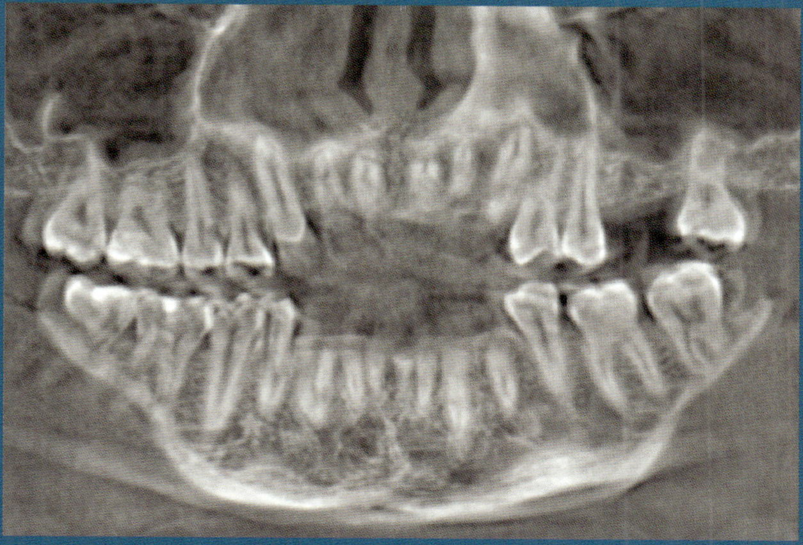

1 Preoperative scout section of CBCT.

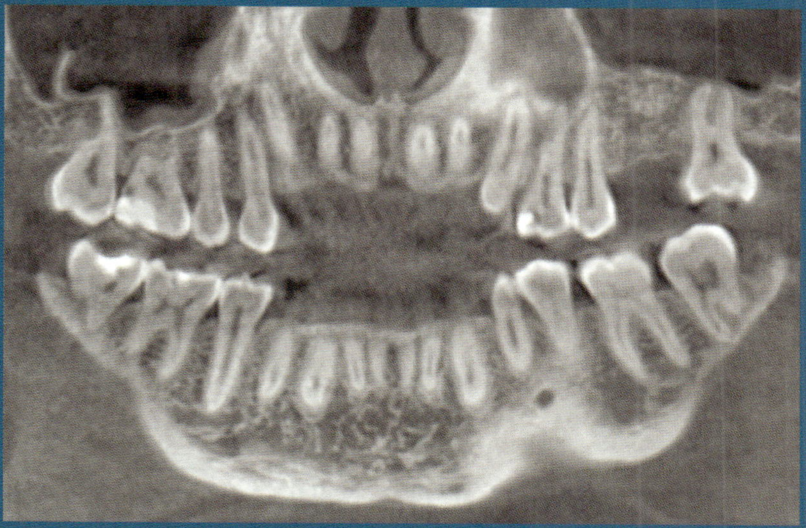

2 CBCT scout section 4 months after sinus lift.

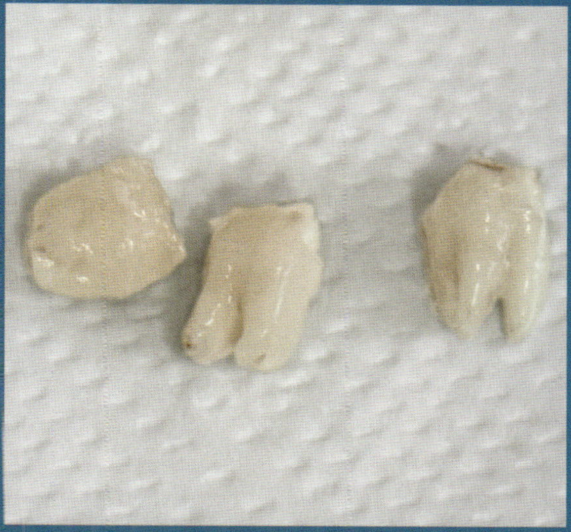

3 The patient's wisdom teeth extracted at the age of 20 and stored in a cardboard box.

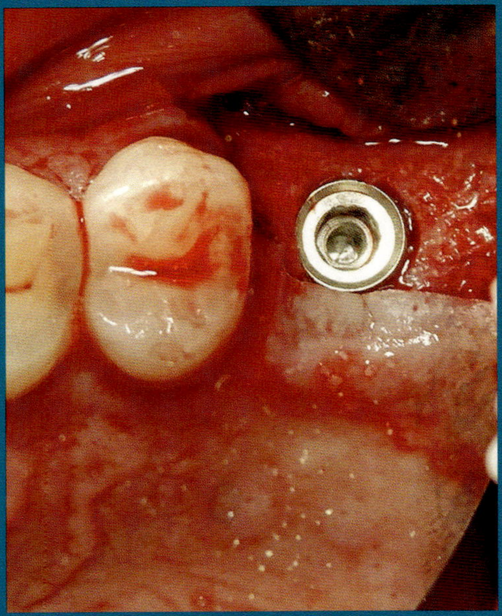

4 Insertion of the implant in the socket, created using a trephine, to histologically analyze the newly formed tissue.

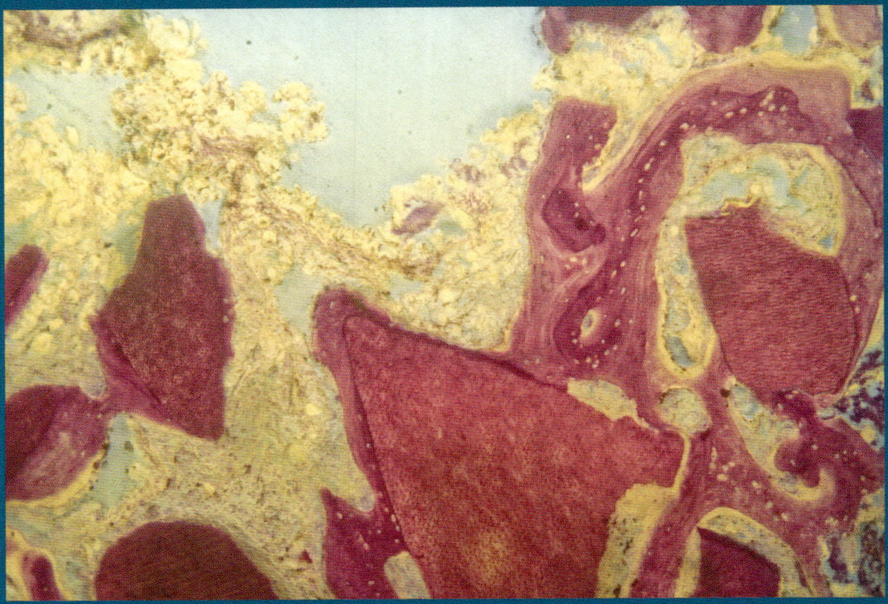

5 Histological sampling. Detail of the sample.

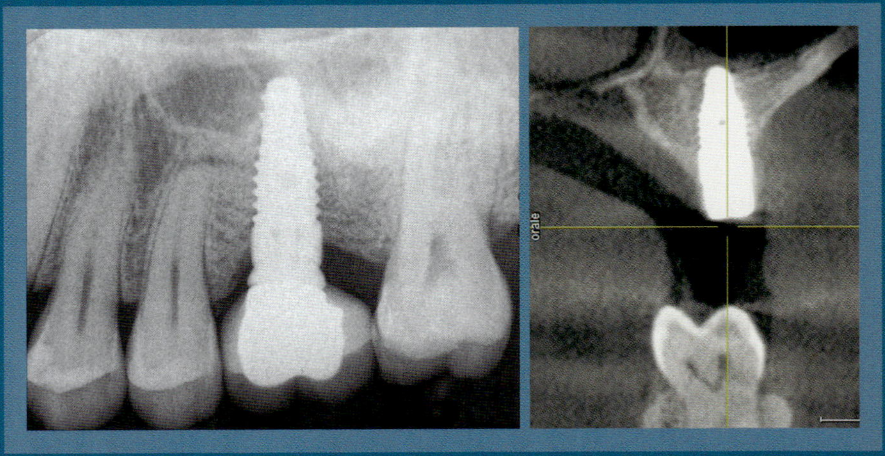

6 CBCT and intraoral X-ray 1 year after loading.

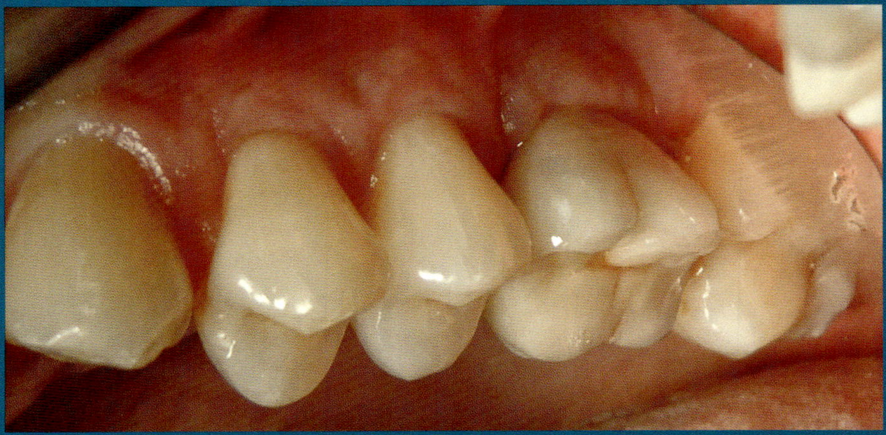

7 Restoration at the follow-up of 54 months.

TUNNEL TECHNIQUE

Clinical case 18

T. Beca Campoy, Madrid, Spain

57-year-old female patient, non-smoker, no previous pathology.

The patient has long-standing edentulism in area 3.6-3.7 and tooth 1.8 which causes pain on chewing. At the CBCT visit, the horizontal bone volume in area 3.6-3.7 is inadequate for implant therapy. It was decided to extract element 1.8 to perform a GBR tunnel technique on the edentulous area and then to be able to insert two ETK implants.

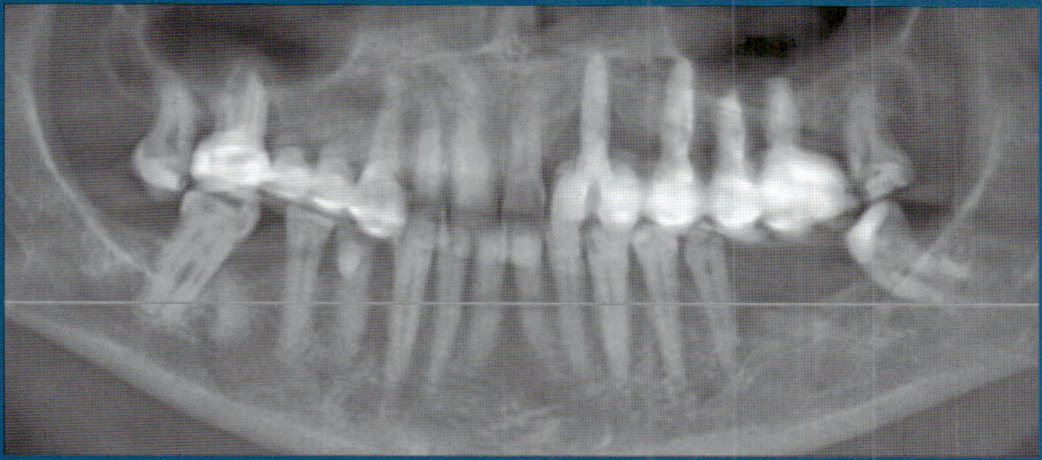

1 OPT preoperative. Note 1.8 and the edentulous area 3.6-3.7.

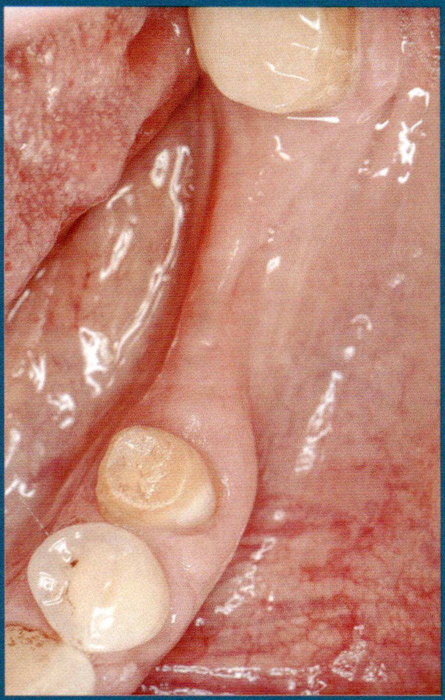

2 Occlusal view of quadrant 4. The loss of thickness of the lingual vestibule is evident.

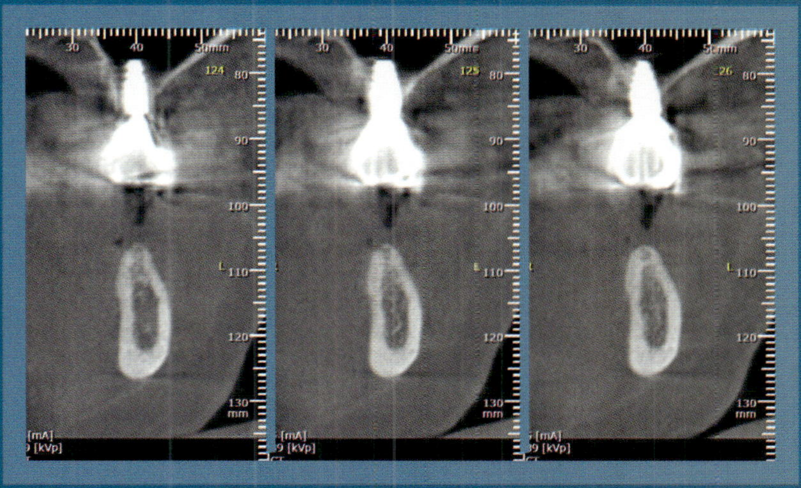

3 CBCT preoperative sagittal section.

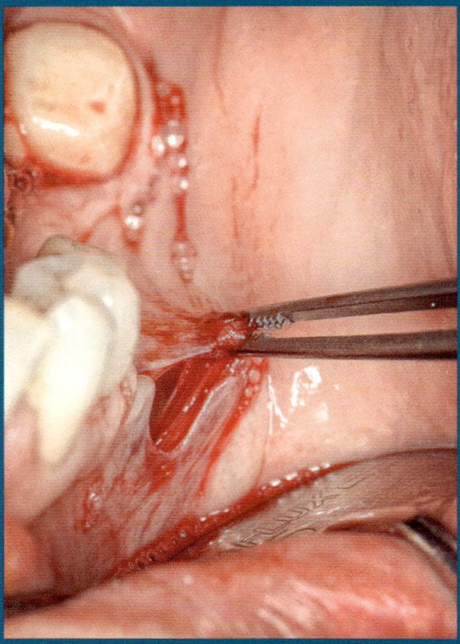

4 Vertical incision of access to the tunnel.

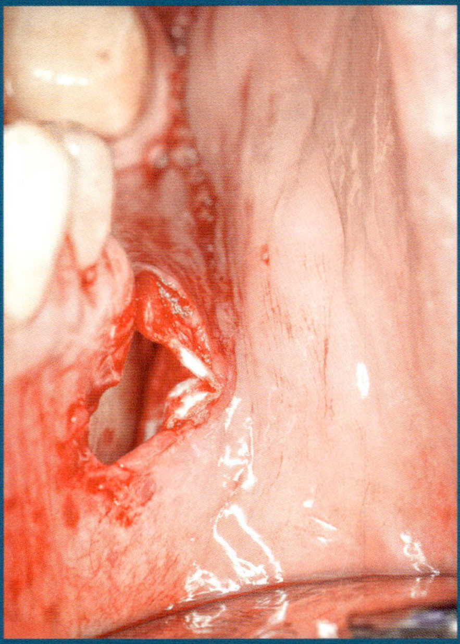

5 Positioning of the subperiosteal membrane inside the tunnel.

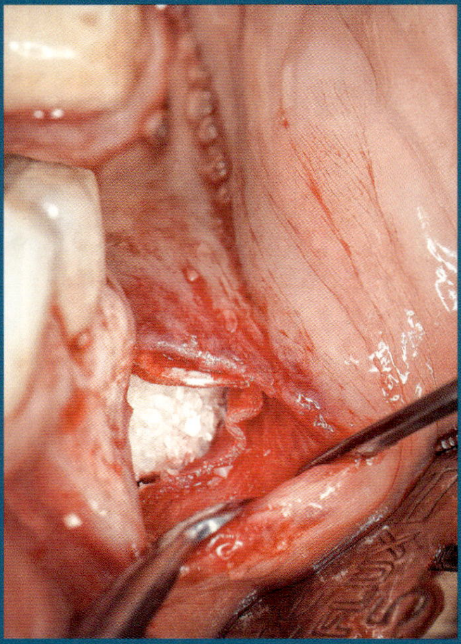

6 Positioning of the preparation of dental origin inserted between the membrane and the bone tissue.

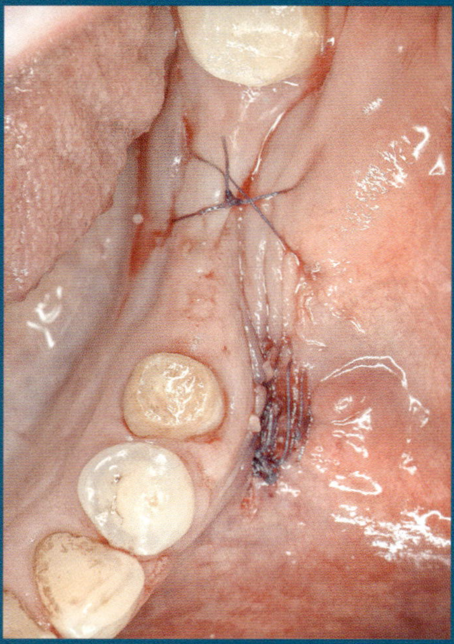

7 Closure of the vertical incision and consolidation of the graft by resorbable suture.

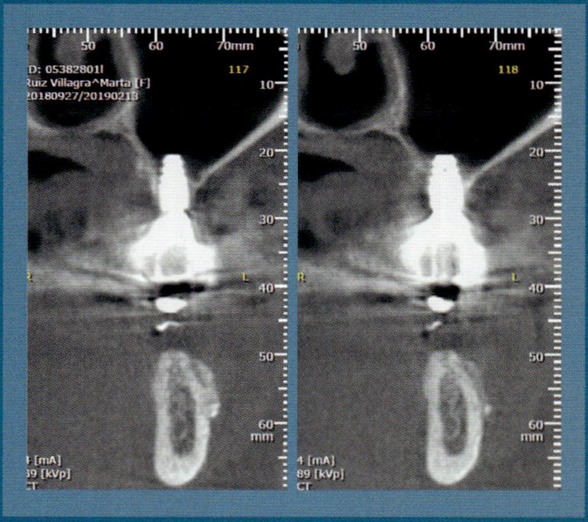

8 Postoperative CBCT. Note the increase in the horizontal dimension.

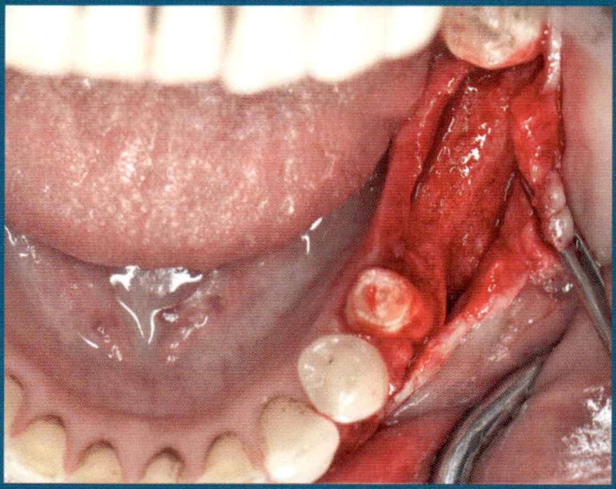

9 Opening of the flap, where it is clearly possible to recognize the graft.

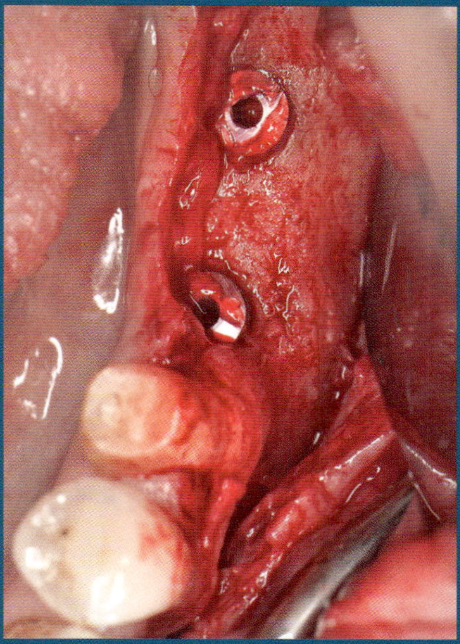

10 Placement of two implants. Thanks to the regeneration they are both correctly inserted.

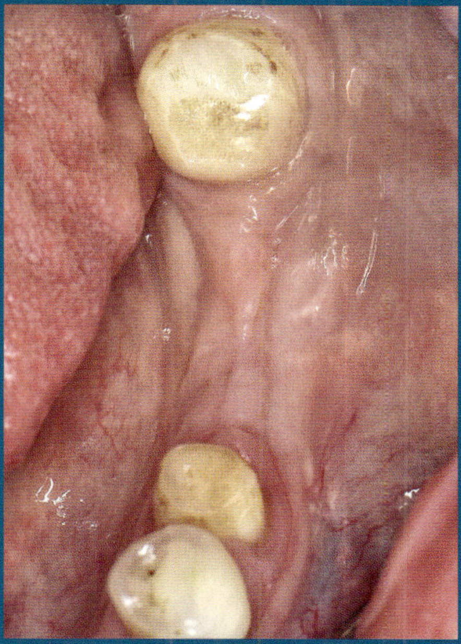

11 Occlusal image 8 months after regeneration. Note the increase in volume.

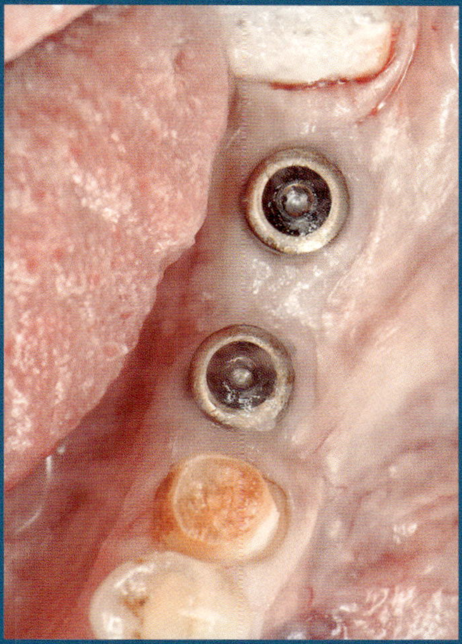

12 Healing of the keratinized mucosa around the healing caps.

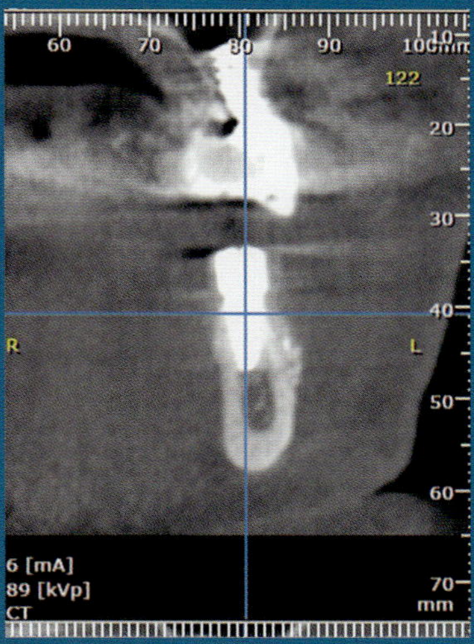

13 CBCT sagittal section after implant healing.

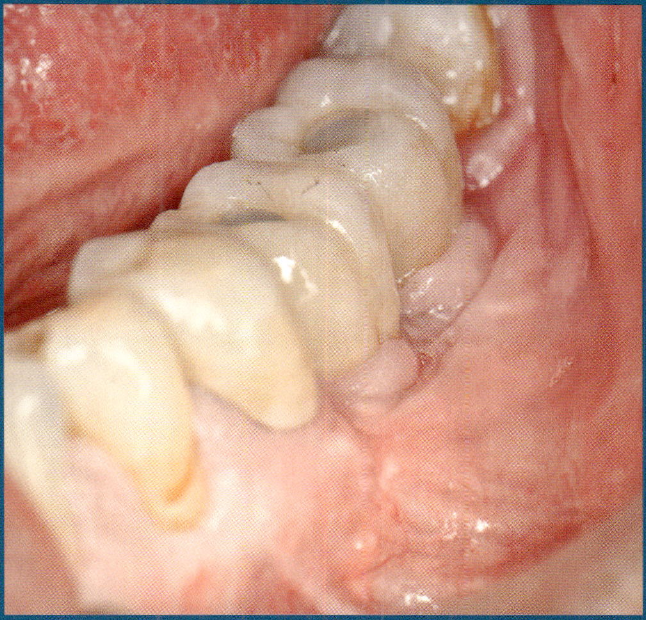

14 Placement of screw-retained implant restorations.

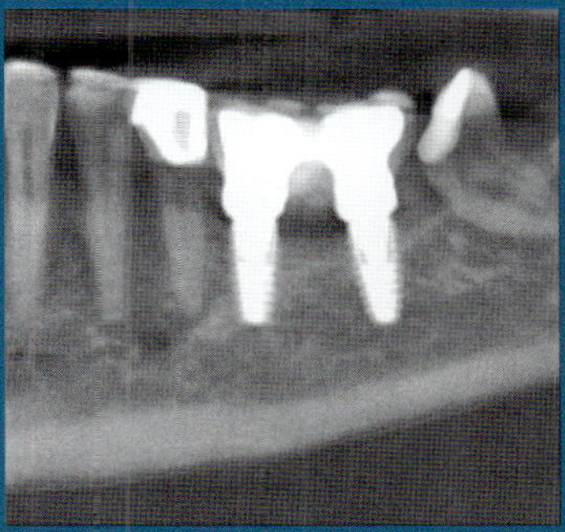

15 Intraoral X-ray at 14 months.

PERIODONTOLOGY

Clinical case 19

J. Schmitz, Milan, Italy

56-year-old male patient with reoccurrent periodontal abscesses and extreme tooth mobility. After the initial preparation, the extractions of the hopeless teeth are confirmed: 1.4, 2.4, 2.6, 2.7, 3.7. Tooth 1.6 is treated endodontically and amputation of the distal root is performed. In area 2.5 there is an unuseful implant that is used to support a long-term provisional, due to the patient's request to avoid removable prostheses. We then proceed to insert a temporary tooth-supported upper arch and two single crowns on the first lower molars. Periodontal interventions are performed to correct interproximal septal defects between 3.3, 3.4, 3.5 and 3.6, 4.5 and 4.6. The implant in zone 1.4 is positioned by filling the excessive gap between the basal bone and the implant surface with TT particles, as well as around implant in zone 2.4 (Biomet 3i), while implant placement in zones 2.6 and 2.7 requires an intervention of large sinus lift.

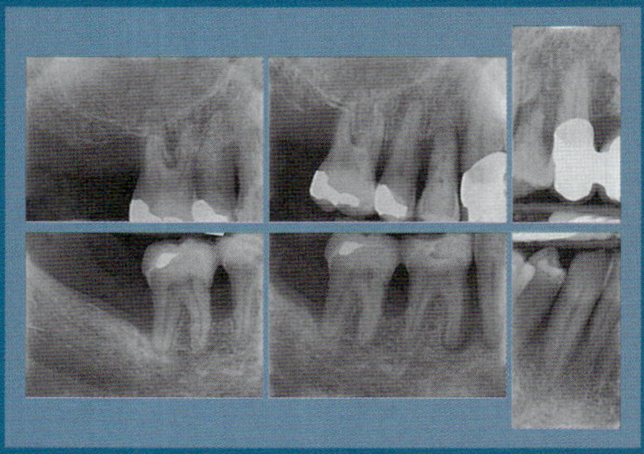

1 Radiographic investigations carried out at the beginning of treatment: very serious and widespread infraosseous periodontal lesions are confirmed, particularly affecting elements 1.4, 4.7, 4.6, 4.5, 4.3.

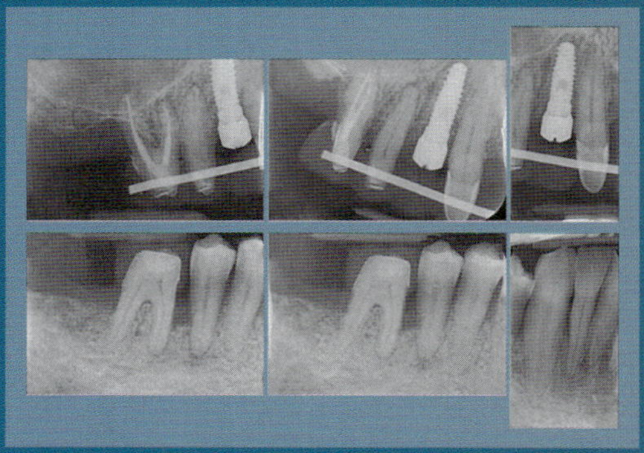

2 Radiographic investigations performed during the provisional phase at the end of the surgery. The 1.4 and 4.7 are extracted and, in a previous phase, the amputation of the distal root is performed.

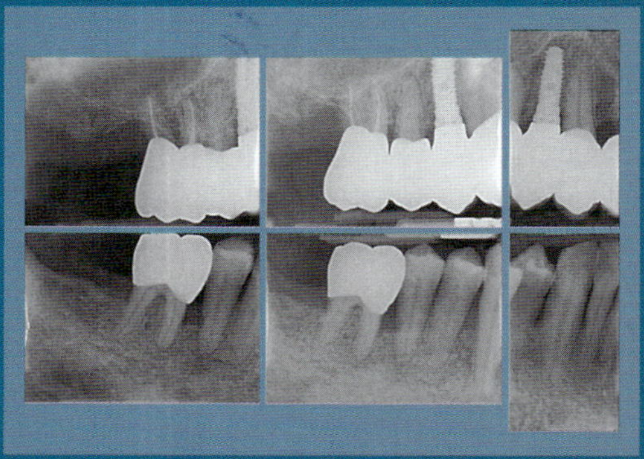

3 Radiographic investigations performed at the delivery of the definitive restorations. Note a sufficient and stable regeneration in the treated areas.

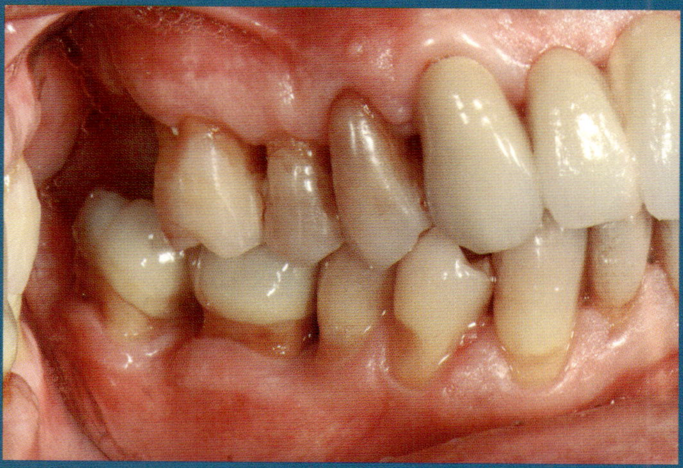

4 Clinical image of the patient at the start of treatment. Note the compromised periodontal picture.

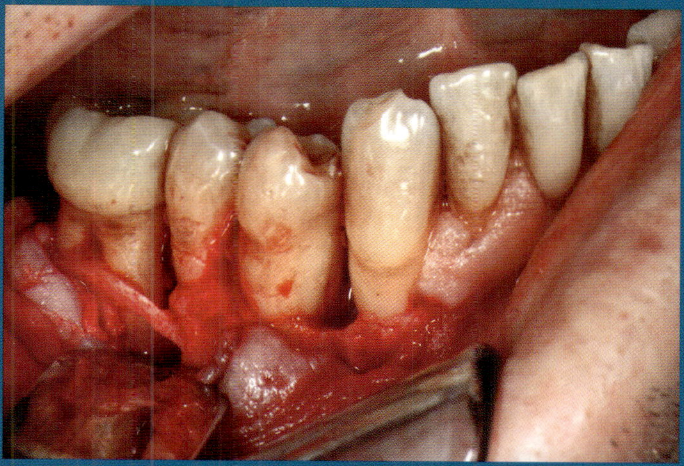

5 After the initial preparation, during which 4.7 is extracted, an intervention is performed to regenerate the interproximal infrabony defects between 4.5 and 4.6 and between 4.3 and 4.4. A bony bridge present apically is preserved in the distal defect.

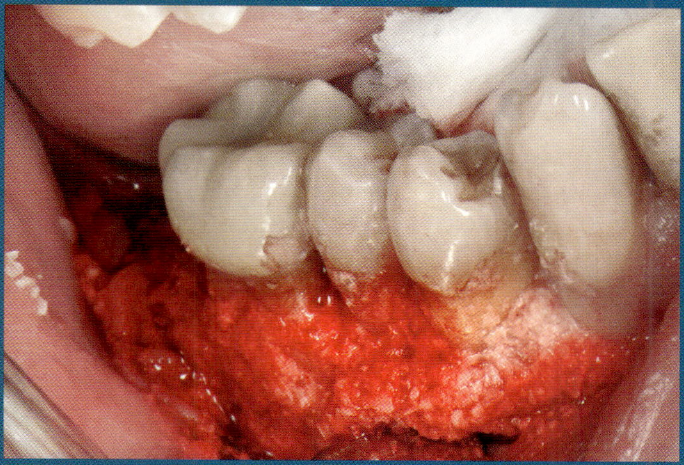

6 Filling of defects with particulates is performed in slight excess with Bio Gide Geistlich membrane covering.

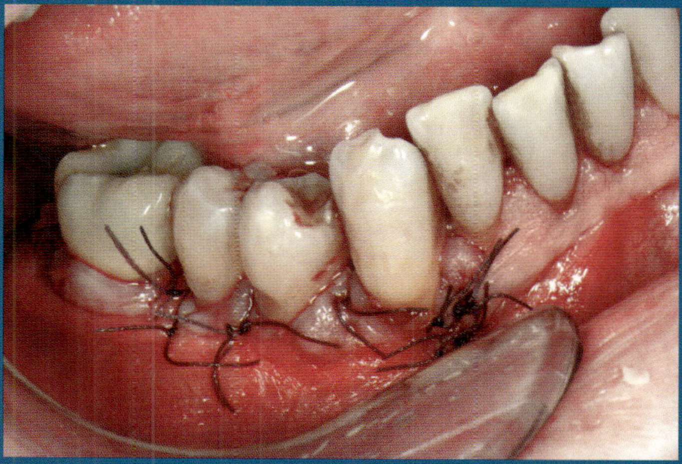

7 Single interrupted sutures with periosteal anchorage.

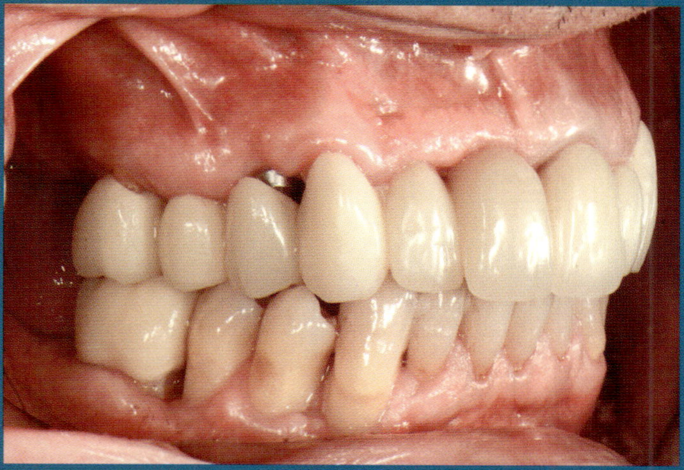

8 Appearance of tissues after healing. In some points, an incomplete maturation is noted.

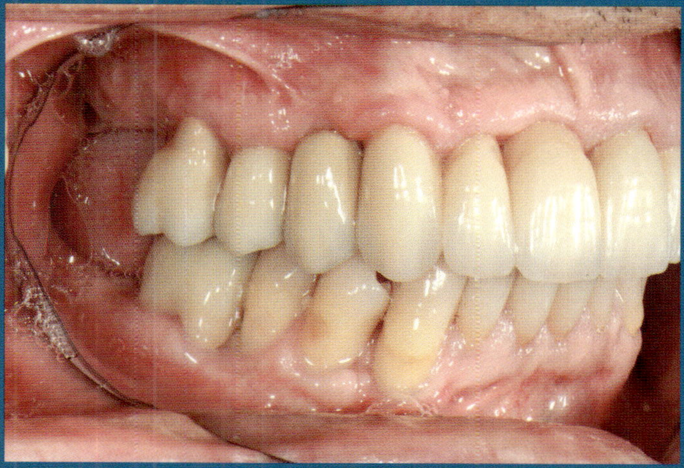

9 Stable appearance of the tissues at the final restoration delivery.

ALVEOLAR PRESERVATION WITH PROTECTIVE POLYPROPYLENE SUPPORT

Clinical case 20

M. Libertucci, Rome, Italy

35-year-old female patient, non-smoker, no previous pathology. In this alveolar preservation, after the extraction of a 2.6, a dental particulate is used with the aid of a polypropylene support to be worn 24 hours a day until obtaining a quick re-epithelialization on the particulate left deliberately exposed. The polypropylene, in addition to protecting the particulate and preventing its dispersion in the oral cavity, "horizontally guides" the connective cells to close the crestal part, minimizing the chance of infiltration of the dental particulate and speeding up the process. When the graft heals, a Biomet 3i implant is placed.

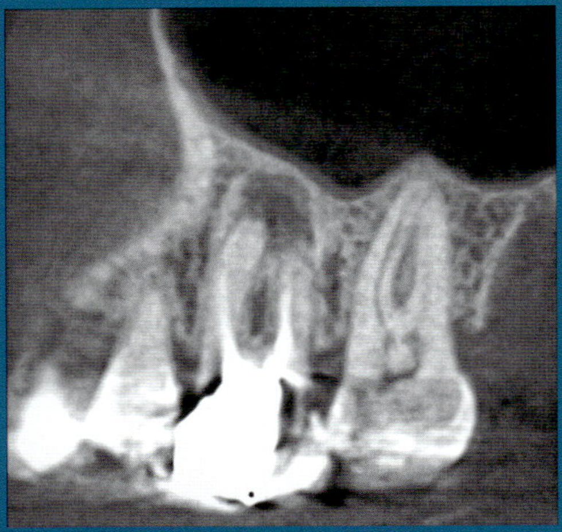

1 Preoperative CBCT.

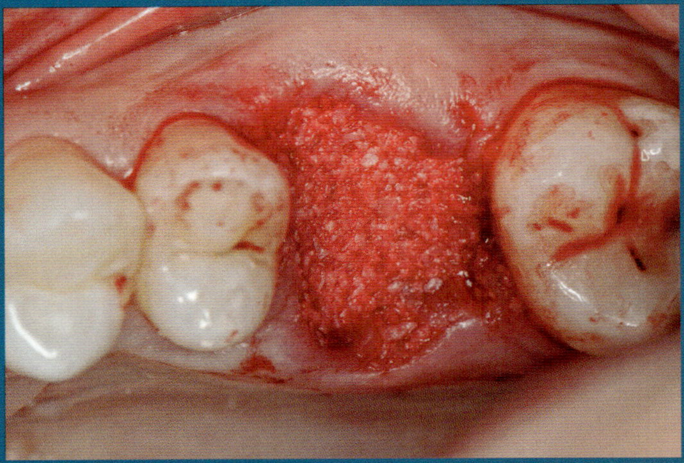

2 Filling of the cavity.

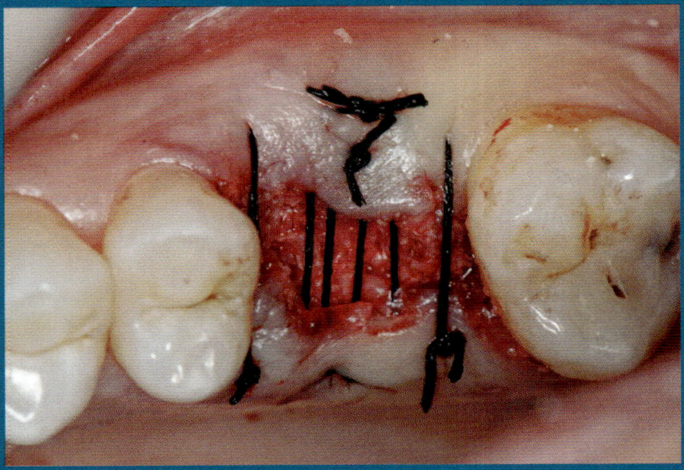

3 Suture of the socket.

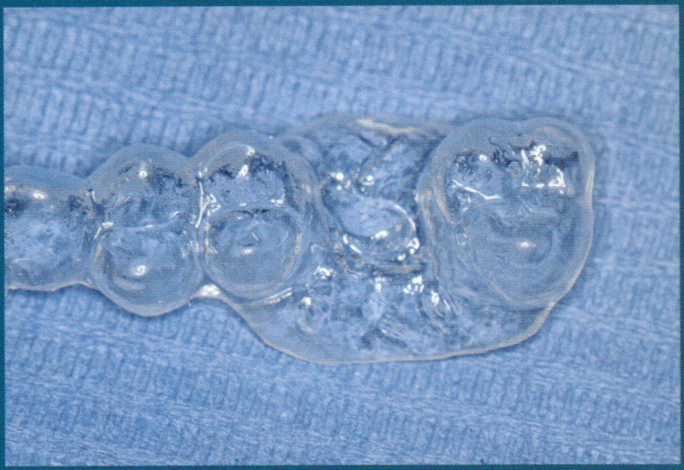

4 Guide in 0.5 mm thick polyethylene.

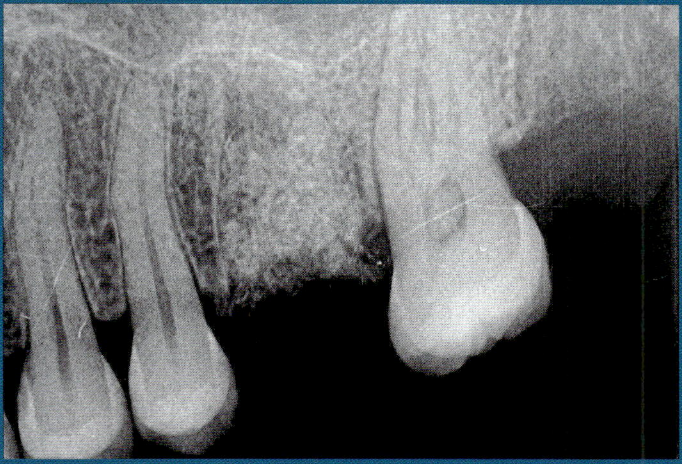

5 Postoperative periapical X-ray.

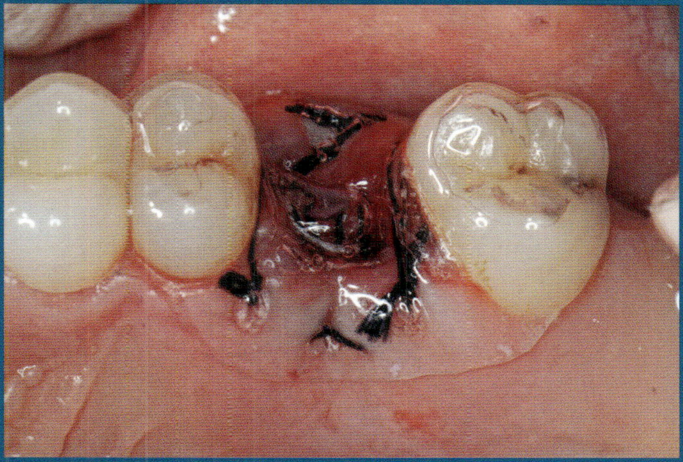

6 Sutured socket with guide in place (24 hours).

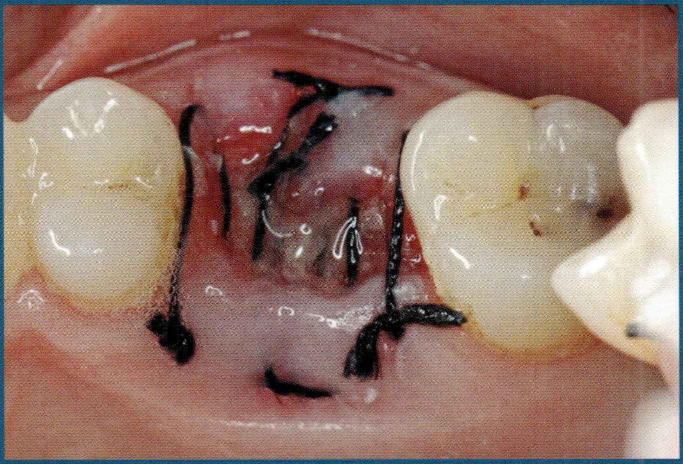

7 Healing after 7 days.

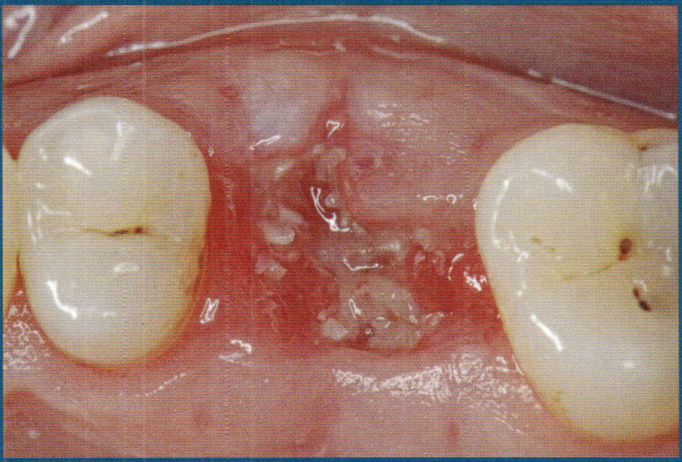

8 Healing after 14 days.

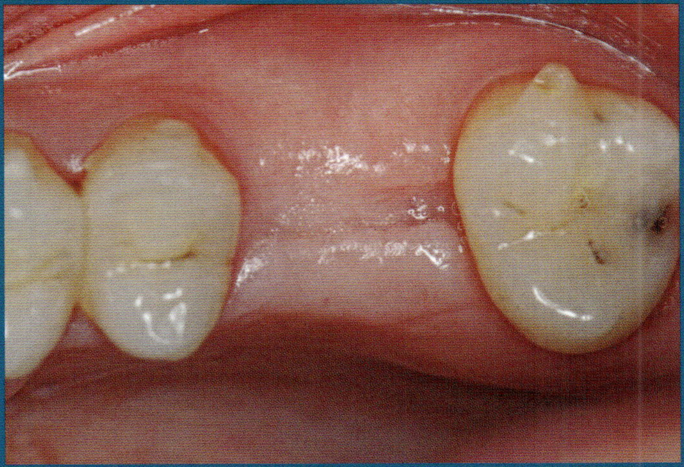

9 Healing at 9 months.

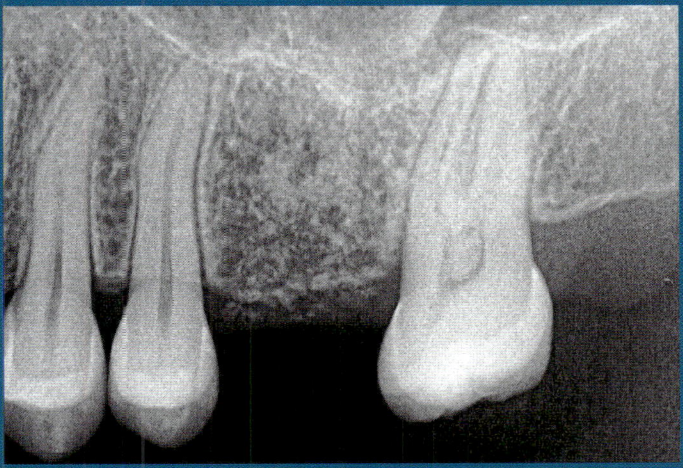

10 Healing at 12 months.

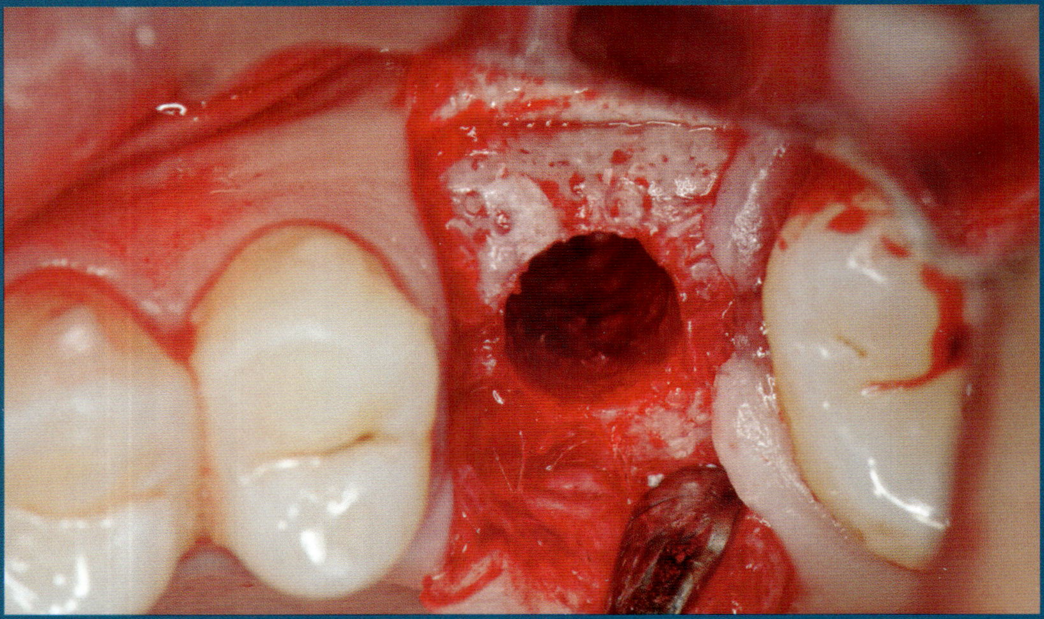

11 Graft well present and consolidated. Osteotomy with trephine and magnetic mallet to allow anchoring on the sinus cortex.

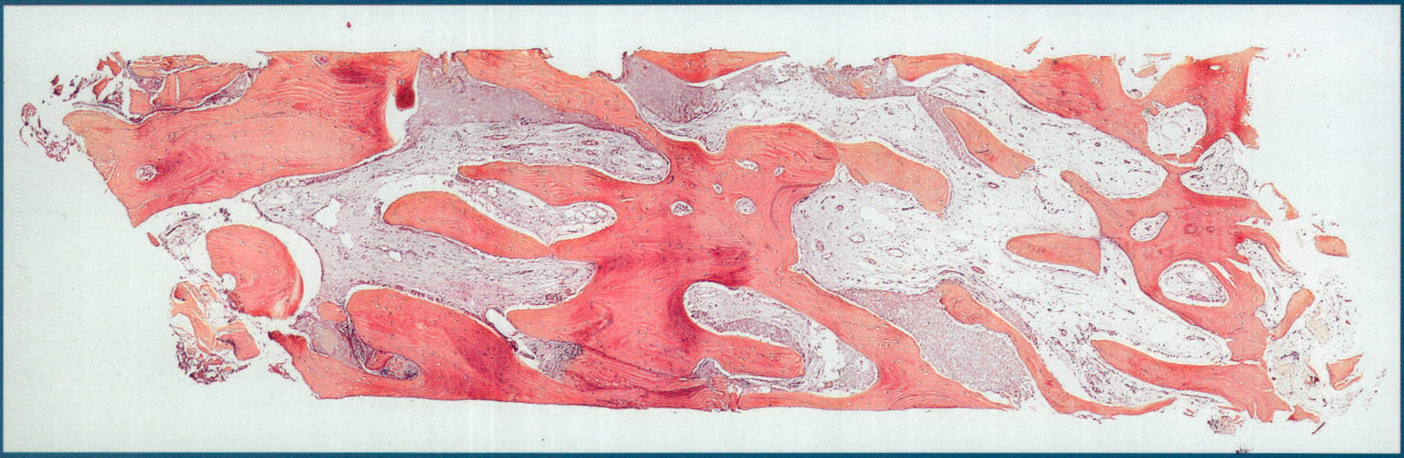

12 Appearance on histological examination of the collected bone sample.

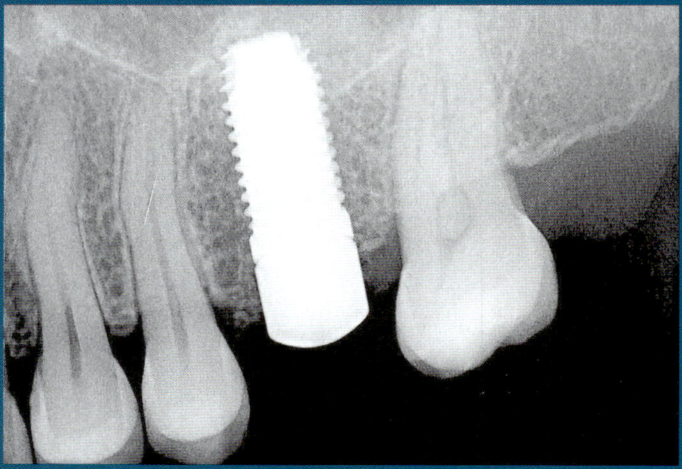

13 Intraoral X-ray after 6 months.

Appendix

In each chapter there are key sentences that briefly allow both to understand the potential of the tooth as a graft and to answer to unclear issues. They are *core points* collected in this Appendix as user friendly summary tables.

Scaffolds must be safe and biocompatible, they must create spaces between the granules where the initial formation of vessels will be possible, they must have surface micropores (100-500 μm) to favour wettability, they must have a correct crystallinity and crystal size and further, they must be easily handled during the surgical phase. All these characteristics are important for the initial stages, the adhesion of osteoblasts and osteoclasts and the deposition of the osteoid.

CHAPTER	3	PAGES	27–28

Cancellous bone tissue is rapidly vascularized, replaced and quickly resorbed.
The cortical bone, thanks to the greater density and the different structure, determines a high mechanical support but is vascularized more slowly.

CHAPTER	3	PAGE	28

All the growth factors are released only when the graft is reabsorbed.

CHAPTER	3	PAGE	28

Two bone substitutes treated with different procedures show very different osteoconductive and resorptive properties in vivo and in vitro.

CHAPTER	3	PAGE	29

Dentin, dental pulp, cementum, periodontal ligament and alveolar bone will be produced starting from the dental follicle.

CHAPTER	4	PAGE	35

The main protein structure of hard tissues of mesenchymal origin is collagen. The fibres are intertwined in the classic three-bundle helical shape and are intimately associated with the mineral deposits. Therefore, in these tissues the proteins of the mesenchymal matrix remain trapped in the mineralized tissue.

CHAPTER	4	PAGE	36

Crystals in mesenchymal tissues (dentin, cementum, bone) measure approximately 5×5×10/50 μm, they are randomly arranged and display a two-dimensional, string-like. Dentin has crystals 10 times larger than bone.[3]
The mature enamel crystals measure approximately 25×25×200 μm and are arranged in a regular three-dimensional manner forming the enamel prisms.

CHAPTER	4	PAGE	38

Physically and chemically, dentin resembles bone.

CHAPTER	4	PAGE	39

Dentin is composed of 65% inorganic material and 35% of organic material similar to bone.

Inorganic component

It consists of $3Ca_3(PO_4)_2Ca(OH)_2$ hydroxyapatite with crystals about 10 times larger thanbone and 300 times smaller than enamel. The dentine crystals are similar to bone and cementum ones.

Organic component

90% of the organic component is made up of collagen: 94% is type 1, 3% type 3 and 3% type 5. The remaining 10% is made up of non-collagen proteins.

CHAPTER 4 PAGE 39

All samples were decalcified using 0.6 M HCl, then washed and sterilized in 70% alcohol before grafting. The grafts were analyzed at 4, 8 and 12 weeks.
In defects filled with decalcified bone, the matrix was resorbed within 4 weeks. Decalcified dentin was better tolerated, but reabsorbed and replaced more slowly than bone. Dentin didn't induce dentinogenesis but osteogenesis.

CHAPTER 4 PAGES 40–41

4.3 The tooth in the books of Histology

Histology by Monesi[25]	Histology and Microscopic Anatomy by Wheater[26]
Chapter 18 – Bone tissue ***18.4 Dentin and tooth cementum*** Dentin and tooth cementum are two specialized forms of bone tissue. Dentin is a special form of bone tissue, harder than compact bone. The substance of the dentin consists of an organic matrix (28%) and an inorganic matrix (72%).	***Chapter 13 – Oral cavity*** ***13.3 Lip and tooth*** Dentin is a mineralized tissue that has a chemical composition similar to that of bone. ***13.4 Structure of the tooth*** Dentin forms most of the crown and roots and is composed of a calcified organic matrix similar to that of bone. The inorganic component is more abundant in dentin than in bone.

CHAPTER 4 PAGE 41

The resorption of the undecalcified dentin was incomplete or delayed. Minerals seemed to make the matrix inaccessible to the action of collagenolytic enzymes. For this reason, undecalcified dentin was not resorbed for 8–12 weeks, much later than the decalcified dentin.

CHAPTER 4 PAGE 41

4.5 Alternatives to HCl tested for demineralization

Preparation	Result
Calcium chloride	It delays the reabsorption and hinders the ostoegenetic reaction
EDTA (ethylenediaminetetraacetic acid) + formic acid + citric acid	It produces bone as with HCl but in a reduced percentage of positive cases
EDTA (ethylenediaminetetraacetic acid) + formic acid + acetic acid	It produces bone as with HCl but in a reduced percentage of positive cases
Lactic acid	Failed to remove all the mineral and a diffuse deposit which remained seemed to increase inflammation and prevent osteogenesis
Heat 70° C	Did not induce bone formation
Nitrous acid + HCl + β-propiolactone	Did not induce bone formation
Nitric acid + HCl + β-propiolactone	Did not induce bone formation
FDNB (dinitrofluorobenzene)	Did not induce bone formation
IAA (iodoacetamide) + HCl	Did not induce bone formation

CHAPTER 4 PAGE 41

Dentin grafts were able to produce bone more easily and to form it more quickly.
The inflammatory response was short and after 5 days the fibroblasts surrounded the grafts.
The decalcified bone and dentin exhibited a brief inflammatory reaction, then they were permeated by mesenchymal cells. Some of the mesenchymal cells transformed into multinucleated giant cells which proceeded by the erosion of tunnels in the matrix enlarging pre-existing cavities. The matrix was immediately recalculated, probably thanks to the diffusion of the ionic residues of the resorption. Then the osteoblasts replaced the multinucleated cells and formed new bone starting from the cementing line.

CHAPTER	4	PAGES	42–43

Different systems have been analyzed to demineralize bone and teeth, but it seems that some procedures may affect the results in the bone tissue production.

CHAPTER	4	PAGE	43

Nade tests on rabbit bone demineralized using HCl or EDTA were also evaluated, observing that some procedures reduced the yield of new bone. In particular, it was noted that the fine particles used by Huggins and colleagues treated as such, could have lost their morphogenetic capabilities. Grafts with EDTA did not result in any morphogenetic activity in guinea pigs. Instead, the use of EDTA at low concentrations for a short time and at low temperatures resulted in a certain morphogenetic activity. Instead, optimal results were obtained if the EDTA was replaced with HCl or H3PO4 (phosphoric acid) at 2° C.

CHAPTER	4	PAGE	43

While for the concentrations between 0.2 and 0.6 the success rates were high (75-85%), with higher concentrations the number of positive outcomes (cases in which bone was generated) was drastically reduced. This seems to indicate that high concentrations of HCl cause changes in the matrix responsible for negative effects on the induction mechanism.

CHAPTER	4	PAGE	43

Proteins have a pile-like structure. If an alteration of the structure occurs by chemical, thermal or mechanical denaturation, the functionality of the proteins is lost. A denatured protein, even if quite similar to the original one, as far as the coarse structure is concerned, is no longer able to perform its biological functions.

CHAPTER	4	PAGE	43

In 1985, Sato and Urist showed that when BMPs were used without any vector, a large amount was needed for an adequate bone induction. Bessho has then shown that the BMPs are very soluble in vivo and, if used without a carrier, they are rapidly washed out, invalidating their action. Based on these observations, the use of an appropriate carrier (collagen) for clinical use was suggested.

CHAPTER	4	PAGE	43

Closed tubules induced chondrogenesis while open tubules induced osteogenesis and the granule sizes of demineralized bone, ranging from 420 to 850 µm, induced more bone using as a carrier vs a powder of about 44-74 µm thinner.

CHAPTER	4	PAGE	43

Koga and colleagues demonstrated that demineralized dentin can be used as a grafting material.

CHAPTER	4	PAGE	43

The granules treated in this way were then grafted into the rat calvaria. Confirming Bang's observations, complete demineralization and the untreated tooth did not result in a greater amount of bone produced. The tooth with partial demineralization and with a particle size between 800 and 1200 µm (as analyzed by Kuboki and colleagues) had the best results at both 4 and 8 weeks. Another aspect analyzed by Koga concerned the in vitro observation of the different reactions of osteoblasts to the untreated surface compared to the demineralized one. In fact, the osteoblasts adhered only to the demineralized surface.

CHAPTER	4	PAGE	44

The SEM images showed that the morphology of the cells was reacting to the nanosurface, with dentinal tubules clearly visible in the DDM image, but not observable on the UDD surface, and only in the DDM the attachment of osteoblast cells to the surface was noticed.

CHAPTER	4	PAGES	44-45

Koga's conclusions were that demineralized dentin can be used as a grafting material, demonstrating a high cellular compatibility and rapid bone regeneration by an optimal balance between the resorption and the production of new bone.

CHAPTER	4	PAGE	45

Therefore, the demineralization process turns out to be a key factor in cell adhesion and in promoting regeneration. Blum, based on an animal model, claimed that, by reducing the mineral part, demineralization facilitates the release of GFs from the bone matrix.

CHAPTER	4	PAGE	45

Demineralization is a necessary process to release various growth factors and proteins, as this is blocked by the presence of hydroxyapatite crystals.

CHAPTER	4	PAGES	45-46

The highly soluble BMPs, have no osteoinductive effect when used alone. The graft material must be used as a carrier for the BMP proteins.

CHAPTER	4	PAGES	45-46

The surfaces, the dissolution of ions and the X-ray diffraction analysis of dentin, dental crown, cortical bone, Bio-Oss, phosphate synthetic biphasic calcium and allograft human bone were also analyzed and compared.

CHAPTER	4	PAGE	46

The thin line in the SDS-PAGE and IEF tests indicated the molecular weight of the sample under analysis.

CHAPTER	4	PAGE	46

Kim, using his own protocol for the use of dentin for regeneration, has also demonstrated the presence of proteins in dentin after a treatment.

CHAPTER	4	PAGE	47

It is interesting that the current analysis was able to demonstrate the invasion of the dentinal tubules by the osteocyte processes and their cytoplasm. Under these conditions, the degree of invasion was approximately 5 µm from the new DDM bone interface. Later the cellular processes of the osteocytes extended into the dentinal tubules and the bone tissue formed and filled the DDM surface.
Therefore demineralization, by increasing the size of the dentinal tubules, supports the adhesion and the activity of the osteoblasts and their total number.

CHAPTER	4	PAGES	47-48

Physio-chemical analyzes, SEM, plasma spectrometry, X-ray analysis, X-ray diffraction and histological and histomorphometric analyses were performed, discovering that deciduous dentin induced bone formation.
This research was innovative and interesting, as the deciduous tooth as a graft material was proposed and analysed for the very first time.

CHAPTER	4	PAGE	48

The conclusions were that the ECM (Extra Cellular Matrix) proteins of the bone and tooth are very well protected. The apatite in which the proteins are embedded, ensures considerable protection from chemical and physical agents even after death. These structures are therefore preserved for thousands of years.

CHAPTER	4	PAGE	54

While the alloplastic mineralized material is known to be only osteoconductive, the osteoinductive factors (that is proteins) contained in the mineralized structure may be usable when the mineralized structure is resorbed during the regeneration process.

CHAPTER	4	PAGE	54

The storage of teeth for 30 months seems not to have any effect on the osteoinductive properties of the teeth.

CHAPTER	4	PAGE	55

5.1 Differences between the two types of grinding in weight and in average percentages of the analyzed samples.

	Weight before (g)	Weight after (g)	% residual
High speed grinding	1.31 ± 0.56	0.56 ± 0.24	43.09% ± 2.17
Low speed grinding	1.51 ± 0.65	1.36 ± 0.61	93.5% ± 2.18

CHAPTER	5	PAGE	62

Upon careful evaluation of the surface of the granules subjected to different treatments, two things were evident:

- the surfaces may appear clean or with residues of various origins;
- the shape and size of the dentinal tubules varies.

One of the focal aspects of this surface variation is the increase in wettability, with an increase in the hydrophilicity of the surface.
The hydrophilic surfaces demonstrated an increase in osteoblast maturation, an increase in the production of local factors and a mineralization compared to the hydrophobic surfaces. Evidently, the maturation of osteoblasts is influenced by microtomography.

CHAPTER	5	PAGE	68

Koga, in 2016, found different sensitivities of osteoblasts to the untreated surface compared to the demineralized one. In fact, the osteoblasts only adhered to the demineralized surface.

CHAPTER	5	PAGE	68

Dentin is recognized by the body as its own bone tissue: it is involved in the same bone remodeling processes and it is treated physiologically by osteoclasts and osteoblasts.

CHAPTER	7	PAGE	108

The quality of newly formed bone is inversely proportional to the amount of residual dentin. This aspect may be quite intuitive and obvious, but unlike the other bone substitutes, which can lead to excellent bone regeneration while retaining their presence, dentin is "converted" into bone, therefore a very good regeneration will have a little residual dentin tissue.

CHAPTER	7	PAGE	111

From these data we can conclude that timewise there is an increase in bone tissue inversely proportional to the amount of the residual material. In fact, in the sample under examination, the values of residual material over time have a decrease of 36% and an increase of about 10% in the quantity of vital bone.

CHAPTER	7	PAGE	112

"The placement of a biomaterial in a post-extraction socket delays the healing; the Bio-Oss particles are not resorbed but surrounded by bone" since the material itself, occupying the space, prevents the growth of further bone.

CHAPTER	7	PAGE	122

The evolution over time of the graft means that the image is very similar to the patient's native bone, also because the tooth is completely reabsorbed and replaced by bone.

CHAPTER	7	PAGE	124

Conclusions

The field of regeneration is totally brand new and the data available are relatively few. Still today there are many questions that have not been answered yet. However, based on the experience we have gained in the recent years and summarized in this volume, the use of the tooth is promising in terms of results both from a qualitative and a quantitative point of view. Clearly the dental sample treatment process is the key point for the success of a regenerative surgery using the autologous tooth. As shown in the book, each single treatment produces a dental particulate which can have different characteristics. Therefore, it is difficult to compare results obtained with different procedures. New studies will likely lead to better tools and treatment options.

The most interesting aspect of the presented methodology is the complete resorbability of the tooth, with total replacement and creation of bone in all respects identical to the patient's native bone. Obviously the considerations made regarding the quantity of residual material must be reconsidered if an autologous material derived from the tooth is used.